Neonatology Questions and Controversies

Hematology and Transfusion Medicine

Neonatology Questions and Controversies
Hematology and Transfusion Medicine

Series Editor
Richard A. Polin, MD
William T. Speck Professor of Pediatrics
College of Physicians and Surgeons
Columbia University
Director, Division of Neonatology
New York Presbyterian
Morgan Stanley Children's Hospital
New York, New York

Other Volumes in the Neonatology Questions and Controversies Series
GASTROENTEROLOGY AND NUTRITION

HEMODYNAMICS AND CARDIOLOGY

INFECTIOUS DISEASE AND PHARMACOLOGY

NEPHROLOGY AND FLUID/ELECTROLYTE PHYSIOLOGY

NEUROLOGY

THE NEWBORN LUNG

Fourth Edition

Neonatology Questions and Controversies

Hematology and Transfusion Medicine

Edited by

Robin K. Ohls, MD
August L Jung Presidential
Professor of Pediatrics
Chief, Division of Neonatology
University of Utah
Salt Lake City, Utah
United States

Akhil Maheshwari, MD, FAAP, FRCP (Edin), FIAH
Professor (Clinical) of Pediatrics, and of Molecular & Cellular Physiology
Chief, Division of Neonatal Medicine
Vice-Chair of Translational Research in Pediatrics
Director
Fellowship Program of Neonatal-Perinatal Medicine
Louisiana State University Health Sciences
   Center – Shreveport
Shreveport, Louisiana
United States

Robert D. Christensen, MD
Professor of Pediatrics
University of Utah
Primary Children's Hospital
Salt Lake City, Utah
United States

Consulting Editor

Richard A. Polin, MD
William T. Speck Professor of Pediatrics
Executive Vice Chair Department of Pediatrics
Vagelos College of Physicians and Surgeons
Columbia University
New York, New York
United States

ELSEVIER

Elsevier
1600 John F. Kennedy Blvd.
Ste 1800
Philadelphia, PA 19103-2899

Content Strategist: Sarah Barth
Senior Content Development Specialist: Vaishali Singh
Content Development Manager: Ranjana Sharma
Publishing Services Manager: Shereen Jameel
Project Manager: Haritha Dharmarajan
Design Direction: Margaret Reid

Printed in India

Last digit is the print number: 9 8 7 6 5 4 3 2 1

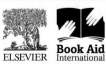

List of Contributors

Archana M. Agarwal, MD
Professor
Department of Pathology
University of Utah/ARUP Laboratories
Salt Lake City, Utah
United States

Timothy M. Bahr, MS, MD
Assistant Professor of Clinical Investigation
Obstetric and Neonatal Operations
Intermountain Healthcare
Murray
Utah
United States
Adjunct Assistant Professor of Pediatrics
Pediatrics
University of Utah
Salt Lake City, Utah
United States

Patrick D. Carroll, MD, MPH
Neonatologist
Women and Newborn Program
St. George Regional Hospital, Intermountain Health
St. George, Utah
United States

Robert D. Christensen, MD
Professor of Pediatrics
Pediatrics
University of Utah
Salt Lake City, Utah
United States

Patricia Davenport, MD
Instructor of Pediatrics
Division of Newborn Medicine
Boston Children's Hospital
Boston, Massachusetts
United States

Emöke Deschmann, MD, MMSc, PhD
Attending Neonatologist, Postdoctor
Department of Women's and Children's Health
Division of Neonatology
Karolinska Institute and Karolinska University
    Hospital
Stockholm
Sweden

Kendell R. German, MD
Assistant Professor
Department of Pediatrics
Division of Neonatology
University of Washington
Seattle, Washington
United States

Sharada H. Gowda, MD
Associate Professor of Pediatrics/Newborns
Baylor College of Medicine
Neonatologist
Texas Children's Hospital
Houston, Texas
United States

Brunetta Guaragni, MD
Chidren's Hospital
Neonatology and Neonatal Intensive Care Unit
ASSAT Spedali Civili di Brescia
Brescia
Italy

Cassandra D. Josephson, MD
Professor (PAR)
Oncology and Pediatrics
Johns Hopkins University School of Medicine
Baltimore, Maryland
United States
Director
Cancer and Blood Disorders Institute
Department of Pediatrics
Director
Blood Bank, Transfusion Medicine, and Apheresis
    Service
Department of Pathology
Johns Hopkins All Children's Hospital
St. Petersburg, Florida
United States

Allison Judkins, MD
Assistant Professor
Pediatrics
University of Utah
Salt Lake City, Utah
United States

Sandra E. Juul, MD, PhD
Professor
Department of Pediatrics
Division of Neonatology
University of Washington
Seattle, Washington
United States

Pamela Jean Kling, MD
Professor
Pediatrics
University of Wisconsin
Madison, Wisconsin
United States

Shelley M. Lawrence, MD, MS
Associate Professor
Department of Pediatrics
Division of Neonatology
University of Utah
Salt Lake City, Utah
United States

Akhil Maheshwari, MD, FAAP, FRCP (Edin), FIAH
Professor (Clinical) of Pediatrics, and of
    Molecular & Cellular Physiology
Chief, Division of Neonatal Medicine
Vice-Chair of Translational Research in Pediatrics
Director
Fellowship Program of Neonatal-Perinatal Medicine
Louisiana State University Health Sciences Center –
    Shreveport
Shreveport, Louisiana
United States

Mario Motta, MD
Neonatology and Neonatal Intensive Care Unit
Ospedale Maggiore
AUSL di Bologna
Emilia-Romagna
Italy

Robin K. Ohls, MD
August L Jung Presidential
Professor of Pediatrics
Chief, Division of Neonatology
University of Utah
Salt Lake City, Utah
United States

Anton Rets, MD, PhD
Assistant Professor
Department of Pathology
University of Utah/ARUP Laboratories
Salt Lake City, Utah
United States

Julie Shakib, DO, MS, MPH
Associate Professor
Pediatrics
University of Utah
Salt Lake City, Utah
United States

Martha C. Sola-Visner, MD
Associate Professor of Pediatrics
Division of Newborn Medicine
Boston Children's Hospital
Boston, Massachusetts
United States

Sarah M. Tweddell, MS, MD
Assistant Professor, Neonatology
Department of Pediatrics
University of Utah
Salt Lake City, Utah
United States

Series Foreword

"To study the phenomena of disease without books is to sail an uncharted sea, while to study books without patients is not to go to sea at all."

"Medicine is learned by the bedside and not in the classroom. Let not your conceptions of disease come from the words heard in the lecture room or read from the book. See and then reason and compare and control. But see first."

William Osler

Before the invention of the movable type by Johannes Gutenberg in the 15th century, physicians learned medicine by serving an apprenticeship with individuals considered experienced. There were no printed textbooks, and medical journals were not published until the beginning of the 19th century. By apprenticing to a physician over a period of years, students learned how to be competent practitioners. Internships in the United States evolved from those apprenticeships in the 18th century. The term *residency* was chosen because the physicians in training had a so-called residence at the hospital. Modern-day internships began at Johns Hopkins Hospital in 1904. The Johns Hopkins Hospital was founded by Osler, Halstead, Welch, and Kelly. Halstead is credited with creating the first surgical residency and coined the phrase "see one, do one, teach one" (SODOTO). That educational philosophy has been adopted by nearly every specialty in medicine, including neonatology.

Modern-day trainees in neonatology still learn how to care for critically ill infants and how to perform procedures by watching, assisting, and listening to more experienced individuals at the bedside. The SODOTO approach is considered a fundamental educational tool; however, over a 3-year period much of education occurs remote from the bedside during teaching rounds and conferences. The teaching is often more theoretical, and by design, rounds in the nursery and conferences are passive learning exercises. In those settings, trainees listen but do not take an active role in the educational process. Learning is always more effective when recipients take an active role in their own education. Ideally, they should be questioning what they hear, reading pertinent literature, and when the opportunity arises teaching others. Unfortunately, much of the information transmitted in those settings is not usually followed by an active phase of questioning and reading by the trainee.

Most graduates of fellowship programs turn out to be excellent practitioners, but once they leave the fellowship program, new information is acquired only intermittently either at conferences or from journals and textbooks. As a source of new information, journals provide access to the most up-to-date information. However, that information is unfiltered, and the conclusions of a study may not be appropriate (or perhaps risky) for a critically ill infant. Textbook series such as *Neonatology Questions and Controversies* offer an opportunity to hear from experts in neonatal-perinatal medicine who have synthesized (and filtered) the existing literature and can provide up-to-date recommendations.

The fourth edition of the *Questions and Controversies* series will also have seven volumes. Each of them has been extensively revised, and we have added several new editors: Terri Inder has joined Jeffrey Perlman for the Neurology volume; James Wynn joined William Benitz and P. Brian Smith as a coeditor for the Infectious Disease, Immunology and Pharmacology volume; and Patrick McNamara is now a coeditor with Martin Kluckow for the Neonatal Hemodynamics volume. The reader will find many completely new chapters; however, like the last edition, each of them is focused on day-to day clinical decisions encountered by neonatologists. Nothing will replace the teaching that occurs at the bedside when confronted with a critically ill neonate, and the SODOTO educational approach still has an important role in education. Procedures are best learned by simulations and guidance by experienced practitioners at the bedside; however, expertise as a practitioner can only be enhanced by reading and incorporating new information into daily practice—once proven safe and effective. Perhaps SODOTO should be changed to LQRT (listen, question, read, and teach). The *Questions and Controversies* series is a unique source to learn from experts in the field who have been through the LQRT process many times. Osler's quotes at the start of this preface suggest that both bedside teaching and journals/textbooks have a synergistic role in physician education, and neither alone is sufficient.

As with all prior editions, I am indebted to an exceptional group of volume editors who chose the content and authors and edited the manuscripts. I also want to thank Sarah Barth (Publisher), as well as Vasowati Shome and Vaishali Singh (Senior Content Development Specialists) at Elsevier, who have guided the development of this series.

RAP

Preface

The developmental constraints of the neonatal hematologic and immune systems are well known, particularly those in the smallest premature infants. Forced to cope with a wide range of physiologic, environmental, and microbial challenges in the extrauterine world, the still-immature fetal hematologic and immunologic systems sometimes can support the healthy development of the fetus, but sometimes cannot. In the fourth edition of this volume of the *Neonatology Questions and Controversies* series, our original goals remain: We seek to update physicians, nurse practitioners, nurses, residents, and students on the most challenging issues in neonatal hematology such as anemia, transfusions, jaundice, leukocyte counts, and thrombocytopenia. The new feature of this edition is the inclusion of several chapters on neonatal transfusion medicine. New chapters include in-depth evaluations of fetal and neonatal iron homeostasis and risk factors for iron deficiency, and improvements in bilirubin assessment and management.

We wish to thank Dr. Richard Polin, the Consulting Editor; Lisa Barnes, our previous Content Development Specialist; and Vaishali Singh, our current Senior Content Development Specialist at Elsevier, for her support and encouragement to write this volume. We are indebted and grateful to the authors of each chapter whose contributions from around the world will be fully appreciated by the readers and to our families for their enduring support.

Finally, we (Akhil Maheshwari and Robin Ohls) again would like to acknowledge Dr. Robert Christensen for his continued participation as author and editor in the fourth edition of this volume; for his ongoing inspiration, enthusiasm, and generosity; and for being the best mentor and role model on the planet.

Robin K. Ohls
Akhil Maheshwari
Robert D. Christensen

Contents

Neonatology Questions and Controversies
Hematology and Transfusion Medicine

Hematology

Chapter 1

Innovations in Screening and Management of Neonatal Hyperbilirubinemia

Julie H. Shakib, DO, MS, MPH, and Timothy M. Bahr, MS, MD

Chapter Outline

Introduction

One of the most significant innovations in the routine management of neonatal hyperbilirubinemia was the publication of the 2004 clinical practice guidelines on the management of hyperbilirubinemia in late preterm and term newborns by the American Academy of Pediatrics (AAP) Subcommittee on Hyperbilirubinemia.[1] These guidelines were largely based on the innovative method of using predischarge total serum bilirubin (TSB) for hour-specific risk stratification developed by Bhutani et al.[2] The 2004 AAP guideline has largely dictated hyperbilirubinemia screening and management practices both in the United States and internationally since publication nearly 20 years ago. Perhaps given the widespread adoption of the guideline, minimal practice change has occurred in the management of hyperbilirubinemia in the nearly 2 decades since its publication.

In this chapter we discuss five practice changes that are areas of active research. These practice changes have been explored, implemented, and studied by various research groups and in various hospitals in the United States and abroad. Each is an attempt to increase the value of the care we provide as we manage hyperbilirubinemia in the newborn; that is, each attempts to decrease the cost or burden on the patient while simultaneously maintaining or increasing the quality of the care provided. These sections are focused on inpatient care of newborns during the birth hospitalization, though outpatient management is also being actively studied.

Eliminating Routine Blood Typing and Direct Antiglobulin Testing for Neonates Born to Blood Group O Mothers

The 2004 AAP guidelines state that if the maternal blood group is O (+), it is an option to test for the infant's blood type and to perform a direct antiglobulin test (DAT), but it is not required to do so provided there is appropriate surveillance for hyperbilirubinemia.[1] Recent studies by our group and others support eliminating routine blood typing and DAT measurement in neonates born to blood group O (+) mothers.[3-6] Specifically, studies utilizing end-tidal carbon monoxide (ETCO) measurement as a marker of hemolysis found that some DAT-positive babies did not have clinically significant hemolysis, and some DAT-negative babies had clinically significant hemolysis, evidenced by elevated ETCO measurements.[7] These findings led us to conclude that the DAT could neither definitively rule in nor rule out hemolysis. We also found that neonates in our health care system who were blood group A or B, born to mothers of group O (+) (and thus the neonates were at some risk for ABO hemolytic disease), did not have a higher incidence of severe neonatal hyperbilirubinemia than neonates of blood group O, born to group O (+) mothers (and thus were at no risk for ABO hemolytic disease). We suggested that this supports our theory that universal bilirubin screening of neonates in the birth hospital identifies those who need phototherapy, including those with significant ABO hemolytic disease, and that this obviates the need for routine neonatal blood type and DAT.[6]

Intermountain Healthcare, a health care system that operates 21 delivery hospitals in the intermountain western region of the United States, discontinued the practice of routine blood typing and DAT measurement in neonates born to blood group O (+) mothers in 2005, the same year universal predischarge hyperbilirubinemia screening was implemented across the health care system. Follow-up data from 2005 to 2016 in 400,000 live births showed that this change did not result in a higher incidence of severe hyperbilirubinemia.[3,6] Other hospitals in the region have also begun implementing this change in practice. The authors' home institution routinely stores cord blood samples during the birth hospitalization and only performs a DAT on these samples if the baby qualifies for phototherapy *and* is found to have hemolytic jaundice by an elevated ETCO (see later).

Universal Screening and the Use of TcB Determinations (and Use of Phototherapy Skin Patches)

Practices to screen for hyperbilirubinemia in newborn nurseries are highly variable. Before the last decade it was common practice for clinicians caring for neonates to attempt to use visual assessment of jaundice to predict bilirubin levels. The inherent appeal of this noninvasive approach, particularly in resource-limited or high-volume nurseries, is self-evident. However, visual assessment has been repeatedly demonstrated to have poor reliability, accuracy, and interobserver agreement.[8-10] A 2008 study by Riskin et al. demonstrated that 62% of term and late preterm neonates with TSB levels in high-risk zones were misclassified by visual assessment.[9]

The potential predictive ability of universal screening for hyperbilirubinemia gained traction in the late 1990s. Expert concerns that the potential for severe hyperbilirubinemia in neonates would be underestimated by busy clinicians due to administrative pressures to reduce the length of hospital admissions and the cost of testing led to studies to evaluate the predictive ability of universal predischarge serum bilirubin screening.[2] In the 2004 AAP guidelines the committee recommended a predischarge bilirubin measurement and/or assessment of clinical risk factors to evaluate the risk of severe hyperbilirubinemia.[11] In 2009 this recommendation was updated by the authors of the 2004 guideline to recommend universal predischarge bilirubin screening using TSB or transcutaneous bilirubin (TcB) measurements.[12] The stated aim of this most recent AAP guideline was to promote a measured approach to both reduce the frequency of severe neonatal hyperbilirubinemia and subsequent bilirubin encephalopathy while also minimizing unintended harms, such as unnecessary treatment, breastfeeding failure, and increased parental anxiety.[12] However, in 2010 the US Preventive Services Task Force and the American Academy of Family Physicians concluded that there was insufficient evidence that universal screening improves adverse outcomes related to hyperbilirubinemia.[13] Despite the lack of evidence regarding the capacity for universal screening to decrease adverse outcomes related to severe hyperbilirubinemia, universal screening has been widely endorsed and adopted likely due to the desire to reduce unintended harms in the newborn period.[14]

TcB screening provides an alternative to serum bilirubin measurements. TcB measurement in late-preterm and term newborns has several important advantages when compared with serum measurement both in the setting of screening and follow-up. TcB screening provides instantaneous results to clinicians without the need for laboratory equipment. As TcB measurement is noninvasive, when implemented in the context of universal screening it eliminates the need for phlebotomy if the result is below standard thresholds for serum confirmation. Several studies have demonstrated that universal TcB screening may decrease the rate of pre-discharge blood draws for TSB.[15-17] Moreover, light-occlusive skin patches have been demonstrated to preserve the validity of TcB determinations during and after phototherapy.[18] Despite these advantages, TcB measurement is not used in some centers because of concerns about accuracy, especially following the initiation of phototherapy. Recently, TcB measurement devices have improved, and studies have confirmed that they correlate with TSB measurements ($r \cong 0.9$) and are typically accurate within 1.5 mg/dL or less.[19-21] Similar to hour-specific risk stratification, we utilize an hour-specific nomogram (see Age-Based Nomogram for Phototherapy Initiation Based on Nearly 400,000 Neonates, next) to determine whether a TcB value warrants a confirmatory TSB measurement. Our review of this process showed that, when newborns with a TcB value that exceeded the 85th percentile received a confirmatory TSB, the risk of obtaining a TcB indicating no TSB is needed, when the simultaneous TSB would have indicated a need for treatment (phototherapy) was close to zero. We conclude that the use of TcB for universal screening for hyperbilirubinemia has high value and is safe.

Age-Based Nomogram for Phototherapy Initiation Based on Nearly 400,000 Neonates

The 1999 Bhutani predischarge, hour-specific serum bilirubin nomogram is widely used and has been very impactful.[2] It was central to developing the 2004 and 2009 AAP clinical guidelines for managing hyperbilirubinemia in the newborn infant 35 weeks and older.[11] Despite this, it was limited by a small sample size, and the data were not sufficiently robust to stratify by sex, or specific gestational ages between 35 and 40 weeks, or race. In addition, later publications recognized several biases in the Bhutani study design.[22,23]

In 2020 our group, in collaboration with Bhutani, developed an updated, statistically rigorous, hour-specific bilirubin nomogram for newborns based on nearly 400,000 newborns. We have used it prospectively as a replacement for the 1999 Bhutani nomogram.[24] This new nomogram (Fig. 1.1) provides robust data in the first 12 hours after birth (which

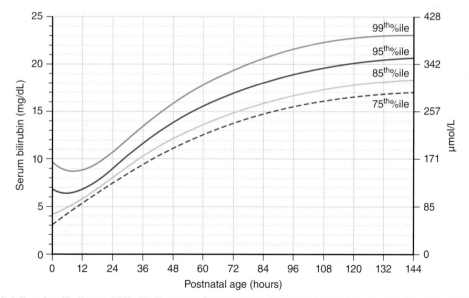

Fig. 1.1 The Utah Hour-Specific Neonatal Bilirubin Nomogram for neonates ≥35 weeks of gestation. The 75th, 85th, 95th, and 99th percentile lines are displayed. In the new Utah Neonatal Bilirubin Management Quality Improvement Program all well-babies have a transcutaneous bilirubin (TcB) performed at 28±8 hours. If the TcB is ≥85th % line, a TSB is obtained by heelstick. If the TSB is ≥95th % line, phototherapy is started and two ETCOc measurements are made.

were not included in the 1999 nomogram); it shows general agreement with the 1999 nomogram for values in the first 60 hours, but higher 75th and 95th percentile TSB values thereafter. This nomogram and its accompanying analysis also showed no difference in TSB between males and females, and higher TSB values among earlier gestation neonates.

In our practice we found high rates of phototherapy use (~10% of neonates ≥35 weeks of gestation). Therefore one of the goals of implementing use of the new nomogram was to decrease unnecessary phototherapy use. In accordance with that goal, the following algorithm was implemented in our newborn nursery: universal screening for hyperbilirubinemia in neonates 35 weeks of gestation and older is first done via TcB. Using the new nomogram, if a TcB value exceeds the 85th percentile, a TSB is ordered. If the TSB exceeds the 95th percentile, we initiate phototherapy.

ETCOc Measurement for Those Receiving Phototherapy to Determine Hemolytic vs. Nonhemolytic Hyperbilirubinemia

When heme is metabolized, carbon monoxide (CO) and bilirubin are produced in equimolar quantities.[25,26] Thus measuring ETCO at the end of an exhaled breath reveals the rate of red blood cell breakdown (hemolysis) and the subsequent rate of bilirubin production. Our group and others have studied ETCOc measurement in newborns and its association with neonatal hyperbilirubinemia. We have shown associations between ETCOc and hyperbilirubinemia risk.[7,26-30]

The 2004 AAP Bilirubin Practice Guideline[11] stated "end-tidal carbon monoxide...levels can confirm the presence or absence of hemolysis... Thus, ETCOc may be helpful in determining the degree of surveillance needed and the timing of intervention. It is not yet known, however, how ETCOc measurements will affect management." This left open the question, "How will ETCOc affect management?"

The largest study of routine use of ETCOc was conducted in 1370 newborns at nine multinational clinical sites. This study evaluated universal screening for risk of hyperbilirubinemia using both predischarge serum bilirubin measurements and ETCOc. The study showed that the addition of an ETCOc measurement

to a serum bilirubin measurement provided insight into the processes that contribute to hyperbilirubinemia (e.g., is severe hemolysis present) but did not improve the predictive ability of an hour-specific TSB.

We studied and implemented the use of ETCOc for newborns receiving phototherapy with the hypothesis that newborns with hemolytic jaundice, evidenced by high ETCOc, would benefit from more aggressive phototherapy and shorter inpatient and outpatient follow-up intervals. In our newborn nursery, newborns who meet criteria for phototherapy and have an ETCOc measurement 2 ppm or greater receive more intensive phototherapy, more frequent bilirubin measurements, and earlier outpatient follow-up. Our initial analysis following implementation (n=170 newborns) showed that higher ETCOc values were associated with earlier institution of phototherapy and longer phototherapy duration. In addition, ETCOc was associated with the number of phototherapy courses needed during the birth hospitalization. Only three newborns required readmission to the hospital for intensive phototherapy following birth hospitalization discharge. While in the nursery all three of these infants who later required readmission had an elevated ETCOc (2.2, 2.6, and 2.9 ppm).

Electronic Health Record Add-On App

To effectively screen and manage hyperbilirubinemia in newborns, clinicians are required to retrieve data from the medical record, synthesize this data for risk classification, and administer phototherapy when bilirubin levels exceed risk-based treatment thresholds. Previous studies have demonstrated that automating low-level cognitive tasks, such as retrieving, organizing, and sorting data, allows clinicians to preserve valuable cognitive resources for more complex tasks.[31,32] In this quality improvement study, an electronic health record add-on app for neonatal bilirubin management saved clinicians a mean of 66 seconds for bilirubin management tasks compared with a commonly used tool. In a retrospective pre-post analysis, the odds of clinically appropriate phototherapy orders during hospitalization increased significantly by 84%. These findings suggest that well designed electronic health record add-on apps may be associated with time savings for physicians and improvements in patient care. Electronic health records

(EHRs) now allow the integration of add-on apps to automate targeted cognitive tasks through a technology known as Substitutable Medical Applications and Reusable Technologies on Fast Healthcare Interoperability Resources (SMART on FHIR).[33]

An EHR add-on app for hyperbilirubinemia management was designed, developed, and implemented in our academic health care system by the authors in collaboration with our informatics team in 2017.[34] It was later updated to include many of the practice changes discussed in this chapter (Fig. 1.2). The add-on app, known as BiliApp, was designed to support bilirubin screening and management by retrieving relevant data, providing a visual data summary, and delivering AAP hyperbilirubinemia guideline-based recommendations for next steps. Approximately 3800 infants 35 weeks or more are born annually at our

institution, and the majority transition to their mother's room (couplet care). Newborns receive care by academic general pediatricians (75% of infants) or family medicine providers (25%).

Prior to app implementation, a stand-alone web-based tool known as BiliTool (BiliTool Inc., Long Beach, CA, USA), which is available as a link in the EHR, was commonly used by our institution's clinicians for bilirubin management.[35] Clinicians would open the BiliTool website and manually enter the time of birth as well as the last total bilirubin level and associated specimen collection time for every newborn. The BiliTool website takes these inputs and provides recommendations for potential risk levels as defined by the AAP guideline (lower, medium, and higher risk).[11] Clinicians would then independently assess the patient-specific risk level described by the 2004

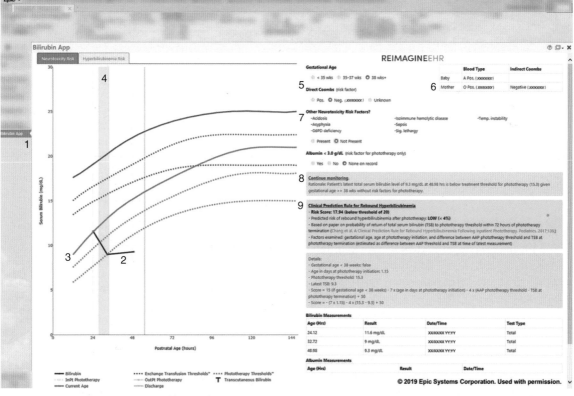

Fig. 1.2 BiliApp, an electronic health record (EHR) add-on app for hyperbilirubinemia management. No additional login outside the EHR is required, and all the information is pulled automatically from the medical record. Clinicians then review the data, including the patient's risk-specific threshold where phototherapy is indicated, history of phototherapy administration, bilirubin levels over time, and patient-specific recommendations on next steps.

AAP guideline for each patient based on each patient's gestational age and direct Coombs test result when available. With the add-on Bili app, no additional login is required, and all the information is pulled automatically from the medical record. Clinicians then review the data, including the patient's risk-specific threshold where phototherapy is indicated, history of phototherapy administration, bilirubin levels over time, and patient-specific recommendations on next steps.

Our implementation team conducted a mixed-methods quality improvement study in 2018 to evaluate the clinical impact of the add-on app for bilirubin management. The app was used 20,516 times by clinicians for 92% of eligible newborns and required a mean of 35 seconds (95% confidence interval [CI] 27–42 sec) per use to complete the bilirubin management tasks compared with 100 seconds (95% CI 89–112 sec) for BiliTool.[34] Furthermore, following the intervention, health care use rates remained stable, while orders for clinically appropriate phototherapy during hospitalization increased for newborns with bilirubin levels above the guideline-recommended threshold (odds ratio, 1.84; 95% CI 1.16–2.90; $P = .009$).[34] This study illustrates that a well-designed EHR hyperbilirubinemia management add-on app not only saves clinician time, but also improves care by helping clinicians more efficiently identify newborns who require phototherapy. This add-on app is currently being prepared for release into EHR app stores as free-to-use software.

Future Directions

Studies on the economic burden of hyperbilirubinemia screening, prevention, and treatment to prevent the development of kernicterus show that the cost of such programs throughout the United States is between $100 and $200 million. Each of the innovations described in this chapter requires further investigation to show efficacy and value sufficient for widespread use. Nevertheless, minimizing unnecessary interventions and cost while improving outcomes is of utmost importance.

Other areas of research in the routine screening, prevention, and management of hyperbilirubinemia that are currently being investigated include the efficacy

and reduction in harm associated with cycling phototherapy off and on (e.g., for 3 hours at a time) during treatment courses,[36] genetic etiologies of mild and severe hyperbilirubinemia,[37,38] and the efficacy of heme-oxygenase inhibitors (especially in cases of severe hyperbilirubinemia).[39-41] In addition, whereas the incidence of kernicterus in the United States is low, in resource-limited countries the incidence of kernicterus is much higher.[42,43] Innovations such as smartphone camera-based bilirubin determinations[44] and TcB determinations[45] show promise as ways to provide low-cost, accessible tools to screen for hyperbilirubinemia.

REFERENCES

1. Subcommittee on Hyperbilirubinemia. Management of hyperbilirubinemia in the newborn infant 35 or more weeks of gestation. *Pediatrics*. 2004;114(1):297-316.
2. Bhutani VK, Johnson L, Sivieri EM. Predictive ability of a pre-discharge hour-specific serum bilirubin for subsequent significant hyperbilirubinemia in healthy term and near-term newborns. *Pediatrics*. 1999;103(1):6-14.
3. Christensen RD, Baer VL, MacQueen BC, et al. ABO hemolytic disease of the fetus and newborn: thirteen years of data after implementing a universal bilirubin screening and management program. *J Perinatol*. 2018;38(5):517-525.
4. Lieberman L, Spradbrow J, Keir A, et al. Use of intravenous immunoglobulin in neonates at a tertiary academic hospital: a retrospective 11-year study: use of IVIG in the NICU. *Transfusion (Paris)*. 2016;56(11):2704-2711.
5. Evanovitch D, Clarke G, Lieberman L, et al. Abstract presentations from the AABB Annual Meeting, San Antonio, Oct 19–22, 2019. *Transfusion*. 2019;59:S3. Available at: https://onlinelibrary.wiley.com/doi/abs/10.1111/trf.15462.
6. Baer VL, Hulse W, Bahr TM, et al. Absence of severe neonatal ABO hemolytic disease at Intermountain Healthcare. Why? *J Perinatol*. 2020;40(2):352-353.
7. Elsaie AL, Taleb M, Nicosia A, et al. Comparison of end-tidal carbon monoxide measurements with direct antiglobulin tests in the management of neonatal hyperbilirubinemia. *J Perinatol*. 2020;40(10):1513-1517.
8. Moyer VA, Ahn C, Sneed S. Accuracy of clinical judgment in neonatal jaundice. *Arch Pediatr Adolesc Med*. 2000;154(4):391-394.
9. Riskin A, Tamir A, Kugelman A, et al. Is visual assessment of jaundice reliable as a screening tool to detect significant neonatal hyperbilirubinemia? *J Pediatr*. 2008;152(6):782-787.e1-e2.
10. Keren R, Tremont K, Luan X, et al. Visual assessment of jaundice in term and late preterm infants. *Arch Dis Child Fetal Neonatal Ed*. 2009;94(5):F317-F322.
11. American Academy of Pediatrics Subcommittee on Hyperbilirubinemia. Management of hyperbilirubinemia in the newborn infant 35 or more weeks of gestation. *Pediatrics*. 2004;114(1):297-316.
12. Maisels MJ, Bhutani VK, Bogen D, et al. Hyperbilirubinemia in the newborn infant > or =35 weeks' gestation: an update with clarifications. *Pediatrics*. 2009;124(4):1193-1198.

13. US Preventive Services Task Force. Screening of infants for hyperbilirubinemia to prevent chronic bilirubin encephalopathy: recommendation statement. *Am· Fam Physician.* 2010;82(4):408-410.

14. Health and Resources and Services Administration. *Newborn Screening for Neonatal Hyperbilirubinemia*: A Summary of the Evidence and Advisory Committee Decision [Internet]. Author; 2012. Available at: https://www.hrsa.gov/sites/default/files/hrsa/advisory-committees/heritable-disorders/hyperbili-27-june-2018.pdf.

15. Nanjundaswamy S, Petrova A, Mehta R, et al. Transcutaneous bilirubinometry in preterm infants receiving phototherapy. *Am J Perinatol.* 2005;22(3):127-131.

16. Kilmartin KC, McCarty EJ, Shubkin CD, et al. Reducing outpatient infant blood draws with transcutaneous measurement of bilirubin. *Pediatr Qual Saf.* 2020;5(4):e335.

17. Hassan Shabuj M, Hossain J, Dey S. Accuracy of transcutaneous bilirubinometry in the preterm infants: a comprehensive meta-analysis. J Matern Fetal Neonatal Med. 2019;32(5):734-741.

18. Fonseca R, Kyralessa R, Malloy M, et al. Covered skin transcutaneous bilirubin estimation is comparable with serum bilirubin during and after phototherapy. *J Perinatol.* 2012;32(2):129-131.

19. Shah MH, Ariff S, Ali SR, et al. Quality improvement initiative using transcutaneous bilirubin nomogram to decrease serum bilirubin sampling in low-risk babies. *BMJ Paediatr Open.* 2019;3(1):e000403.

20. Maisels MJ, DeRidder JM, Kring EA, et al. Routine transcutaneous bilirubin measurements combined with clinical risk factors improve the prediction of subsequent hyperbilirubinemia. *J Perinatol.* 2009;29(9):612-617.

21. Taylor JA, Burgos AE, Flaherman V, et al. Discrepancies between transcutaneous and serum bilirubin measurements. *Pediatrics.* 2015;135(2):224-231.

22. Maisels MJ, Newman TB. Predicting hyperbilirubinemia in newborns: the importance of timing. *Pediatrics.* 1999;103(2):493-494.

23. Fay DL, Schellhase KG, Suresh GK. Bilirubin screening for normal newborns: a critique of the hour-specific bilirubin nomogram. *Pediatrics.* 2009;124(4):1203-1205.

24. Bahr TM, Henry E, Christensen RD, et al. A new hour-specific serum bilirubin nomogram for neonates ≥35 weeks of gestation. *J Pediatr.* 2021;236:28-33.e1.

25. Tidmarsh GF, Wong RJ, Stevenson DK. End-tidal carbon monoxide and hemolysis. *J Perinatol.* 2014;34(8):577-581.

26. Maisels MJ, Kring E. The contribution of hemolysis to early jaundice in normal newborns. *Pediatrics.* 2006;118(1):276-279.

27. Christensen RD, Malleske DT, Lambert DK, et al. Measuring end-tidal carbon monoxide of jaundiced neonates in the birth hospital to identify those with hemolysis. *Neonatology.* 2016;109(1):1-5.

28. Bhutani VK, Maisels MJ, Schutzman DL, et al. Identification of risk for neonatal haemolysis. *Acta Paediatr.* 2018;107(8):1350-1356.

29. Christensen RD, Lambert DK, Henry E, et al. End-tidal carbon monoxide as an indicator of the hemolytic rate. *Blood Cells Mol Dis.* 2015;54(3):292-296.

30. Bhutani VK, Srinivas S, Castillo Cuadrado ME, et al. Identification of neonatal haemolysis: an approach to predischarge management of neonatal hyperbilirubinemia. *Acta Paediatr.* 2016;105(5):e189-e194.

31. Ericsson KA, Hoffman RR, Kozbelt A, et al. *The Cambridge Handbook of Expertise and Expert Performance.* Cambridge, United Kingdom: Cambridge University Press; 2018.

32. Camos V. Domain-specific versus domain-general maintenance in working memory: reconciliation within the time-based resource sharing model. *Psychol Learn Motiv.* 2017;67:135-171.

33. Mandel JC, Kreda DA, Mandl KD, et al. SMART on FHIR: a standards-based, interoperable apps platform for electronic health records. *J Am Med Inform Assoc.* 2016;23(5):899-908.

34. Kawamoto K, Kukhareva P, Shakib JH, et al. Association of an electronic health record add-on app for neonatal bilirubin management with physician efficiency and care quality. *JAMA Netw Open.* 2019;2(11):e1915343.

35. Longhurst C, Turner S, Burgos AE. Development of a web-based decision support tool to increase use of neonatal hyperbilirubinemia guidelines. *Jt Comm J Qual Patient Saf.* 2009;35(5):256-262.

36. Arnold C, Tyson JE, Pedroza C, et al. Cycled phototherapy dose-finding study for extremely low-birth-weight infants: a randomized clinical trial. *JAMA Pediatr.* 2020;174(7):649.

37. Rets A, Clayton AL, Christensen RD, et al. Molecular diagnostic update in hereditary hemolytic anemia and neonatal hyperbilirubinemia. *Int J Lab Hematol.* 2019;41(S1):95-101.

38. Christensen RD, Nussenzveig RH, Yaish HM, et al. Causes of hemolysis in neonates with extreme hyperbilirubinemia. *J Perinatol.* 2014;34(8):616-619.

39. Fujioka K, Kalish F, Wong RJ, et al. Inhibition of heme oxygenase activity using a microparticle formulation of zinc protoporphyrin in an acute hemolytic newborn mouse model. *Pediatr Res.* 2016;79(2):251-257.

40. Bhutani VK, Poland R, Meloy LD, et al. Clinical trial of tin mesoporphyrin to prevent neonatal hyperbilirubinemia. *J Perinatol.* 2016;36(7):533-539.

41. Rosenfeld WN, Hudak ML, Ruiz N, et al. Stannsoporfin with phototherapy to treat hyperbilirubinemia in newborn hemolytic disease. *J Perinatol.* 2022;42(1):110-115.

42. Thielemans L, Peerawaranun P, Mukaka M, et al. High levels of pathological jaundice in the first 24 hours and neonatal hyperbilirubinaemia in an epidemiological cohort study on the Thailand-Myanmar border. *PloS One.* 2021;16(10):e0258127.

43. Mabogunje CA, Olaifa SM, Olusanya BO. Facility-based constraints to exchange transfusions for neonatal hyperbilirubinemia in resource-limited settings. *World J Clin Pediatr.* 2016;5(2):182-190.

44. Taylor JA, Stout JW, de Greef L, et al. Use of a smartphone app to assess neonatal jaundice. *Pediatrics.* 2017;140(3):e20170312.

45. Olusanya BO, Emokpae AA. Use of transcutaneous bilirubin to determine the need for phototherapy in resource-limited settings. *Neonatology.* 2017;111(4):324-330.

Chapter 2

The Pivotal Role of Macrophages in the Pathogenesis of Necrotizing Enterocolitis

Sharada H. Gowda, MD and Akhil Maheshwari, MD, FAAP, FRCP (Edin), FIAH

Chapter Outline

Introduction: Necrotizing Enterocolitis

Necrotizing enterocolitis (NEC) is an inflammatory bowel necrosis seen in infants who are either born extremely premature or are critically ill with multiple organ dysfunction syndrome (MODS).[1-3] The intestinal injury in NEC begins in the mucosa and progresses outwards, and in severe cases, may result in transmural necrosis and perforation.[4,5] Unfortunately, despite major progress in most outcomes, this disease continues to be a leading cause of morbidity and mortality in neonates born between 22 and 28 weeks' gestation.[6,7] The pathophysiology also remains unclear; epidemiologic studies show modest associations with a wide range of seemingly disparate genetic,[8-19] ethnic,[20-23] geographical,[24-27] seasonal (more in April/May), temporal (decadal variations),[28-30] and clinical factors.[2,24,31-62] The clinical associations may span across the pre-, peri-, and post-natal periods, but it is unclear whether these events truly cause NEC or are just epiphenomena related to the overall severity of illness. These clinical variables include intrauterine growth retardation, placental abruption, prolonged rupture of membranes, chorioamnionitis, perinatal asphyxia, congenital cardiac defects, bacterial dysbiosis, patency of the *ductus arteriosus* and/or its treatment with non-steroidal anti-inflammatory drugs, histamine receptor 2 blockers, formula feedings, bovine fortifiers of human milk, certain viral infections, feed thickeners, and severe anemia and/or subsequent red blood cell transfusions.[2,24,31-65] Thrombocytopenia been noted as a risk-factor for NEC in some reports, but the drop in platelet counts could just be a part of the MODS during NEC and not actually cause it.[66,67]

We,[32,67-72] and others,[6,73-85] have described the inflammatory response in NEC lesions. Histopathologically, NEC lesions are marked mainly by intestinal inflammation marked by mucosal edema and leukocyte infiltration, and foci of infarction. Most of these infiltrating leukocytes are macrophages. The specific findings can range from mucosal injury to full-thickness bowel necrosis and perforation.[86] The terminal ileum and colon are involved in most cases, although the entire gastrointestinal tract can be affected in severe cases. Gas-filled bubbles (*pneumatosis*) are seen in affected tissues in 50%; most of these lesions are seen in the submucosa but can extend to other layers in about 50%.[87,88] These changes can be seen both on the mesenteric and the antimesenteric sides.[89] Most of the earlier studies, particularly those on older patients, suggested that *pneumatosis* represented dilated lymphatic vessels,[90-92] but newer descriptions suggest gases entrapped in damaged tissues may be a more likely cause. Microthrombi and microhemorrhages are seen, although vascular thrombi are rare.[93] As the gut heals, bowel wall thickening, fibrinous adhesions, and areas of stenosis can be seen.[94,95]

Macrophages constitute 60% to 70% of the leukocytes in these inflammatory lesions, although there can be some variability between individual patients and sometimes even between noncontiguous lesions in tissues excised from the same patient.[32,67-70,96,97] These changes were seen as indicative as a sign of chronic inflammation. However, in our murine models, macrophage, not neutrophil, infiltration was an initiating sign of inflammation in NEC-like injury.[32,71,72,87,98] Pender et al.[99] have also noted increased CD68+ macrophages in NEC lesions. Managlia et al. noted the role of inflammatory activation of monocytes in experimental NEC.[100] In another study, Tanner and coworkers collated the information in existing studies of NEC and also emphasized the role of macrophages.[101] In preterm infants, peritoneal macrophages also show similar immaturity with hyperinflammatory characteristics.[102] Most NEC lesions also show 20% to 40% neutrophils, but the total number of lymphocytes (about 10%) does not seem to change over unaffected bowel loops.[68]

Macrophage Ontogeny

The name "macrophages" or "big eaters" came from the Greek words, *makros* or large, and *phagein* or eat. These cells have large nuclei with abundant cytoplasm that is sometimes vacuolated. Functionally, macrophages are highly motile, phagocytic, and can also modulate the function of other immune cells. During development, macrophages develop either in (1) the yolk sac from primary progenitors on day 18 or the erythromyeloid progenitors (EMPs) on day 30[103]; and (2) the aorta-gonad-mesonephros (AGM) zone, from CD34+ CD45+ hematopoietic stem cells

(HSCs) (Fig. 2.1).[104] On day 32, these HSCs migrate and differentiate in either the (1) liver during 8 to 32 weeks' gestation or (2) bone marrow. The stages of differentiation can be identified more clearly in the marrow.[105] HSCs mature into common myeloid progenitors, granulocyte-monocyte precursors, common monocyte and dendritic cell (DC) precursors (MDP), premonocytes, and monocytes.[106] After birth, liver HSCs migrate to the bone marrow.[107] HSCs mature into common myeloid progenitors (CMPs) and then differentiate either directly into tissue macrophages or pass through the aforementioned stages to differentiate into monocytes.[108] There are 3 subsets of monocytes: (1) nearly 90% are the classical CD14++ inflammatory monocytes; (2) 10% are the non-classical CD16++ type that patrol the vasculature to assess endothelial integrity, and produce cytokines at intermediate levels; and (3) a few cells that express CD14, CD16, and MHC-II; present antigens; and might activate T lymphocytes.

There are two major subgroups of macrophages that can be differentiated by surface markers, tissue localization, intracellular signaling, and function. The proinflammatory M1 macrophages are regulated by cytokines such as the tumor necrosis factor (TNF) and interferon-γ, bacterial lipopolysaccharide (LPS), and the granulocyte-macrophage colony-stimulating factor (GM-CSF). These cells express surface markers such as CD54, CD80, CD86, and CD197.[109,110] M1 macrophages quickly "inhibit" and kill pathogens as a host defense mechanism.[111] The second class is comprised of the immunoregulatory M2 macrophages responds to interleukin-4 (IL-4), IL-10, IL-13, and IL-21, and to glucocorticoids. M2 macrophages express scavenger receptors such as CD163, CD204, and the mannose receptor, CD206.[109,110] These macrophages are active in immunoregulation, maintain tissue integrity following injuries and in chronic infections, and promote angiogenesis.[111] There is some variability in this nomenclature, although the heterogeneity in the M2 macrophages is being recognized (M2a, M2b, M2c, M2d, and M2f) (Fig. 2.2).[112,113]

In the intestine, EMPs fade away at birth. Macrophages differentiate either from primary progenitors or from circulating monocytes.[114] Unlike the non-inflammatory macrophages in the mature intestine,

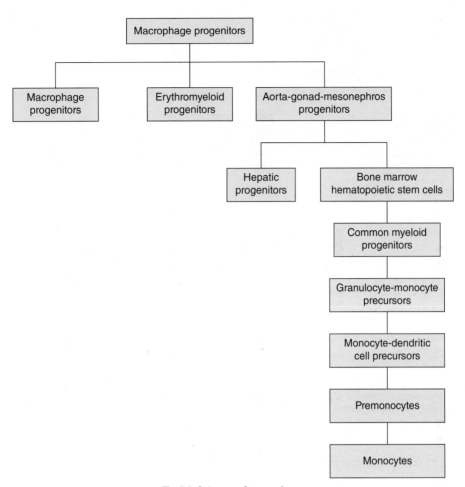

Fig. 2.1 Ontogeny of macrophages.

these cells are still in the process of tissue-specific differentiation and may resemble those in other tissues with inflammatory M1 and various M2 polarization.[115,116]

Macrophages show considerable functional diversity.[117] In premature infants, macrophages express high levels of CD11b, chemokine receptors CCR1, CCR2, CCR5, CXCR1, CXCR2, molecules such as CD115, triggering receptors expressed on myeloid cells (TREM), and 6-sulfo N-acetyllactosamine (LacNAc) glycans. Neonatal macrophages respond both to exogenous chemicals, microbial products, and microparticles[118]; and endogenous stimulants such as cytokines; oxidized lipids; reactive oxygen (ROS) and

nitrogen species (RNS); metabolic products, heat-shock proteins (HSPs), and damage-associated molecular patterns (DAMPs).[118]

MDMs and mDCs show important differences.[119] Ex vivo, monocytes differentiate into macrophages upon exposure to M-CSF, and into mDCs following treatment with GM-CSF and IL-4. Both macrophages and DCs share the phenotypic markers CD11b, CD11c, CD80, CD86, CD163, CD209, and MHC-II. However, macrophages typically express CD68 (macrosialin) and CD33 (siglec-3) with some specificity; DCs may express intercellular adhesion molecule-3-grabbing nonintegrin (DC-SIGN/CD209), CD1c, and CD141.[120]

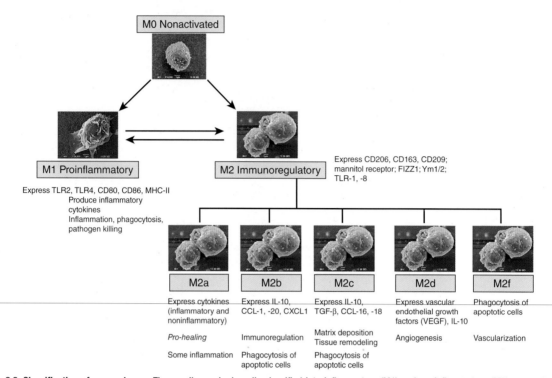

Fig. 2.2 Classification of macrophages. These cells can be broadly classified into inflammatory (M1) and noninflammatory (M2) macrophages. Increasing information now suggests that the M2 cells are comprised of multiple subclasses that may play distinct roles in development, homeostasis, and healing. *IL-10*, Interleukin 10; *MHC-II*, major histocompatibility complex class 2; *TGF*, transforming growth factor; *TLR*, Toll-like receptor.

Maintenance of Macrophage Pools

In the neonatal intestine, gut macrophages are maintained at low levels through continuous local production and recruitment of monocytes, but the pool is expanded during stress, infection, and inflammation. Macrophage subsets may also be altered in resolving inflammation.[121] In other instances, macrophages recruited during the healing phases may promote atypical/chronic inflammation following accumulation of cellular débris,[122-124] microvascular changes,[124-126] or focal apoptosis.[122,123]

M1 macrophages can recognize nucleic acids released from dying cells.[127] TLR3 recognizes double stranded RNA.[128] TLR9 (CD289) can recognize double stranded DNA, DNA: RNA hybrids, and unmethylated CpG.[128] Once activated, TLR9 moves from endoplasmic reticulum to the Golgi apparatus and lysosomes, where it induces MyD88-dependent signaling. TLR7 and the closely related TLR8 respond to purine-rich single-stranded ribonucleic acid.[129] Intracellular

proteins released from dying cells such as IFN-γ, and bacterial components such as peptidoglycan and lipopolysaccharides are also recognized by M1 macrophages.[130] These macrophages express CD86, reactive oxygen species, and proinflammatory cytokines, such as IL-1, IL-6, TNF, and IFN-γ.

Neonatal Gut Macrophages Are yet to Develop the Inflammatory Anergy Seen in Adults

In the adult intestine, macrophages show robust chemotactic and phagocytic responses upon exposure to bacteria and bacterial products but do not produce inflammatory mediators.[131] With this unique dichotomy of function, these macrophages eliminate the invading microorganisms without any unnecessary inflammation and collateral tissue damage. This non-inflammatory differentiation of gut macrophages occurs following exposure to various epithelial and stromal cell-derived peptide growth factors, such as the transforming growth factor (TGF)-β, which are stored in the extracellular matrix (ECM).[131-133]

The premature intestine is developmentally deficient in TGF-β, particularly in its most potent isoform TGF-$β_2$.[32,68-70,98,134] Consequently, neonatal gut macrophages differentiating either from local resident precursors or from newly-recruited hepatic/circulating monocytes are yet to be fully matured and lack the tolerance to bacterial products seen in macrophages in the mature intestine.[68,69,71,98,100,135-139] In neonates, macrophages present in the peritoneal cavity are also hyperresponsive to bacterial products.[140,141] Consequently, any damage to the gut mucosal barrier and bacterial infiltration can trigger a disproportionately intense inflammatory response and cause tissue damage typical of NEC.[32,68-70,98,134]

Macrophages in the Intestinal Mucosa and in Necrotizing Enterocolitis (NEC)

As briefly described above, macrophages comprise up to two-thirds of the leukocyte infiltrates in NEC and play an important role in its pathogenesis (Fig. 2.3).[68,88] Circulating monocyte-derived M1 macrophages with a proinflammatory profile are recruited to NEC lesions, but these cells do not undergo the normal TGF-β-induced hypoinflammatory differentiation.[68,69] These macrophages damage the epithelial barrier and promote bacterial ingress and inflammation in the intestine.[142] The active recruitment of circulating monocytes to NEC lesions is reflected in decreased absolute monocyte counts (AMCs) in peripheral blood; this acute drop in AMCs may be a useful early diagnostic marker of NEC.[143] Consistent with these findings, the severity of necrosis in NEC lesions can be reduced in animal models by inhibiting macrophage recruitment by (1) using specific antibodies against the chemokine ligands or the cognate receptors; (2) using pharmacologic inhibitors; or (3) depleting macrophages in genetically modified mice.[68,69,136,144] Epithelial-derived CXC-motif chemokine ligand 5 (CXCL5)/epithelial-derived neutrophil-activating peptide 78 (ENA-78) and its cognate receptor, CXC-receptor 2 (CXCR2), on macrophages seem to be particularly important in macrophage recruitment.[145] During NEC, the TLR-mediated activation of the nuclear transcription factor NF-kB plays an important role in the recruitment, differentiation, and M1- activation of macrophages in the affected intestine.[146] Interferon regulatory factor 5 (IRF5) can activate M1 genes and promote the immune differentiation and TLR-mediated signal transduction.[147,148] In this context, recent findings that TGF-β and heparin-binding EGF-like growth factor (HB-EGF) can promote an M2-like polarization in macrophages are exciting.[68,69,142]

Microarray Profiles of Human NEC: We compared gene expression datasets from human NEC and uninflamed human neonatal intestine by principal components analysis (PCA). In NEC, PCA accounted for 75.7% of the variability in gene expression. The comparison of gene-expression using fold-change cutoffs of ±1.5, p-value <0.05 (in analysis of variance), and a false discovery rate of 5%, 1377 genes out of a total of 33,297 probe sets were differentially expressed. Of these, 324 genes were upregulated in NEC, whereas 1053 genes were overexpressed in the uninflamed neonatal intestine. The top five upregulated pathways are listed in Table 2.1. A complete listing of the DEGs in NEC has been previously reported.[70,149] The top immune system processes were leukocyte migration (enrichment score of 19.39) and immune response (enrichment scores of 7.95).

Disease-Related Pathways Active in NEC: Consistent with our findings in inflammation and macrophage infiltration, the most important top disease-related pathways[150] were TNF-activated signaling, hematopoietic cell signaling, and cytokine-cytokine receptor interaction. The most important genes were IL-1α, IL-1β, IL-1 receptor 1 (IL1R1), IL1R2, IL-6, TNF receptor superfamily member 1B (TNFRSF1B)/TNFR2, TNFα-induced protein 3 (TNFAIP3)/A20, IL18R1, TGF-$β_3$, TNF superfamily, member 10 (TNFSF10)/TNF-related apoptosis-inducing ligand (TRAIL); chemokines CXC-motif ligand (CXCL)-1, CXCL2, CXCL3, CXCL5, CC-motif ligand (CCL)-2, CCL3, leukocyte receptors CD14, integrin alpha M (ITGAM)/CD11b, colony stimulating factor receptor (CSFR)-2b; the transcription factor CCAAT/enhancer binding protein (C/EBP)-β, enzymes such as prostaglandin-endoperoxide synthase 2 (PTGS2) and alanyl aminopeptidase (ANPEP), and signaling mediators such as suppressor of cytokine signaling 3 (SOCS3), and nuclear factor of kappa light

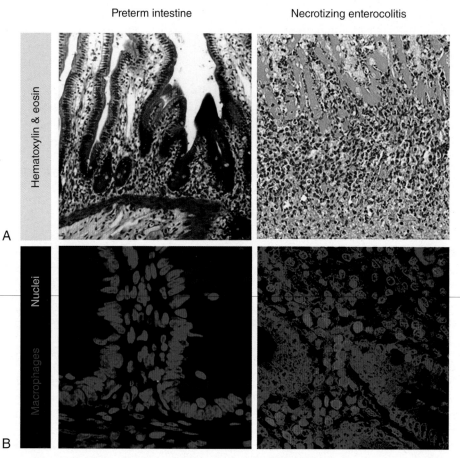

Fig. 2.3 Intestinal loops affected by necrotizing enterocolitis (NEC) show intense leukocyte infiltration. (A) Photomicrographs on the *top* show tissue samples stained with hematoxylin & eosin. Images on *left* show normal-appearing margins of ileum resected for intestinal atresia, and the one on *right* shows a NEC lesion in ileum with marked inflammation. Magnification 100x; **(B)** Fluorescence immunohistochemistry of these lesions (*bottom*; red staining for the macrophage-specific HAM56 antigen) shows that macrophages may comprise up to two-thirds of the infiltrating leukocytes. Nuclei are stained in blue. Magnification 1000x.

TABLE 2.1 Top Canonical Pathways in Necrotizing Enterocolitis		
Name	**p-value**	**Overlap**
Lipopolysaccharide/interleukin-1-mediated inhibition of retinoid X receptor, which affects other nuclear hormone receptors	1.4E-17	35.7% (79/221 genes)
Genes associated with neutrophil and macrophage function	5.74E-16	37.3% (66/177 genes)
Farnesoid X receptor, a member of the nuclear receptor superfamily of ligand-activated transcription factors that regulates bile acid, cholesterol, lipid, and glucose metabolism	8.61E-12	37.3% (47/126 genes)
Xenobiotic metabolism, conversion of relatively lipophilic compounds into more readily excreted hydrophilic metabolites	1.66E-11	28.6% (78/273 genes)
Monocyte (and lymphocyte) adhesion and diapedesis	3.2E-10	30.7% (58/189 genes)

polypeptide gene enhancer in B-cells inhibitor, alpha (NFKBIA)/inhibitor of kappa B-alpha (IκBα).

The top immune system process in NEC was leukocyte migration.[68,88,151] Several cytokines and chemokines were upregulated, including IL-1α, IL-1β, IL-6, CXCL1, CXCL2, CXCL5, CCL2, and CCL3. These findings are consistent with existing data from preclinical and clinical studies on cytokine expression in plasma and tissue samples.[68,152-154] Monocyte/macrophage infiltration in NEC lesions explained upregulation of leukocyte receptors CD14 and CD11b.[68,88,151,155] Increased NF-κB1 and IκB expression was consistent with existing information that single nucleotide polymorphisms (SNPs) of NF-κB1 (g.-24519delATTG) and IκB (g.-1004A>G) were overrepresented, consistent with the dysregulated inflammatory reaction seen in NEC.[156]

LPS-induced Transcriptional Networks: The identification of LPS as the top upstream transcriptional regulator was consistent with the well-documented role of gram-negative bacteria in NEC pathogenesis. We further examined the transcriptional networks associated with LPS exposure. There was an upregulation of IL-1β, IL-6, TNF, and IFN-γ, which, in turn, activated the transcription factors nuclear factor-kappa B-1 (NF-κB1), signal transducer and activator of transcription (STAT)-3, and *c*-Jun. STAT1 and IκBα were predicted to dampen these inflammatory cascades. C/EBP-β activation was identified to be important. Glucocorticoid receptor (nuclear receptor subfamily 3, group C, member 1/NR3C1) was identified as a likely inhibitor in human NEC.

These findings are consistent with existing clinical and laboratory findings in NEC. Infants who develop NEC display a microbial dysbiosis that antedates the onset of NEC, with overrepresentation of gammaproteobacteria (including *Enterobacteriaceae and Pseudomonadaceae*).[49,157] The role of bacteria in NEC pathogenesis is also evident from the occurrence of NEC always after postnatal bacterial colonization and never in the sterile uterine microenvironment prior to birth.[158] Histopathologically, bacterial overgrowth and signatures of bacterial activity such as *pneumatosis*, the accumulation of gaseous products of bacterial fermentation in the bowel wall, are readily evident in NEC.[88,159] Finally, the pathogenic role of gram-negative bacteria in NEC is supported

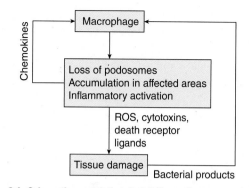

Fig. 2.4. Schematic postulating that inflammatory macrophages play an important pathophysiologic role in necrotizing enterocolitis (NEC). Histopathologic and transcriptional studies show that macrophage infiltration is a prominent finding in NEC. In preterm infants, focal injuries in the gut mucosa can promote bacterial translocation. And stimulated by bacterial products, the still-immature, hyperinflammatory macrophages present in the developing intestine can accentuate the mucosal damage by producing toxic mediators such as reactive oxygen species *(ROS)*, cytotoxins, and death receptor ligands. These changes result in a feed-forward loop of intestinal injury, bacterial translocation, inflammation, and then more injury. Many of these at-risk infants also show gut microbial dysbiosis with increased coliform bacteria, the products or components of which may further accentuate the inflammatory changes.

by evidence that enteral antibiotics such as aminoglycosides can protect against NEC and related mortality.[160] We have combined findings from histopathologic and transcriptional studies with the likely effects of bacterial products in a schematic in Fig. 2.4.

Mechanistic Studies to Study the Role of Gut Macrophages in NEC

(a) Loss of TGF-β-mediated gut macrophage differentiation. To study the role of developmentally-regulated normal, noninflammatory differentiation of gut macrophages in protecting against NEC, we used transgenic mice where TGF-β signaling could be suppressed in gut macrophages. These mice expressed an inducible, dominant-negative truncated version of the TGF-β type II receptors (TGF-β RII) that was nonfunctional.[161] This transgene was expressed in macrophages and carried a metallothionein-like promoter that was inducible upon subcutaneous zinc administration (50 µg/g/day administered for 3 days partially, and for 7 days completely inhibited TGF-β signaling). NEC-like gut injury was induced using a established model, where platelet-activating factor (PAF) and lipopolysaccharide (LPS) were administered intraperitoneally on postnatal day (P) 10.[162,163] Partial and complete abrogation of TGF-β signaling to block normal noninflammatory differentiation of gut macrophages resulted in increasingly severe NEC-like injury.[98,161] Mice were sacrificed 2 hours after PAF and LPS administration, and mucosal injury was graded on a 5-point scale; grade 0: no injury; grade 1: mild separation of *lamina propria*; grade 2: moderate separation of submucosa; grade 3: severe separation and/or edema in submucosa; grade 4: transmural injury.[164]

(b) Intestinal injury by formula feeding and repeated exposures to hypoxia and hypothermia. In these models,[75, 80-82, 164-166] rat or mouse pups were separated from the dam and were fed every 3 hours with formula prepared by mixing 15 grams Similac 60/40 (Abbott Laboratories, Abbott Park, IL) in 75 ml of Esbilac canine milk replacer (PetAg, Hampshire, IL); 200 µL/5 grams weight by gavage. These pups are exposed to hypoxia (5% oxygen for 2 min) and hypothermia (4° Celsius for 10 minutes) twice daily prior to feedings. Pups were sacrificed after 4 days, and intestinal injury was measured as above. Several variants of this protocol have been used, including without the hypothermia,[98] the duration limited to 72 hours, or with gut colonization with bacteria and/or LPS.[100] In another modification of the rat model,[167] *Cronobacter sakazakii* (10^5 cfu/dose) added to the formula caused bacteremia and increased the severity of intestinal injury. In these conditions, leukocyte depletion worsened the outcomes.

Halpern et al.[168] have shown that NEC is associated with macrophage recruitment and activation in NEC through increased expression of IL-18. When they subjected wild type and IL-18 knockout mice to the formula feeding-hypoxia-hypothermia protocol for 72 hours, the incidence and severity of gut injury was significantly reduced in IL-18$^{-/-}$ mice.

Wei *et al.*[11] have also shown proinflammatory M1 macrophages to promote NEC injury. They showed that human NEC was associated with increased expression of interferon regulatory factor 5 (IRF5), which promotes proinflammatory M1 polarization in macrophages.[169] They have also confirmed M1 polarization with upregulation of IRF5 in macrophages in murine NEC. Myeloid-specific deficiency of Irf5 reduced M1 macrophage polarization and systematic inflammation, and prevented experimental NEC. IRF5 bound the promoters of M1 macrophage-associated genes Ccl4, Ccl5, Tnf, and Il12b. The ablation of Irf5 in myeloid cells also suppressed intestinal epithelial cell apoptosis and intestinal barrier dysfunction in experimental NEC.

(c) Observational model for NEC in neonatal baboons. Premature baboons delivered at 67% gestation were treated per current norms for human preterm infants. NEC lesions resembled human NEC with coagulative necrosis, inflammation, hemorrhages, and vascular congestion. There was a deficiency of gut epithelial expression of TGF-$β_2$,[71] which was consistent with our findings on the role of these pathways on macrophage maturation in the gastrointestinal tract.

(d) Risk of Inflammatory Mucosal Injury during Specific Phases of Gut Development. Epidemiologic studies show that the most premature infants who develop NEC do so at a relatively later postnatal age. Computation of the postmenstrual age (PMA; gestational age at birth + postnatal age) showed that the occurrence of NEC peaks at PMA of 32 weeks' gestation.[170-172] Since the clinical risk factors of NEC seem unusually diverse, we hypothesized that NEC represents a generic response to tissue injury during a particular phase of gut development, not to specific causative triggers.[68,151] These possibilities were again consistent with our thinking about the role of immature macrophages in the pathophysiology of NEC. We standardized a mouse model with acute, immune-mediated intestinal injury by enteral administration of the oxidizing organic acid 2, 4, 6-trinitrobenzene sulfonic acid (TNBS; two doses of 0.05 mg/g weight dissolved in 30% ethanol; intragastric and per rectum). Despite a suggestive name, TNBS, which is a derivative of picric acid, does not act like a corrosive to cause a chemical burn on the gut mucosa. The instilled volumes of the TNBS solution are small (1.5 μL/g body weight), aqueous TNBS solutions are not injurious, and no intestinal injury is seen in germ-free animals. TNBS causes intestinal injury in pups through the recruitment and inflammatory activation of gut macrophages resembling that in NEC.[68] This macrophage activation and the relative paucity of lymphocytes differs from that in adult animals where the intestinal injury resembles inflammatory bowel disease with increased Th1-Th17 lymphocytes.[173]

In the neonatal intestine, monocyte recruitment and differentiation into mucosal macrophages normally contributes to mucosal immunity.[132,174] These macrophages display near normal phagocytic and bactericidal properties, but unlike in adults, develop tolerance to bacterial products characteristic of the mature intestine only to some extent.[98] These changes are known to occur under the influence of TGF-beta (TGF-β), particularly the isoform TGF-$β_2$, present in the local extracellular matrix (ECM).[131] In the midgestation intestine, the ECM stores and the bioavailability of TGF-β are still in development.[175] Interestingly, low circulating TGF-β concentrations even on the first postnatal day may predict later occurrence of NEC.[152] In addition to the immaturity of the microenvironment, neonatal intestinal macrophages are also relatively resistant to the hypoinflammatory effects of TGF-β because the downstream signaling pathways are still in development.[68,98,132,176,177] One explanation for both the developmental deficiency of TGF-$β_2$ and the resistance to its intracellular effects is in increased levels of the signaling inhibitor smad7, which in turn, are related to low levels of the ski-like (SKIL) oncoprotein that normally represses the Smad7 promoter,[178,179] Besides blocking TGF-β signaling, smad7 also inhibits the autocrine expression of TGF-$β_2$ in the intestinal epithelium through increased demethylation of lysine 9 on the histone H3 nucleosome (H3K9) and consequent transcriptional silencing.[180] Smad7 may also suppress TGF-β signaling by (1) binding histone deacetylase 1, silent mating type information regulation-1 (SIRT1), and acetyltransferase p300, all of which compete with the activating Smads; (2) promoting the degradation of the TGF-β receptor I (TBRI) either through direct binding or via the formation of a ternary complex with the bone morphogenetic *protein* and activin membrane-bound inhibitor (BAMBI); (3) binding the phosphatase growth-arrest and DNA-damage-inducible protein 34 (GADD34)-protein phosphatase 1c (PP1c) complex to promote TBRI dephosphorylation.[181-183]

(e) NEC-like injury in severely-anemic infants who receive RBC transfusions: Premature infants are a heavily transfused population.[184,185] Unfortunately, red blood cell (RBC) transfusions can be associated with necrotizing enterocolitis (NEC); 25% to 40% of infants who develop NEC may have received an RBC transfusion in the previous 48 hours.[186] The association of transfusions with subsequent NEC has been noted in numerous clinical studies[186-208] and in meta-analysis of data recorded in these studies.[188,209-211]

Our research team developed a murine model of transfusion and anemia-associated NEC (taa-NEC).[136] Macrophages were noted to play a significant role in the pathogenesis of taa-NEC. We examined mouse pups in 4 groups: (1) naïve control; (2) transfusion control; (3) anemic control; and (4) anemic-transfused mice. In preliminary studies, our mice showed near-absence of *Gammaproteobacteria* in their intestines, and therefore we examined some mice after introducing *Serratia marcescens* isolated from a human infant with NEC (10⁴ colony-forming units; gavage) in all groups.[82] This approach has been used in earlier studies to examine the effects of bacterial colonization on NEC.[46] The bacterial colonization did not change the outcomes in our murine model.

The naïve controls were observed without further intervention. Anemic control and anemic-transfused groups were rendered anemic by repeated phlebotomy on P2, P4, P6, P8, and P10. In phlebotomized mice, the hematocrit dropped from 49.2±1% on P2 to 21.7±0.4% after the 5th phlebotomy on P10. The anemic control and anemic-transfused pups showed normal physical activity, no weight gain, and on autopsy, no hepatic venous congestion, indicating that these animals did not develop congestive heart failure due to severe anemia. Transfusion controls and anemic-transfused pups were given an allogeneic RBC transfusion[212] on P11 with leukoreduced, packed RBCs (20 mL/kg RBCs obtained from FVB/NJ donors, injected into the retro-orbital venous plexus). These transfused RBCs had been previously leukoreduced by buffy coat removal[213] to eliminate >99% leukocytes and platelets, packed to a hematocrit of 70%, and stored at 4°C for 7 days. Animals were sacrificed on P13, or earlier if they developed physical distress. Intestinal injury was seen in anemic-transfused mice and was graded as above.[68] Histopathologic findings of necrosis, inflammation, and interstitial hemorrhages indicated a strong resemblance to human NEC.[88]

Both anemic and the anemic-transfused mice showed monocyte/macrophage infiltration in the affected intestine.[214] RBC transfusions contained free hemoglobin and heme,[215] which activated the newly-recruited monocytes and macrophages in the intestine by activating Toll-like receptor 4 (TLR4)-mediated signaling, redox cycling,[216] and downstream NF-κB pathways.[217] The role of TLR4 in NEC pathogenesis has been noted in other NEC models,[218] and these seminal findings in transfusion and anemia-associated NEC (taa-NEC) highlighted the importance of these pathways as a unifying mechanism in NEC. The requirement of macrophages in (taa-NEC) was notable because macrophage depletion prior to transfusions was protective. Blocking the NF-κB pathway in macrophages by administering specific inhibitory nanoparticles was also protective against (taa-NEC).[136]

The severity of anemia was important in murine taa-NEC. Mouse pups defined to have severe anemia (hematocrit 20% to 24%) developed more severe bowel injury as compared to those with moderate anemia (hematocrit 25% to 30%). The duration of anemia was also important; mice transfused on P10 (soon after the last phlebotomy) sustained less bowel damage than those transfused 24 hours later, on P11. If the transfused RBCs were leukoreduced, washed, and resuspended in saline prior to storage, the severity of taa-NEC was decreased. Pups that received multiple transfusions showed more severe injury. However, the duration of RBC storage (7 days vs. 14 days) prior to transfusions did not change the severity of taa-NEC.

Conclusions and Future Directions: Existing information indicates that inflammatory macrophages play a deleterious role in the development of neonatal intestinal injury. However, our understanding of the pathophysiology of NEC has considerable limitations. Macrophages, with agile movement, phagocytosis, activation, and application of molecular pathways involving ROS, and TLR4- and NF-κB-activated signaling cascades, have been noted to serve both protective and pathologic roles, depending on the activating stimuli.[219-222] There could well be a context- and stage-dependent dichotomy in the impact of these cells.

In NEC, a disease that affects the tiniest of infants, nearly all histopathologic information has been obtained from tissue samples obtained from surgery or autopsies. There could well be a bias in our understanding of this disease towards the severe end of its spectrum. Consequently, the animal models that have been developed to simulate our observations may also reflect severe disease. In this context, early detection of NEC by bedside tools such as portable sonography[45] and in-vivo imaging of inflammatory mediators, including activated macrophages,[223] can help in the development of diagnostic biomarkers. The note of caution is that these bedside tools for detecting markers such as *pneumatosis* may detect only 50% of all patients. We may also need to re-evaluate our animal models. With improving survival of the most premature infants, the age at onset of NEC is moving to later postnatal chronological ages, and traditional models such as those based on formula feeding-hypoxia-hypothermia in the first 3-4 postnatal days may need re-evaluation. There is a need for cautious interpretation and validation of laboratory findings, and possibly for less reluctance in developing/testing/evaluating new models.

With an incidence as low as 2% to 3% of very-low-birth-weight infants, it is difficult to design adequately-powered clinical studies with an appropriate number of patients with NEC. In all studies focused on diseases defined by histopathology or limited markers, there is a need for caution in the interpretation of results.[224] Just as cirrhosis of the liver can occur following exposure to diverse causes of injury including alcohol, chemicals, and viruses, conditions such as NEC could well be a conglomeration of disorders rather than a single condition.[225] There have been commendable efforts to design multicentric studies to recruit larger samples, but considering the variability in the incidence of NEC in various centers, which indicate that genetic, geographic, and practice-related factors may be important, even these numbers may not be adequate. In our (unpublished) e-mail surveys, the incidence of NEC varied between 3% to 12% in the largest academic centers. There are hospitals that claimed near-nil incidence, but the number of extremely-low-birth-weight infants in these centers seemed low. We need to continue these efforts to obtain accurate epidemiologic information.

The variability in clinical practice in various neonatal centers is also an important issue. Improvements in clinical management of NEC may have reduced the need for surgical excision only to the most severely-afflicted infants, but this limits the information from a scientific standpoint. Because NEC remains an idiopathic disease, the preclinical/animal models are at best an approximation to simulate the disease in the laboratory and may not always capture the complexity and temporal progression of this natural, multifactorial disease. Studies in small animals may also overlook the physiologic covariates such as blood pressures and perfusion of vascular watershed areas, feeding experience, comorbidities, and microbial flora. Nevertheless, our findings indicate a clear opportunity to re-evaluate the role of a subset of leukocytes, the macrophages, in the pathogenesis of NEC. This information may also allow better understanding of these cells in other disease processes.

REFERENCES

1. Xiong T, Maheshwari A, Neu J, Ei-Saie A, Pammi M. An overview of systematic reviews of randomized-controlled trials for preventing necrotizing enterocolitis in preterm infants. *Neonatology.* 2020;117:46-56.
2. Pammi M, De Plaen IG, Maheshwari A. Recent advances in necrotizing enterocolitis research: strategies for implementation in clinical practice. *Clin Perinatol.* 2020;47:383-397.
3. Garg PM, Hitt MM, Blackshear C, Maheshwari A. Clinical determinants of postoperative outcomes in surgical necrotizing enterocolitis. *J Perinatol.* 2020;40:1671-1678.
4. Frost BL, Jilling T, Caplan MS. The importance of pro-inflammatory signaling in neonatal necrotizing enterocolitis. *Semin Perinatol.* 2008;32:100-106.
5. Henry MC, Moss LR. Necrotizing enterocolitis. *Annu Rev Med.* 2008;60:111-124. doi:10.1146/annurev.med.60.050207.092824.
6. Neu J, Walker WA. Necrotizing enterocolitis. *N Engl J Med.* 2011; 364:255-264.
7. Patel RM, Kandefer S, Walsh MC, et al. Causes and timing of death in extremely premature infants from 2000 through 2011. *N Engl J Med.* 2015;372:331-340.
8. O'Neill Jr JA, Stahlman MT, Meng HC. Necrotizing enterocolitis in the newborn: operative indications. *Ann Surg.* 1975;182:274-279.
9. Tremblay E, Ferretti E, Babakissa C, et al. IL-17-related signature genes linked to human necrotizing enterocolitis. *BMC Res Notes.* 2021;14:82.
10. Kosik K, Szpecht D, Al-Saad SR, et al. Single nucleotide vitamin D receptor polymorphisms (FokI, BsmI, ApaI, and TaqI) in the pathogenesis of prematurity complications. *Sci Rep.* 2020;10: 21098.
11. Wei J, Tang D, Lu C, et al. Irf5 deficiency in myeloid cells prevents necrotizing enterocolitis by inhibiting M1 macrophage polarization. *Mucosal Immunol.* 2019;12:888-896.
12. Cuna A, George L, Sampath V. Genetic predisposition to necrotizing enterocolitis in premature infants: current knowledge, challenges, and future directions. *Semin Fetal Neonatal Med.* 2018;23:387-393.
13. Chen G, Li Y, Su Y, et al. Identification of candidate genes for necrotizing enterocolitis based on microarray data. *Gene.* 2018;661:152-159.
14. Sampath V, Bhandari V, Berger J, et al. A functional ATG16L1 (T300A) variant is associated with necrotizing enterocolitis in premature infants. *Pediatr Res.* 2017;81:582-588.
15. Jung K, Koh I, Kim JH, et al. RNA-Seq for gene expression profiling of human necrotizing enterocolitis: a pilot study. *J Korean Med Sci.* 2017;32:817-824.
16. Banyasz I, Bokodi G, Vásárhelyi B, et al. Genetic polymorphisms for vascular endothelial growth factor in perinatal complications. *Eur Cytokine Netw.* 2006;17:266-270.
17. Bhandari V, Bizzarro MJ, Shetty A, et al. Familial and genetic susceptibility to major neonatal morbidities in preterm twins. *Pediatrics.* 2006;117:1901-1906.
18. Barak S, Riskin A, Kugelman A, et al. Necrotizing enterocolitis in a premature infant as the presenting symptom of familial dysautonomia in the neonatal period: case report and review of the literature. *Am J Perinatol.* 2005;22:353-355.
19. Heninger E, Treszl A, Kocsis I, et al. Genetic variants of the interleukin-18 promoter region (-607) influence the course of necrotising enterocolitis in very low birth weight neonates. *Eur J Pediatr.* 2002;161:410-411.
20. Cuna A, Sampath V, Khashu M. Racial disparities in necrotizing enterocolitis. *Front Pediatr.* 2021;9:633088.
21. Uauy RD, Fanaroff AA, Korones SB, et al. Necrotizing enterocolitis in very low birth weight infants: biodemographic and clinical correlates. National Institute of Child Health and Human Development Neonatal Research Network. *J Pediatr.* 1991;119:630-638.
22. Anderson JG, Rogers EE, Baer RJ, et al. Racial and ethnic disparities in preterm infant mortality and severe morbidity: a population-based study. *Neonatology.* 2018;113:44-54.
23. Jammeh ML, Adibe OO, Tracy ET, et al. Racial/ethnic differences in necrotizing enterocolitis incidence and outcomes in premature very low birth weight infants. *J Perinatol.* 2018;38: 1386-1390.
24. Sankaran K, Puckett B, Lee DS, et al. Variations in incidence of necrotizing enterocolitis in Canadian neonatal intensive care units. *J Pediatr Gastroenterol Nutr.* 2004;39:366-372.
25. Alsaied A, Islam N, Thalib L. Global incidence of Necrotizing Enterocolitis: a systematic review and meta-analysis. *BMC Pediatr.* 2020;20:344.
26. Su BH, Hsieh WS, Hsu CH, et al. Neonatal outcomes of extremely preterm infants from Taiwan: comparison with Canada, Japan, and the USA. *Pediatr Neonatol.* 2015;56:46-52.

27. Guner YS, Friedlich P, Wee CP, et al. State-based analysis of necrotizing enterocolitis outcomes. *J Surg Res.* 2009;157:21-29.

28. Ahle M, Drott P, Andersson RE. Epidemiology and trends of necrotizing enterocolitis in Sweden: 1987-2009. *Pediatrics.* 2013; 132:e443-e451.

29. Javidi D, Wang Z, Rajasekaran S, Hussain N. Temporal and seasonal variations in incidence of stage II and III NEC-a 28-year epidemiologic study from tertiary NICUs in Connecticut, USA. *J Perinatol.* 2021;41:1100-1109.

30. Meinzen-Derr J, Morrow AL, Hornung RW, et al. Epidemiology of necrotizing enterocolitis temporal clustering in two neonatology practices. *J Pediatr.* 2009;154:656-661.

31. Kasivajjula H, Maheshwari A. Pathophysiology and current management of necrotizing enterocolitis. *Indian J Pediatr.* 2014;81: 489-497.

32. MohanKumar K, Namachivayam K, Song T, et al. A murine neonatal model of necrotizing enterocolitis caused by anemia and red blood cell transfusions. *Nat Commun.* 2019;10(1):3494.

33. Rao PS. Single ventricle-A comprehensive review. *Children (Basel).* 2021;8(6):441.

34. Papneja K, Laks J, Szabo AB, Grosse-Wortmann L. Low descending aorta flow is associated with adverse feeding outcomes in neonates with small left-sided structures. *Int J Cardiovasc Imaging.* 2021;37:269-273.

35. Minocha PK, Phoon C. *Tricuspid Atresia.* In: StatPearls [Internet]. Treasure Island (FL): StatPearls Publishing; 2023 Jan.

36. Kelleher ST, McMahon CJ, James A. Necrotizing enterocolitis in children with congenital heart disease: a literature review. *Pediatr Cardiol.* 2021;42(8):1688-1689. doi:10.1007/s00246-021-02691-1.

37. Gunadi, Sirait DN, Fauzi AR, et al. Challenge in diagnosis of late onset necrotizing enterocolitis in a term infant: a case report. *BMC Pediatr.* 2021;21:152.

38. Talavera MM, Jin Y, Zmuda EJ, et al. Single nucleotide polymorphisms in the dual specificity phosphatase genes and risk of necrotizing enterocolitis in premature infant. *J Neonatal Perinatal Med.* 2020;13:373-380.

39. Spinner JA, Morris SA, Nandi D, et al. Necrotizing enterocolitis and associated mortality in neonates with congenital heart disease: a multi-institutional study. *Pediatr Crit Care Med.* 2020;21:228-234.

40. O'Connor G, Brown KL, Taylor AM. Faecal calprotectin concentrations in neonates with CHD: pilot study. *Cardiol Young.* 2020;30:624-628.

41. Klinke M, Wiskemann H, Bay B, et al. Cardiac and inflammatory necrotizing enterocolitis in newborns are not the same entity. *Front Pediatr.* 2020;8:593926.

42. Jones IH, Hall NJ. Contemporary outcomes for infants with necrotizing Enterocolitis-A systematic review. *J Pediatr.* 2020; 220:86-92.e3.

43. Lau PE, Cruz SM, Ocampo EC, et al. Necrotizing enterocolitis in patients with congenital heart disease: a single center experience. *J Pediatr Surg.* 2018;53:914-917.

44. ElHassan NO, Tang X, Gossett J, et al. Necrotizing enterocolitis in infants with hypoplastic left heart syndrome following stage 1 palliation or heart transplant. *Pediatr Cardiol.* 2018;39:774-785.

45. Cuna AC, Lee JC, Robinson AL, et al. Bowel ultrasound for the diagnosis of necrotizing enterocolitis: a meta-analysis. *Ultrasound Q.* 2018;34:113-118.

46. Pammi M, Cope J, Tarr PI, et al. Intestinal dysbiosis in preterm infants preceding necrotizing enterocolitis: a systematic review and meta-analysis. *Microbiome.* 2017;5:31.

47. Lu Q, Cheng S, Zhou M, Yu J. Risk factors for necrotizing enterocolitis in neonates: a retrospective case-control study. *Pediatr Neonatol.* 2017;58:165-170.

48. Hyung N, Campwala I, Boskovic DS, et al. The relationship of red blood cell transfusion to intestinal mucosal injury in premature infants. *J Pediatr Surg.* 2017;52:1152-1155.

49. Warner BB, Deych E, Zhou Y, et al. Gut bacteria dysbiosis and necrotising enterocolitis in very low birthweight infants: a prospective case-control study. *Lancet.* 2016;387(10031):1928-1936. doi:10.1016/S0140-6736(16)00081-7.

50. Lin HC, Su BH, Chen AC. H2-blocker therapy and necrotizing enterocolitis for very low birth weight preterm infants. *Pediatrics.* 2006;118:1794-1795; author reply 1795-1796.

51. Guillet R, Stoll BJ, Cotten CM, et al. Association of H2-blocker therapy and higher incidence of necrotizing enterocolitis in very low birth weight infants. *Pediatrics.* 2006;117:e137-e142.

52. Lodha A, de Silva N, Petric M, Moore AM. Human torovirus: a new virus associated with neonatal necrotizing enterocolitis. *Acta Paediatr.* 2005;94:1085-1088.

53. Kenton AB, O'Donovan D, Cass DL, et al. Severe thrombocytopenia predicts outcome in neonates with necrotizing enterocolitis. *J Perinatol.* 2005;25:14-20.

54. Giannone PJ, Luce WA, Nankervis CA, Hoffman TM, Wold LE. Necrotizing enterocolitis in neonates with congenital heart disease. *Life Sci.* 2008;82:341-347.

55. Goelz R, Hamprecht K, Klingel K, Poets CF. Intestinal manifestations of postnatal and congenital cytomegalovirus infection in term and preterm infants. *J Clin Virol.* 2016;83:29-36.

56. Yu VY, Tudehope DI. Neonatal necrotizing enterocolitis: 2. Perinatal risk factors. *Med J Aust.* 1977;1:688-693.

57. Kliegman RM, Hack M, Jones P, Fanaroff AA. Epidemiologic study of necrotizing enterocolitis among low-birth-weight infants. Absence of identifiable risk factors. *J Pediatr.* 1982;100:440-444.

58. Martinez-Tallo E, Claure N, Bancalari E. Necrotizing enterocolitis in full-term or near-term infants: risk factors. *Biol Neonate.* 1997;71:292-298.

59. Kosloske AM, Ulrich JA. A bacteriologic basis for the clinical presentations of necrotizing enterocolitis. *J Pediatr Surg.* 1980; 15:558-564.

60. Carbonaro CA, Clark DA, Elseviers D. A bacterial pathogenicity determinant associated with necrotizing enterocolitis. *Microb Pathog.* 1988;5:427-436.

61. Clark DA, Fornabaio DM, McNeill H, et al. Contribution of oxygen-derived free radicals to experimental necrotizing enterocolitis. *Am J Pathol.* 1988;130:537-542.

62. Stoll BJ, Kanto Jr WP, Glass RI, Nahmias AJ, Brann Jr AW. Epidemiology of necrotizing enterocolitis: a case control study. *J Pediatr.* 1980;96:447-451.

63. Sharma R, Garrison RD, Tepas JJ III, et al. Rotavirus-associated necrotizing enterocolitis: an insight into a potentially preventable disease? *J Pediatr Surg.* 2004;39:453-457.

64. van Acker J, de Smet F, Muyldermans G, et al. Outbreak of necrotizing enterocolitis associated with Enterobacter Sakazakii in powdered milk formula. *J Clin Microbiol.* 2001;39: 293-297.

65. Warren S, Schreiber JR, Epstein MF. Necrotizing enterocolitis and hemolysis associated with Clostridium perfringens. *Am J Dis Child.* 1984;138:686-688.

66. Kenton AB, Hegemier S, Smith EO, et al. Platelet transfusions in infants with necrotizing enterocolitis do not lower mortality but may increase morbidity. *J Perinatol.* 2005;25:173-177.

67. Namachivayam K, MohanKumar K, Shores DR, et al. Targeted inhibition of thrombin attenuates murine neonatal necrotizing enterocolitis. *Proc Natl Acad Sci U S A.* 2020;117:10958-10969.

68. MohanKumar K, Kaza N, Jagadeeswaran R, et al. Gut mucosal injury in neonates is marked by macrophage infiltration in contrast to pleomorphic infiltrates in adult: evidence from an

animal model. *Am J Physiol Gastrointest Liver Physiol.* 2012;303: G93-G102.

69. MohanKumar K, Namachivayam K, Chapalamadugu KC, et al. Smad7 interrupts TGF-β signaling in intestinal macrophages and promotes inflammatory activation of these cells during necrotizing enterocolitis. *Pediatr Res.* 2016;79:951-961.

70. MohanKumar K, Namachivayam K, Cheng F, et al. Trinitrobenzene sulfonic acid-induced intestinal injury in neonatal mice activates transcriptional networks similar to those seen in human necrotizing enterocolitis. *Pediatr Res.* 2016;81:99-112.

71. Namachivayam K, Blanco CL, MohanKumar K, et al. Smad7 inhibits autocrine expression of TGF-beta2 in intestinal epithelial cells in baboon necrotizing enterocolitis. *Am J Physiol Gastrointest Liver Physiol.* 2013;304:G167-G180.

72. Namachivayam K, MohanKumar K, Garg L, Torres BA, Maheshwari A. Neonatal mice with necrotizing enterocolitis-like injury develop thrombocytopenia despite increased megakaryopoiesis. *Pediatr Res.* 2017;81:817-824.

73. Amer MD, Hedlund E, Rochester J, Caplan MS. Platelet-activating factor concentration in the stool of human newborns: effects of enteral feeding and neonatal necrotizing enterocolitis. *Biol Neonate.* 2004;85:159-166.

74. Caplan MS, Amer M, Jilling T. The role of human milk in necrotizing enterocolitis. *Adv Exp Med Biol.* 2002;503:83-90.

75. Caplan MS, Hedlund E, Adler L, Hsueh W. Role of asphyxia and feeding in a neonatal rat model of necrotizing enterocolitis. *Pediatr Pathol.* 1994;14:1017-1028.

76. Caplan MS, Hedlund E, Adler L, Lickerman M, Hsueh W. The platelet-activating factor receptor antagonist WEB 2170 prevents neonatal necrotizing enterocolitis in rats. *J Pediatr Gastroenterol Nutr.* 1997;24:296-301.

77. Caplan MS, Hsueh W. Necrotizing enterocolitis: role of platelet activating factor, endotoxin, and tumor necrosis factor. *J Pediatr.* 1990;117:S47-S51.

78. Caplan MS, Jilling T. Neonatal necrotizing enterocolitis: possible role of probiotic supplementation. *J Pediatr Gastroenterol Nutr.* 2000;30 suppl 2:S18-S22.

79. Caplan MS, MacKendrick W. Necrotizing enterocolitis: a review of pathogenetic mechanisms and implications for prevention. *Pediatr Pathol.* 1993;13:357-369.

80. Caplan MS, Sun XM, Hsueh W. Hypoxia, PAF, and necrotizing enterocolitis. *Lipids.* 1991;26:1340-1343.

81. De Plaen IG, Liu SX, Tian R, et al. Inhibition of nuclear factor-kappaB ameliorates bowel injury and prolongs survival in a neonatal rat model of necrotizing enterocolitis. *Pediatr Res.* 2007;61:716-721.

82. Jilling T, Simon D, Lu J, et al. The roles of bacteria and TLR4 in rat and murine models of necrotizing enterocolitis. *J Immunol.* 2006;177:3273-3282.

83. Nanthakumar NN, Fusunyan RD, Sanderson I, Walker WA. Inflammation in the developing human intestine: a possible pathophysiologic contribution to necrotizing enterocolitis. *Proc Natl Acad Sci U S A.* 2000;97:6043-6048.

84. Neu J, Chen M, Beierle E. Intestinal innate immunity: how does it relate to the pathogenesis of necrotizing enterocolitis. *Semin Pediatr Surg.* 2005;14:137-144.

85. Nowicki PT. Ischemia and necrotizing enterocolitis: where, when, and how. *Semin Pediatr Surg.* 2005;14:152-158.

86. Yu L, Tian J, Zhao X, et al. Bowel perforation in premature infants with necrotizing enterocolitis: risk factors and outcomes. *Gastroenterol Res Pract.* 2016;2016:6134187.

87. Garg PM, Bernieh A, Hitt MM, et al. Incomplete resection of necrotic bowel may increase mortality in infants with necrotizing enterocolitis. *Pediatr Res.* 2021;89:163-170.

88. Remon JI, Amin SC, Mehendale SR, et al. Depth of bacterial invasion in resected intestinal tissue predicts mortality in surgical necrotizing enterocolitis. *J Perinatol.* 2015;35:755-762.

89. Feczko PJ, Mezwa DG, Farah MC, White BD. Clinical significance of pneumatosis of the bowel wall. *Radiographics.* 1992;12:1069-1078.

90. Haboubi NY, Honan RP, Hasleton PS, et al. Pneumatosis coli: a case report with ultrastructural study. *Histopathology.* 1984;8:145-155.

91. Gui X, Zhou Y, Eidus L, et al. Is pneumatosis cystoides intestinalis gas-distended and ruptured lymphatics? Reappraisal by immunohistochemistry. *Arch Pathol Lab Med.* 2014;138:1059-1066.

92. Koreishi A, Lauwers GY, Misdraji J. Pneumatosis intestinalis: a challenging biopsy diagnosis. *Am J Surg Pathol.* 2007;31:1469-1475.

93. Edison P, Arunachalam S, Baral V, Bharadwaj S. Varying clinical presentations of umbilical venous catheter extravasation: a case series. *J Paediatr Child Health.* 2021;57:1123-1126.

94. Janik JS, Ein SH, Mancer K. Intestinal stricture after necrotizing enterocolitis. *J Pediatr Surg.* 1981;16:438-443.

95. Kosloske AM, Burstein J, Bartow SA. Intestinal obstruction due to colonic stricture following neonatal necrotizing enterocolitis. *Ann Surg.* 1980;192:202-207.

96. Mezu-Ndubuisi OJ, Maheshwari A. Role of macrophages in fetal development and perinatal disorders. *Pediatr Res.* 2020;90(3):513-523. doi:10.1038/s41390-020-01209-4.

97. MohanKumar K, Namachivayam K, Sivakumar N, et al. Severe neonatal anemia increases intestinal permeability by disrupting epithelial adherens junctions. *Am J Physiol Gastrointest Liver Physiol.* 2020;318:G705-G716.

98. Maheshwari A, Kelly DR, Nicola T, et al. TGF-β2 suppresses macrophage cytokine production and mucosal inflammatory responses in the developing intestine. *Gastroenterology.* 2011;140:242-253.

99. Pender SL, Braegger C, Gunther U, et al. Matrix metalloproteinases in necrotizing enterocolitis. *Pediatr Res.* 2003;54:160-164.

100. Managlia E, Liu SXL, Yan X, et al. Blocking NF-kappaB activation in Ly6c(+) monocytes attenuates necrotizing enterocolitis. *Am J Pathol.* 2019;189:604-618.

101. Tanner SM, Berryhill TF, Ellenburg JL, et al. Pathogenesis of necrotizing enterocolitis: modeling the innate immune response. *Am J Pathol.* 2015;185:4-16.

102. Agrawal V, Jaiswal MK, Ilievski V, et al. Platelet-activating factor: a role in preterm delivery and an essential interaction with Toll-like receptor signaling in mice. *Biol Reprod.* 2014;91:119.

103. Stremmel C, Schuchert R, Wagner F, et al. Yolk sac macrophage progenitors traffic to the embryo during defined stages of development. *Nat Commun.* 2018;9:75.

104. Mariani SA, Li Z, Rice S, et al. Pro-inflammatory aorta-associated macrophages are involved in embryonic development of hematopoietic stem cells. *Immunity.* 2019;50:1439-1452.e5.

105. McGrath KE, Frame JM, Fegan KH, et al. Distinct sources of hematopoietic progenitors emerge before HSCs and provide functional blood cells in the mammalian embryo. *Cell Rep.* 2015;11:1892-1904.

106. Kelemen E, Janossa M. Macrophages are the first differentiated blood cells formed in human embryonic liver. *Exp Hematol.* 1980;8:996-1000.

107. Palis J, Yoder MC. Yolk-sac hematopoiesis: the first blood cells of mouse and man. *Exp Hematol.* 2001;29:927-936.

108. Sinka L, Biasch K, Khazaal I, Peault B, Tavian M. Angiotensin-converting enzyme (CD143) specifies emerging lympho-hematopoietic progenitors in the human embryo. *Blood.* 2012;119:3712-3723.

109. Martinez FO, Gordon S. The M1 and M2 paradigm of macrophage activation: time for reassessment. *F1000Prime Rep.* 2014;6:13.

110. Wang N, Liang H, Zen K. Molecular mechanisms that influence the macrophage M1–M2 polarization balance. *Front Immunol.* 2014;5:614.

111. Mills CD, Ley K. M1 and M2 macrophages: the chicken and the egg of immunity. *J Innate Immun.* 2014;6:716-726.

112. Yao Y, Xu XH, Jin L. Macrophage polarization in physiological and pathological pregnancy. *Front Immunol.* 2019;10:792.

113. Hong H, Tian XY. The role of macrophages in vascular repair and regeneration after ischemic injury. *Int J Mol Sci.* 2020;21(17):6328.

114. Perdiguero EG, Geissmann F. The development and maintenance of resident macrophages. *Nat Immunol.* 2016;17:2-8.

115. Wynn TA, Chawla A, Pollard JW. Macrophage biology in development, homeostasis and disease. *Nature.* 2013;496:445-455.

116. Dreschers S, Ohl K, Schulte N, Tenbrock K, Orlikowsky TW. Impaired functional capacity of polarised neonatal macrophages. *Sci Rep.* 2020;10:1-12.

117. Winterberg T, Vieten G, Meier T, et al. Distinct phenotypic features of neonatal murine macrophages. *Eur J Immunol.* 2015;45:214-224.

118. de la Paz Sánchez-Martínez M, Blanco-Favela F, Mora-Ruiz MD, et al. IL-17-differentiated macrophages secrete proinflammatory cytokines in response to oxidized low-density lipoprotein. *Lipids Health Dis.* 2017;16:196.

119. Merad M, Sathe P, Helft J, Miller J, Mortha A. The dendritic cell lineage: ontogeny and function of dendritic cells and their subsets in the steady state and the inflamed setting. *Annu Rev Immunol.* 2013;31:563-604.

120. Geissmann F, Manz MG, Jung S, et al. Development of monocytes, macrophages, and dendritic cells. *Science.* 2010;327:656-661.

121. Murray PJ. Macrophage polarization. *Annu Rev Physiol.* 2017;79:541-566.

122. Hashimoto D, Chow A, Noizat C, et al. Tissue-resident macrophages self-maintain locally throughout adult life with minimal contribution from circulating monocytes. *Immunity.* 2013;38:792-804.

123. Blériot C, Dupuis T, Jouvion G, et al. Liver-resident macrophage necroptosis orchestrates type 1 microbicidal inflammation and type-2-mediated tissue repair during bacterial infection. *Immunity.* 2015;42:145-158.

124. Yang X, Chang Y, Wei W. Emerging role of targeting macrophages in rheumatoid arthritis: focus on polarization, metabolism and apoptosis. *Cell Prolif.* 2020;53(7):e12854.

125. Graney P, Ben-Shaul S, Landau S, et al. Macrophages of diverse phenotypes drive vascularization of engineered tissues. *Sci Adv.* 2020;6:eaay6391.

126. Liu YC, Zou XB, Chai YF, Yao YM. Macrophage polarization in inflammatory diseases. *Int J Biol Sci.* 2014;10:520.

127. Krzyszczyk P, Schloss R, Palmer A, Berthiaume F. The role of macrophages in acute and chronic wound healing and interventions to promote pro-wound healing phenotypes. *Front Physiol.* 2018;9:419.

128. Alexopoulou L, Holt AC, Medzhitov R, Flavell RA. Recognition of double-stranded RNA and activation of NF-kappaB by Toll-like receptor 3. *Nature.* 2001;413:732-738.

129. Diebold SS, Kaisho T, Hemmi H, Akira S, Reis e Sousa C. Innate antiviral responses by means of TLR7-mediated recognition of single-stranded RNA. *Science.* 2004;303:1529-1531.

130. Ferrante CJ, Leibovich SJ. Regulation of macrophage polarization and wound healing. *Adv Wound Care.* 2012;1:10-16.

131. Smythies LE, Sellers M, Clements RH, et al. Human intestinal macrophages display profound inflammatory anergy despite avid phagocytic and bacteriocidal activity. *J Clin Invest.* 2005;115:66-75.

132. Smythies LE, Maheshwari A, Clements R, et al. Mucosal IL-8 and TGF-beta recruit blood monocytes: evidence for crosstalk between the lamina propria stroma and myeloid cells. *J Leukoc Biol.* 2006;80:492-499.

133. Maheshwari A, Smythies LE, Wu X, et al. Cytomegalovirus blocks intestinal stroma-induced down-regulation of macrophage HIV-1 infection. *J Leukoc Biol.* 2006;80:1111-1117.

134. Maheshwari A. Immunologic and hematological abnormalities in necrotizing enterocolitis. *Clin Perinatol.* 2015;42:567-585.

135. Prince LR, Maxwell NC, Gill SK, et al. Macrophage phenotype is associated with disease severity in preterm infants with chronic lung disease. *PLoS One.* 2014;9:e103059.

136. MohanKumar K, Namachivayam K, Song T, et al. A murine neonatal model of necrotizing enterocolitis caused by anemia and red blood cell transfusions. *Nat Commun.* 2019;10:3494.

137. Kalymbetova TV, Selvakumar B, Rodríguez-Castillo JA, et al. Resident alveolar macrophages are master regulators of arrested alveolarization in experimental bronchopulmonary dysplasia. *J Pathol.* 2018;245:153-159.

138. Liu F, McCullough LD. Inflammatory responses in hypoxic ischemic encephalopathy. *Acta Pharmacol Sin.* 2013;34:1121-1130.

139. He YM, Li X, Perego M, et al. Transitory presence of myeloid-derived suppressor cells in neonates is critical for control of inflammation. *Nat Med.* 2018;24:224-231.

140. Winterberg T, Vieten G, Meier T, et al. Distinct phenotypic features of neonatal murine macrophages. *Eur J Immunol.* 2015;45:214-224.

141. Winterberg T, Vieten G, Feldmann L, et al. Neonatal murine macrophages show enhanced chemotactic capacity upon toll-like receptor stimulation. *Pediatr Surg Int.* 2014;30:159-164.

142. Wei J, Besner GE. M1 to M2 macrophage polarization in heparin-binding epidermal growth factor-like growth factor therapy for necrotizing enterocolitis. *J Surg Res.* 2015;197:126-138.

143. Remon J, Kampanatkosol R, Kaul RR, et al. Acute drop in blood monocyte count differentiates NEC from other causes of feeding intolerance. *J Perinatol.* 2014;34:549-554.

144. Namachivayam K, MohanKumar K, Shores DR, et al. Targeted inhibition of thrombin attenuates murine neonatal necrotizing enterocolitis. *Proc Natl Acad Sci U S A.* 2020;117(20):10958-10969. doi:10.1073/pnas.1912357117.

145. Hernandez M, Gamonal J, Salo T, et al. Reduced expression of lipopolysaccharide-induced CXC chemokine in Porphyromonas gingivalis-induced experimental periodontitis in matrix metalloproteinase-8 null mice. *J Periodontal Res.* 2011;46:58-66.

146. Managlia E, Liu SXL, Yan X, et al. Blocking NF-κB activation in Ly6c+ monocytes attenuates necrotizing enterocolitis. *Am J Pathol.* 2019;189:604-618.

147. Wei J, Tang D, Lu C, et al. Irf5 deficiency in myeloid cells prevents necrotizing enterocolitis by inhibiting M1 macrophage polarization. *Mucosal Immunol.* 2019;12:888-896.

148. Kaur A, Lee LH, Chow SC, Fang CM. IRF5-mediated immune responses and its implications in immunological disorders. *Int Rev Immunol.* 2018;37:229-248.

149. Ashburner M, Ball CA, Blake JA, et al. Gene ontology: tool for the unification of biology. The Gene Ontology Consortium. *Nat Genet.* 2000;25:25-29.

150. Huang da W, Sherman BT, Lempicki RA. Systematic and integrative analysis of large gene lists using DAVID bioinformatics resources. *Nat Protoc.* 2009;4:44-57.

151. MohanKumar K, Namachivayam K, Chapalamadugu KC, et al. Smad7 interrupts TGF-β signaling in intestinal macrophages and promotes inflammatory activation of these cells during necrotizing enterocolitis. *Pediatr Res.* 2016;79(6):951-961. doi:10.1038/pr.2016.18.

152. Maheshwari A, Schelonka RL, Dimmitt RA, et al. Cytokines associated with necrotizing enterocolitis in extremely-low-birth-weight infants. *Pediatr Res.* 2014;76:100-108.

153. Harris MC, Costarino Jr AT, Sullivan JS, et al. Cytokine elevations in critically ill infants with sepsis and necrotizing enterocolitis. *J Pediatr.* 1994;124:105-111.

154. Ng PC, Li K, Wong RP, et al. Proinflammatory and anti-inflammatory cytokine responses in preterm infants with systemic infections. *Arch Dis Child Fetal Neonatal Ed.* 2003;88:F209-F213.

155. Remon J, Kampanatkosol R, Kaul RR, et al. Acute drop in blood monocyte count differentiates NEC from other causes of feeding intolerance. *J Perinatol.* 2014;34:549-554.

156. Sampath V, Le M, Lane L, et al. The NFKB1 (g.-24519de-lATTG) variant is associated with necrotizing enterocolitis (NEC) in premature infants. *J Surg Res.* 2011;169:e51-e57.

157. Wang Y, Hoenig JD, Malin KJ, et al. 16S rRNA gene-based analysis of fecal microbiota from preterm infants with and without necrotizing enterocolitis. *ISME J.* 2009;3:944-954.

158. Hsueh W, Caplan MS, Tan X, MacKendrick W, Gonzalez-Crussi F. Necrotizing enterocolitis of the newborn: pathogenetic concepts in perspective. *Pediatr Dev Pathol.* 1998;1:2-16.

159. Bucher BT, McDuffie LA, Shaikh N, et al. Bacterial DNA content in the intestinal wall from infants with necrotizing enterocolitis. *J Pediatr Surg.* 2011;46:1029-1033.

160. Bury RG, Tudehope D. Enteral antibiotics for preventing necrotizing enterocolitis in low birthweight or preterm infants. *Cochrane Database Syst Rev.* 2001;(1):CD000405.

161. Serra R, Johnson M, Filvaroff EH, et al. Expression of a truncated, kinase-defective TGF-beta type II receptor in mouse skeletal tissue promotes terminal chondrocyte differentiation and osteoarthritis. *J Cell Biol.* 1997;139:541-552.

162. Hsueh W, Gonzalez-Crussi F, Arroyave JL. Platelet-activating factor: an endogenous mediator for bowel necrosis in endotoxemia. *FASEB J.* 1987;1:403-405.

163. Sun X, Rozenfeld RA, Qu X, et al. P-selectin-deficient mice are protected from PAF-induced shock, intestinal injury, and lethality. *Am J Physiol.* 1997;273:G56-G61.

164. Musemeche C, Caplan M, Hsueh W, Sun X, Kelly A. Experimental necrotizing enterocolitis: the role of polymorphonuclear neutrophils. *J Pediatr Surg.* 1991;26:1047-1049; discussion 1049-1050.

165. Caplan MS, Sun XM, Hsueh W, Hageman JR. Role of platelet activating factor and tumor necrosis factor-alpha in neonatal necrotizing enterocolitis. *J Pediatr.* 1990;116:960-964.

166. Jilling T, Lu J, Jackson M, Caplan MS. Intestinal epithelial apoptosis initiates gross bowel necrosis in an experimental rat model of neonatal necrotizing enterocolitis. *Pediatr Res.* 2004;55:622-629.

167. Emami CN, Mittal R, Wang L, Ford HR, Prasadarao NV. Role of neutrophils and macrophages in the pathogenesis of necrotizing enterocolitis caused by Cronobacter Sakazakii. *J Surg Res.* 2012;172:18-28.

168. Halpern MD, Khailova L, Molla-Hosseini D, et al. Decreased development of necrotizing enterocolitis in IL-18-deficient mice. *Am J Physiol Gastrointest Liver Physiol.* 2008;294:G20-G26.

169. Kaur A, Lee LH, Chow SC, Fang CM. IRF5-mediated immune responses and its implications in immunological disorders. *Int Rev Immunol.* 2018;37:229-248.

170. Sharma R, Hudak ML, Tepas JJ III, et al. Impact of gestational age on the clinical presentation and surgical outcome of necrotizing enterocolitis. *J Perinatol.* 2006;26:342-347.

171. Yee WH, Soraisham AS, Shah VS, et al. Incidence and timing of presentation of necrotizing enterocolitis in preterm infants. *Pediatrics.* 2012;129:e298-e304.

172. Llanos AR, Moss ME, Pinzòn MC, et al. Epidemiology of neonatal necrotising enterocolitis: a population-based study. *Paediatr Perinat Epidemiol.* 2002;16:342-349.

173. Alex P, Zachos NC, Nguyen T, et al. Distinct cytokine patterns identified from multiplex profiles of murine DSS and TNBS-induced colitis. *Inflamm Bowel Dis.* 2009;15:341-352.

174. Maheshwari A, Kurundkar AR, Shaik SS, et al. Epithelial cells in fetal intestine produce chemerin to recruit macrophages. *Am J Physiol Gastrointest Liver Physiol.* 2009;297:G1-G10.

175. Namachivayam K, Coffing HP, Sankaranarayanan NV, et al. Transforming growth factor-beta2 is sequestered in preterm human milk by chondroitin sulfate proteoglycans. *Am J Physiol Gastrointest Liver Physiol.* 2015;309:G171-G180.

176. MohanKumar K, Namachivayam K, Ho TT, et al. Cytokines and growth factors in the developing intestine and during necrotizing enterocolitis. *Semin Perinatol.* 2016;41:52-60.

177. Namachivayam K, MohanKumar K, Arbach D, et al. All-trans retinoic acid induces TGF-beta2 in intestinal epithelial cells via RhoA- and p38alpha MAPK-mediated activation of the transcription factor ATF2. *PLoS One.* 2015;10:e0134003.

178. Tecalco-Cruz AC, Sosa-Garrocho M, Vázquez-Victorio G, Ortiz-García L, Domínguez-Hüttinger E, Macías-Silva M. Transforming growth factor-β/SMAD Target gene SKIL is negatively regulated by the transcriptional cofactor complex SNON-SMAD4. *J Biol Chem.* 2012;287:26764-76.

179. Jahchan NS, Luo K. SnoN in mammalian development, function and diseases. *Curr Opin Pharmacol.* 2010;10:670-675.

180. Strahl BD, Allis CD. The language of covalent histone modifications. *Nature.* 2000;403:41-45.

181. Yan X, Lin Z, Chen F, et al. Human BAMBI cooperates with Smad7 to inhibit transforming growth factor-beta signaling. *J Biol Chem.* 2009;284:30097-30104.

182. Zhang S, Fei T, Zhang L, et al. Smad7 antagonizes transforming growth factor beta signaling in the nucleus by interfering with functional Smad-DNA complex formation. *Mol Cell Biol.* 2007;27:4488-4499.

183. Ovcharenko I, Loots GG, Giardine BM, et al. Mulan: multiple-sequence local alignment and visualization for studying function and evolution. *Genome Res.* 2005;15:184-194.

184. Aucott SW, Maheshwari A. To transfuse or not transfuse a premature infant: the new complex question. *J Perinatol.* 2019;39:351-353.

185. Strauss RG. Practical issues in neonatal transfusion practice. *Am J Clin Pathol.* 1997;107:S57-S63.

186. Christensen RD, Lambert DK, Henry E, et al. Is "transfusion-associated necrotizing enterocolitis" an authentic pathogenic entity? *Transfusion.* 2009;50:1106-1112.

187. Amin SC, Remon JI, Subbarao GC, Maheshwari A. Association between red cell transfusions and necrotizing enterocolitis. *J Matern Fetal Neonatal Med.* 2012;25:85-89.

188. Mohamed A, Shah PS. Transfusion associated necrotizing enterocolitis: a meta-analysis of observational data. *Pediatrics.* 2012;129:529-540.

189. Hyung N, Campwala I, Boskovic DS, et al. The relationship of red blood cell transfusion to intestinal mucosal injury in premature infants. *J Pediatr Surg.* 2017;52(7):1152-1155. doi:10.1016/j.jpedsurg.2016.10.049.

190. Demirel G, Celik IH, Aksoy HT, et al. Transfusion-associated necrotising enterocolitis in very low birth weight premature infants. *Transfus Med.* 2012;22:332-337.

191. Stritzke AI, Smyth J, Synnes A, Lee SK, Shah PS. Transfusion-associated necrotising enterocolitis in neonates. *Arch Dis Child Fetal Neonatal Ed.* 2013;98:F10-F14.

192. Christensen RD, Lambert DK, Gordon PV, et al. Neonates presenting with bloody stools and eosinophilia can progress to two different types of necrotizing enterocolitis. *J Perinatol.* 2012;32:874-879.

193. El-Dib M, Narang S, Lee E, Massaro AN, Aly H. Red blood cell transfusion, feeding and necrotizing enterocolitis in preterm infants. *J Perinatol.* 2011;31:183-187.

194. Patel RM, Knezevic A, Shenvi N, et al. Association of red blood cell transfusion, anemia, and necrotizing enterocolitis in very low-birth-weight infants. *JAMA.* 2016;315:889-897.

195. Josephson CD, Wesolowski A, Bao G, et al. Do red cell transfusions increase the risk of necrotizing enterocolitis in premature infants? *J Pediatr.* 2010;157:972-978.

196. Garg PM, Ravisankar S, Bian H, Macgilvray S, Shekhawat PS. Relationship between packed red blood cell transfusion and severe form of necrotizing enterocolitis: a case control study. *Indian Pediatr.* 2015;52:1041-1045.

197. AlFaleh K, Al-Jebreen A, Baqays A, et al. Association of packed red blood cell transfusion and necrotizing enterocolitis in very low birth weight infants. *J Neonatal Perinatal Med.* 2014;7:193-198.

198. Baxi AC, Josephson CD, Iannucci GJ, Mahle WT. Necrotizing enterocolitis in infants with congenital heart disease: the role of red blood cell transfusions. *Pediatr Cardiol.* 2014;35:1024-1029.

199. Derienzo C, Smith PB, Tanaka D, et al. Feeding practices and other risk factors for developing transfusion-associated necrotizing enterocolitis. *Early Hum Dev.* 2014;90:237-240.

200. Christensen RD, Wiedmeier SE, Baer VL, et al. Antecedents of Bell stage III necrotizing enterocolitis. *J Perinatol.* 2010;30:54-57.

201. Christensen RD, Baer VL, Del Vecchio A, Henry E. Unique risks of red blood cell transfusions in very-low-birth-weight neonates: associations between early transfusion and intraventricular hemorrhage and between late transfusion and necrotizing enterocolitis. *J Matern Fetal Neonatal Med.* 2013;26 suppl 2:60-63.

202. Bak SY, Lee S, Park JH, Park KH, Jeon JH. Analysis of the association between necrotizing enterocolitis and transfusion of red blood cell in very low birth weight preterm infants. *Korean J Pediatr.* 2013;56:112-115.

203. Singh R, Visintainer PF, Frantz ID III, et al. Association of necrotizing enterocolitis with anemia and packed red blood cell transfusions in preterm infants. *J Perinatol.* 2011;31:176-182.

204. Elabiad MT, Harsono M, Talati AJ, Dhanireddy R. Effect of birth weight on the association between necrotising enterocolitis and red blood cell transfusions in ≤1500 g infants. *BMJ Open.* 2013;3:e003823.

205. Mally P, Golombek SG, Mishra R, et al. Association of necrotizing enterocolitis with elective packed red blood cell transfusions in stable, growing, premature neonates. *Am J Perinatol.* 2006;23:451-458.

206. Marin T, Moore J, Kosmetatos N, et al. Red blood cell transfusion-related necrotizing enterocolitis in very-low-birthweight infants: a near-infrared spectroscopy investigation. *Transfusion.* 2013;53:2650-2658.

207. Paul DA, Mackley A, Novitsky A, et al. Increased odds of necrotizing enterocolitis after transfusion of red blood cells in premature infants. *Pediatrics.* 2011;127:635-641.

208. Blau J, Calo JM, Dozor D, et al. Transfusion-related acute gut injury: necrotizing enterocolitis in very low birth weight neonates after packed red blood cell transfusion. *J Pediatr.* 2011;158:403-409.

209. Tao HK, Tang Q, Hei MY, Yu B. [Meta-analysis of post-transfusion necrotizing enterocolitis in neonates]. *Zhonghua Er Ke Za Zhi.* 2013;51:336-339.

210. Hay S, Zupancic JA, Flannery DD, Kirpalani H, Dukhovny D. Should we believe in transfusion-associated enterocolitis? Applying a GRADE to the literature. *Semin Perinatol.* 2017;41:80-91.

211. Nickel RS, Josephson CD. Neonatal transfusion medicine: five major unanswered research questions for the twenty-first century. *Clin Perinatol.* 2015;42:499-513.

212. Hod EA, Zhang N, Sokol SA, et al. Transfusion of red blood cells after prolonged storage produces harmful effects that are mediated by iron and inflammation. *Blood.* 2010;115:4284-4292.

213. Yang J, Gonon AT, Sjoquist PO, Lundberg JO, Pernow J. Arginase regulates red blood cell nitric oxide synthase and export of cardioprotective nitric oxide bioactivity. *Proc Natl Acad Sci U S A.* 2013;110:15049-15054.

214. Zaynagetdinov R, Sherrill TP, Kendall PL, et al. Identification of myeloid cell subsets in murine lungs using flow cytometry. *Am J Respir Cell Mol Biol.* 2013;49:180-189.

215. Zhong H, Yin H. Role of lipid peroxidation derived 4-hydroxynonenal (4-HNE) in cancer: focusing on mitochondria. *Redox Biol.* 2015;4:193-199.

216. Gladwin MT, Kanias T, Kim-Shapiro DB. Hemolysis and cell-free hemoglobin drive an intrinsic mechanism for human disease. *J Clin Invest.* 2012;122:1205-1208.

217. Belcher JD, Chen C, Nguyen J, et al. Heme triggers TLR4 signaling leading to endothelial cell activation and vaso-occlusion in murine sickle cell disease. *Blood.* 2014;123:377-390.

218. Leaphart CL, Cavallo J, Gribar SC, et al. A critical role for TLR4 in the pathogenesis of necrotizing enterocolitis by modulating intestinal injury and repair. *J Immunol.* 2007;179:4808-4820.

219. Raza A, Crothers JW, McGill MM, et al. Anti-inflammatory roles of p38alpha MAPK in macrophages are context dependent and require IL-10. *J Leukoc Biol.* 2017;102:1219-1227.

220. Formentini L, Santacatterina F, Núñez de Arenas C, et al. Mitochondrial ROS production protects the intestine from inflammation through functional M2 macrophage polarization. *Cell Rep.* 2017;19:1202-1213.

221. Meshkibaf S, Martins AJ, Henry GT, Kim SO. Protective role of G-CSF in dextran sulfate sodium-induced acute colitis through generating gut-homing macrophages. *Cytokine.* 2016;78:69-78.

222. Araki A, Kanai T, Ishikura T, et al. MyD88-deficient mice develop severe intestinal inflammation in dextran sodium sulfate colitis. *J Gastroenterol.* 2005;40:16-23.

223. Eisenblatter M, Ehrchen J, Varga G, et al. In vivo optical imaging of cellular inflammatory response in granuloma formation using fluorescence-labeled macrophages. *J Nucl Med.* 2009;50:1676-1682.

224. Knijn N, Simmer F, Nagtegaal ID. Recommendations for reporting histopathology studies: a proposal. *Virchows Arch.* 2015;466:611-615.

225. Oxford AE, Stewart ES, Rohn TT. Clinical trials in Alzheimer's Disease: a hurdle in the path of remedy. *Int J Alzheimers Dis.* 2020;2020:5380346.

Chapter 3

Nucleated Red Blood Cells in Neonatal Medicine

Robert D. Christensen, MD

Chapter Outline

Introduction

It is distinctly uncommon and definitely pathologic to have nucleated red blood cells (NRBCs) in the circulating blood.[1] This statement is true for all humans—in fact, for all mammals—with the singular exception of newborn infants, where small numbers of NRBCs can be a normal finding on the day of birth and perhaps for a day or two thereafter.[2] However, some human newborn infants, particularly those with severe hemolytic disease, severe intrauterine growth restriction, or severe intrauterine hypoxia, have very large numbers of NRBCs in the blood. The explanation for and the implications of this finding are the focuses of this chapter.

Erythroid Development in the Human Fetus

Erythropoiesis is the process whereby RBCs are produced in the bone marrow as well as in the fetal liver of mid- and late-trimester fetuses. The erythropoietic process is a continuous one, but it can be instructive to consider it as occurring in a series of four definable stages: (1) the commitment of pluripotent stem cells into erythroid progenitors, (2) the early erythropoietin-independent stage of clonal expansion of early committed erythroid progenitors, (3) the erythropoietin-dependent late phase involving further clonal expansion and initiation of hemoglobin synthesis, and (4) nuclear condensation, enucleation, and reticulocyte release into the blood.[3]

As shown in Fig. 3.1, early hematopoietic progenitors, which have the capacity to generate clones of multiple lineages, can be recognized by their capacity to give rise in cell culture systems to colonies that contain mixtures of granulocytes, erythrocytes, macrophages, and megakaryocytes. Colonies containing such a mixture of cell types are derived from a single progenitor cell termed a colony-forming-unit (CFU)–GEMM. Further erythroid commitment of pluripotent hematopoietic progenitors produces a cell capable of generating large clones consisting exclusively of

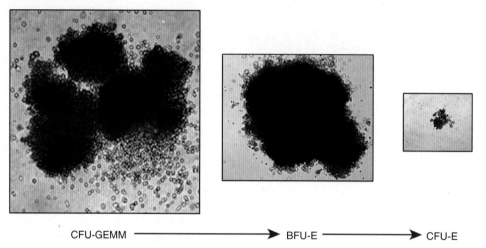

CFU-GEMM ——————————————→ BFU-E ——————→ CFU-E

Fig. 3.1 Committed erythrocyte progenitors, identified by the cells they clonally generate in culture. *BFU-E,* Burst-forming unit–erythroid; *CFU-E,* colony-forming unit–erythroid; *CFU-GEMM,* colony-forming unit–granulocyte, erythrocyte, megakaryocyte, macrophage.

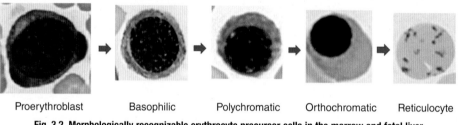

Proerythroblast   Basophilic   Polychromatic   Orthochromatic   Reticulocyte

Fig. 3.2 Morphologically recognizable erythrocyte precursor cells in the marrow and fetal liver.

erythrocytes. These progenitors are termed burst forming units–erythroid (BFU-E), which are found primarily in the marrow and fetal liver but also in the circulating blood, where they appear morphologically like an immature blast with a large nucleus containing nucleoli. CFU-GEMM and BFU-E express Epo receptors but at very low densities. BFU-E, after about 14 days in culture, produce colonies containing 500 to perhaps 50,000 hemoglobinized erythroblasts. The early stages of BFU-E proliferation are Epo independent.

The next stage in erythroid development is termed the CFU-E, or colony-forming unit–erythroid. Such progenitors, in culture for 2 or 3 days, generate colonies composed of 8 to about 32 hemoglobinized cells. Most CFU-E are in an active stage of DNA synthesis. Epo receptors are expressed densely on the surface of CFU-E and proerythroblasts. Since those states have the highest density of Epo receptors, they are considered to be the principle hematopoietic targets of Epo

and are the most responsive to Epo of any cells. Consequently, high Epo concentrations result in marked expansion of the CFU-E compartment. CFU-E also have a high cell-surface expression of the transferrin receptor (CD 71), as a means of importing iron that will be needed for hemoglobin production required for generating mature erythrocytes.

After the CFU-E stage, maturing erythrocyte precursors can be recognized as morphologically distinct cell types in the marrow and fetal liver (Fig. 3.2). The first is the proerythroblast, a moderate to large oval or round cell with a relatively large nucleus with prominent nucleoli and a rim of basophilic cytoplasm. The next more mature red cell precursor is the basophilic erythroblast, which is slightly smaller with a nucleus that lacks nucleoli. Next, the polychromatic erythroblast is recognized by a mixture of blue and pink cytoplasm (thus polychromatic), the pink color signifying hemoglobin. The nuclear chromatin of that cell type is becoming condensed and smaller. Once the cytoplasm is almost completely pink and the nucleus has become pyknotic and small, the cell is termed an orthochromatic erythroblast. It is at this stage that enucleation occurs, thereby producing a reticulocyte, lacking a nucleus but retaining organelles.

Enucleation of Orthochromatic Erythroblasts

Circulating RBCs of fish and amphibians have nuclei.[4] Perhaps this enables their erythrocytes to be at least somewhat transcriptionally active and thereby might provide the animals with some survival advantage. However, if that is so, why was erythrocyte enucleation selected for during mammalian evolution? At least three possibilities have been suggested: (1) Enucleation provides more room in erythrocytes for hemoglobin, (2) enucleation likely improves blood circulation by preventing potential flow impedance in capillaries by erythrocytes that have a large and stiff nucleus, thus rendering them less deformable. Deformation and reformation of RBC occurs repeatedly during the circulation when they pass through spaces narrower than 7.5 μm.[5] (3) Reducing blood viscosity by erythrocyte enucleation might reduce cardiac workload.

The mechanisms involved in mammalian erythrocyte enucleation involve several concomitant processes. These include simultaneous nuclear chromatin condensation and increased hemoglobin production.

Chromatin condensation is controlled by upregulating histone deacetylases with parallel downregulation of histone transferases. Time-lapse photography of enucleating erythroblasts show that the nucleus migrates to one side of the cytoplasm and lies in close apposition to the erythroblast plasma membrane by a process that involves a ring of actin around the nucleus. The erythroblast submembrane cytoskeletal proteins, such as ankyrin, spectrin, actin, and protein 4.1, move away from the membrane in the area where the nucleus is being extruded. The entire process appears to occur quickly with resealing of the plasma membrane followed by reorganization of the cytoskeletal proteins (Fig. 3.3). Micro RNA species that posttranscriptionally modulate expression of a variety of genes are involved in this intricate process, but clearer definition of the exact processes is needed. The extruded nucleus is termed a pyrenocyte, from Greek *pyren*, the pit of a stone fruit. Macrophages in the marrow or liver interact with and engulf the pyrenocyte. However, in tissue culture, even in the absence of macrophages, enucleation occurs. Therefore presumably macrophages are not critical to the enucleation process other than to recover the pyrenocyte and recycle its elements.

Regulating NRBC Release From Production Sites

Little definitive information is available regarding the mechanisms regulating release of reticulocytes from

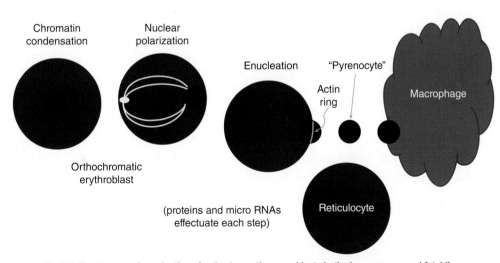

Fig. 3.3 The process of enucleation of orthochromatic normoblasts in the bone marrow and fetal liver.

the bone marrow (and fetal liver) into the circulating blood. Reticulocytes do not express cell-surface Epo receptors; therefore it is not likely that Epo directly interacts with reticulocytes in the marrow or fetal liver to induce their release into the circulation. However, endothelial cells express Epo-R.[6] Whether endothelial cells in the bone marrow or the fetal liver in some way gate the release of reticulocytes into the blood, or gate the premature release of NRBC under some circumstances, is uncertain. It is also uncertain whether the process regulating release of erythrocytes differs between marrow and liver. If there are indeed differences, perhaps these explain why neonates (who have an element of hepatic erythropoiesis) are much more likely to release NRBC prematurely than are older children or adults who have no hepatic erythropoiesis.

Once in the circulation, reticulocytes can be sequestered temporarily (perhaps for a day) in the spleen, where additional maturation may occur. As reticulocytes mature they lose the capacity to synthesize hemoglobin, and their size shrinks by about 20%. Thus the reticulocyte changes over a day or two into the morphologically recognizable mature circulating erythrocyte.

Reference Ranges for NRBC Counts in Neonates, According to Gestational Age

Using the large clinical laboratory dataset of Intermountain Healthcare, we reported an average of 1000 NRBC/μL, or 6 NRBC/100 white blood cells (WBCs), during the first 24 hours after birth of late preterm and term infants, with a 95th percentile upper reference interval of 2900 NRBC/μL or 18 NRBC/100 WBCs.[2] However, we found that the reference interval for NRBC at birth is highly dependent on gestational age. The nomograms for NRBC counts on the day of birth, expressed as a function of gestational age (Fig. 3.4).

NRBC in Small for Gestational Age Neonates and in Neonates Following Significant Birth Asphyxia

We observed that among 3650 neonates who were small for gestational age (SGA, birth weight <10th percentile for GA), 2981 had a NRBC/μL recorded on the day of birth, and the NRBC count inversely correlated with the

blood neutrophil count (Fig. 3.5) (P<0.001). Those SGA neonates who were most severely weight restricted (those <1st percentile) had the highest NRBC counts and the lowest neutrophil counts. We speculated that fetal hypoxia resulted in elevated fetal Epo levels, which increased RBC production with a subsequent reduction in platelet and neutrophil production.[7]

Several reports focused on NRBC counts in neonates after birth asphyxia, which was defined quite variably in the different reports.[8-16] A correlation between birth asphyxia and elevated NRBC counts was shown in three reports from India[12-14] and one from Iran.[15] Also, among 375 neonates with an umbilical cord blood gas definition of perinatal asphyxia (pH <7 and base deficit ≥16 mm/L), we found an inverse relationship between the NRBC count and the platelet count (Fig. 3.6). As with SGA neonates, we speculated that some neonates with a cord gas definition of asphyxia had chronic intrauterine hypoxia, and these were more likely to have low platelet counts and elevated NRBC counts.[16]

NRBC Counts in Neonates With Hemolytic Disease

The original name for hemolytic disease of the fetus and neonate (HDFN) was erythroblastosis fetalis, later identified as Rh hemolytic disease. That original name was derived from the markedly increased number of NRBCs in the circulation of these infants, including not only orthochromatic erythroblasts but also polychromatic and basophilic erythroblasts. In contrast to HDFN resulting from maternal immunization to the Rh D antigen, HDFN from ABO, Kell, Duffy, Kidd, MNSs, Lutheran, Diego, Xg, P, Ee, and Cc antigen systems sometimes results in orthochromatic erythroblasts in the circulation, but rarely are polychromatic and basophilic erythroblasts seen in those conditions.

How Long Does It Take for Fetal Hypoxia to Result in an Elevated NRBC Count in the Blood?

The answer to this question has important pathogenic implications, and perhaps it sometimes has medicolegal implications. The latter being related to adverse outcomes following hypoxic-ischemic encephalopathy

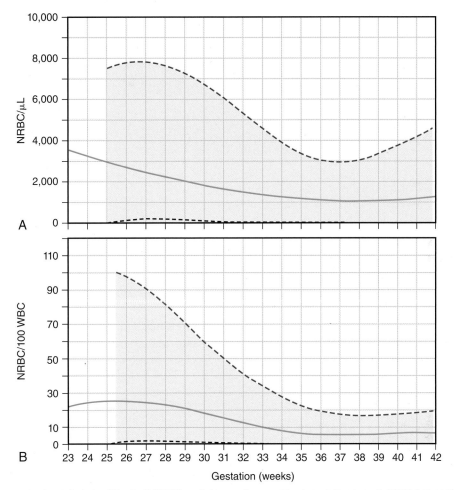

Fig. 3.4 Reference ranges for nucleated red blood cell *(NRBC)* **counts in neonates, according to gestational age. A,** NRBC/μL blood. **B,** NRBC/100WBC. In both panels the *solid line* represents the average value, and the *dashed lines* represent the 5th and 95th percentile lower and upper reference intervals. The *shaded area* incorporates all values that fall within the reference range for gestational age. *WBC,* White blood cell. (Modified from Christensen RD et al. Reference ranges for blood concentrations of nucleated red blood cells in neonates. *Neonatology,* 2011;99:289-294.)

(HIE) and attempts to identify the time at which the fetal hypoxic insult occurred. Namely, did the hypoxia occur minutes, hours, or days before birth? Moreover, if the baby had been delivered minutes or hours sooner, would this have likely prevented the damage?

The fetal NRBC emergence time is defined as the interval between the onset of significant hypoxia in utero and the first appearance of NRBC in the blood in sufficient quantities to elevate the NRBC count into the abnormal range.[2] Attempts to measure the NRBC emergence time have taken several approaches, using experimental models of newborn rodents,[17,18] models

using fetal and neonatal sheep,[19,20] and observational studies of human neonates.[21-25]

Blackwell et al. modeled acute fetal hypoxia by placing timed-pregnant rats into a chamber containing a hypoxic gas mixture of 9% O_2 and 3% CO_2 for a period of 2 hours, vs. a sham chamber containing room air.[17] Groups were sacrificed immediately after the chamber exposure, or 4, 12, 24, 36, 48, or 60 hours after the exposure. The first appearance of NRBCs in the blood was at 12 hours, with higher concentrations at 24 hours. NRBC counts were not elevated by 36 hours; presumably they had been cleared

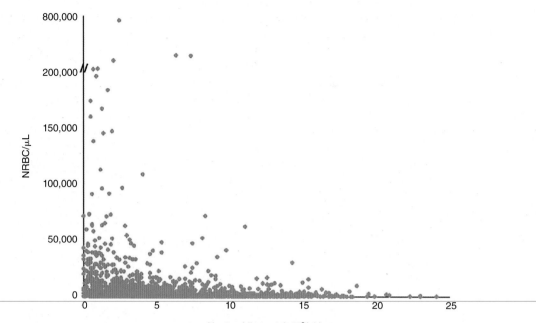

Fig. 3.5 Relationship between blood neutrophil count (horizontal axis) and nucleated red blood cell count (*NRBC*; vertical axis) among neonates who are small for gestational age. (Modified from Christensen RD et al. Early-onset neutropenia in small-for-gestational-age infants. *Pediatrics.* 2015;136(5):e1259-e1267.)

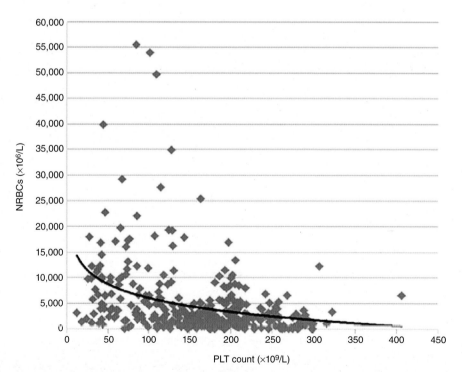

Fig. 3.6 Relationship between platelet count, *PLT*; (horizontal axis) and nucleated red blood cell count, *NRBCs*; (vertical axis) among neonates with an umbilical cord blood gas pH <7 and BE, Base Excess >16. (Modified from Christensen RD et al. Thrombocytopenia in late preterm and term neonates after perinatal asphyxia. *Transfusion.* 2015;55(1):187-196.)

from the blood by the spleen and liver by 36 hours. The researchers concluded that in their model, the NRBC emergence time after fetal hypoxia began after a delay of 12 hours and was clearly established by 24 hours.[17] Thirteen years later, Minior et al. reported somewhat similar experiments, but they varied the time of hypoxic exposure, including 2, 6, 12, 24, 48, and 120 hours of hypoxia, and then they delivered the pups by hysterotomy. They found that a longer duration of hypoxia was associated with a higher elevation in NRBC counts. The NRBC emergence time was 24 hours, and hypoxia exceeding 24 hours resulted in reduced fetal body weight and reduced liver weight.[18]

Widness et al. produced acute hypoxia in fetal lambs by infusing sodium nitrite into the mother's circulation, causing methemoglobinemia and a predictable incremental fall in maternal and fetal arterial oxygen content. By measuring Epo in the catheterized fetuses before and at intervals after the hypoxic insult, they found that 4 to 5 hours was required, after fetal hypoxia, before the Epo levels began to increase.[19] The mechanism by which hypoxia causes an increase in Epo involve the specific species of hypoxia-inducing factor (HIF) called HIF-1α, which is stabilized by hypoxia and results in up to a 1000-fold increase in Epo gene transcription and production.[26] The next question to be settled was how long, after an elevation in hypoxia-induced endogenous Epo levels, does it take before NRBCs are released from the fetal liver/bone marrow, thus elevating the NRBC count to abnormal levels?

Our group sought to provide an experimental answer to that question by administering recombinant Epo (darbepoetin alfa) (or a vehicle placebo control) to newborn lambs, then drawing blood from indwelling lines to measure NRBC counts and reticulocyte counts every 12 hours × 2 and then daily for the next 4 days (Fig. 3.7). We found that NRBC and reticulocytes increased by 24 hours, peaked by 48 to 72 hours, then fell by 96 hours.[20]

Observational studies in human neonates, aimed at defining the NRBC emergence time, leave several unanswered questions. Blackwell et al. reviewed over 36,000 singleton term deliveries at Hutzel Hospital in Detroit, finding 45 with early-onset (within 72 hours of birth) seizures. They found their NRBC counts to be significantly higher than controls. They concluded that neurologic injury leading to early-onset seizures typically occurs before the intrapartum period because fetal hypoxia, resulting in the seizures, most likely occurred 24 hours or so before birth.[21]

Hermansen disagreed with Blackwell's interpretation and sited data from neonates who had elevated NRBC counts within 1 or 2 hours of an hypoxic event, including uterine rupture and umbilical cord prolapse.[22] He concluded:

It may require 48 hours of hypoxia to result in de novo *erythropoietic activity. However, increased circulation of NRBC occurs rapidly after hypoxia, not from new erythropoiesis but from a release of previously stored*

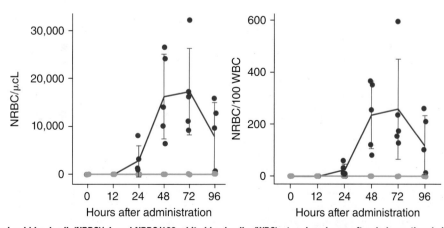

Fig. 3.7 Nucleated red blood cell *(NRBC)*/µL **and NRBC/100 white blood cells** *(WBC)*, **at various hours after darbepoetin administration (10 µg/ kg) to newborn lambs.** *Red lines* and *red circles* indicate values obtained from darbepoetin recipients, and *green lines* and *green circles* are from **placebo control recipients.** (Modified from Bahr TM et al. Nucleated red blood cell emergence-time in newborn lambs following a dose of darbepoetin alfa. *Cur Pediatr Rev.* 2022.)

NRBC. Basic evidence indicates that this rapid release is caused by erythropoietin-induced increases in marrow blood flow and an increase in the porous infrastructure of the marrow that allows easy escape of nucleated red blood cells.... Published basic research and clinical data indicate that NRBC counts can rise within 1 hour of severe hypoxia.[22]

Our group reported 31 preterm neonates who received darbepoetin at the decision of their clinician to prevent RBC transfusions.[23] Twenty-six of the 31 had a complete blood count (CBC) within 24 hours of their darbepoetin dose, and none had an elevated NRBC count. The first appearance of NRBC in this group was between 24 and 36 hours following the darbepoetin dose. We speculated that following a fetal hypoxic insult 4 to 5 hours was required to increase Epo production after which another 24 hours likely elapsed before NRBC appeared in the blood, making an estimated NRBC emergence time of about 28 to 29 hours.

We observed four tragic cases where a pregnant mother, nearing term gestation, had sudden death (such as a motor vehicle accident). In each case paramedics applied cardiopulmonary resuscitation (CPR) while she was transported to an emergency department, where the baby was delivered by cesarean section. In each case (1–4 hours after the accident) the cord blood showed profound acidosis, but NRBC counts were normal. All four babies lived, and all four mothers died after CPR was stopped. We concluded that a period of 1 to 4 hours after severe fetal hypoxia was not sufficiently long for NRBC to emerge from the liver/bone marrow into the circulating blood.[24]

Recently we investigated associations between NRBC counts of neonates with HIE, acute perinatal sentinel events, and neurodevelopmental outcomes.[25] We also examined the mechanism causing the elevated NRBC counts. It was a retrospective analysis from three of our neonatal intensive care units (NICUs), involving neonates with HIE treated with hypothermia and receiving neurodevelopmental testing at 24±6 months. Of 152 such neonates, 95 (63%) had normal NRBC counts, while 57 (37%) had elevated counts. Those with a documented sentinel event during labor resulting in emergent delivery (i.e., acute abruption, cord prolapse, uterine rupture) (n=79) almost always had a normal NRBC count (odds ratio

257; 95% confidence interval [CI], 33–1988). Of the 152 infants, 134 infants (88%) survived to discharge. When the first NRBC count was normal, the odds of surviving were threefold greater (95% CI, 1.1–8.3) than when it was elevated. Normal NRBC counts were moderately predictive of a normal neurodevelopmental evaluation at 2 years (p<0.001). The NRBC half-life ($t_{1/2}$) was longer in those with elevated (60 hours) vs. normal NRBC counts (39 hours) (p<0.01). This suggested that the elevated counts were due in part to defective removal of NRBCs from the blood by the spleen and liver, perhaps from hypoxic damage.

From that study we concluded that among neonates with HIE, a normal NRBC count after birth was highly associated with having had an acute intrapartum event necessitating emergent delivery. Normal counts were modestly predictive of better prognosis. We speculate that elevated NRBC counts occur from hypoxia that occurred earlier or chronically and that impaired clearance of NRBC from the blood is one mechanistic explanation for the high counts.[25]

Implications of Finding an Elevated NRBC Count in a Nonneonatal Child

Hypoxia increases erythropoietin levels in healthy adults.[26] When a CBC of a child beyond the neonatal period identifies circulating NRBCs, the finding invokes the possibility of a malignancy, bone marrow dysfunction, or some other serious disorder. Pedersen et al. found that of 2065 admissions to their children's hospital in Edmonton, 368 had NRBC detectible on a CBC, and that this finding was associated with both ICU admission and hospital mortality.[27] Children with sickle cell disease hospitalized with acute chest syndrome sometimes have NRBC identified. Ballantine et al. found that an increase in NRBC during a hospitalization for acute chest syndrome was a useful biomarker for predicting complications such as a fall in hemoglobin or need for transfusion.[28]

Finding NRBC in hospitalized or ill children can be the result of hyposplenism because NRBC that escape from the marrow are normally cleared rapidly from the blood by the spleen.[29] Children with myeloproliferative disorders can overload the spleen, incapacitate splenic function, and lead to NRBCs in the circulation. In children with cardiopulmonary disorders, NRBCs might suggest an unfavorable prognosis.[30] Extramedullary hematopoiesis with hepatosplenomegaly can also result in NRBC perhaps because the enucleation process that normally occurs with erythropoiesis within the bone marrow is less efficient when erythropoiesis occurs in other tissues such as the spleen and liver. Another worrisome possibility to explain NRBC in children is invasion of the bone marrow by tumor cells or infectious diseases.

Implications of Finding an Elevated NRBC Count in a Neonate

Many authors have reported a relationship between high NRBC counts in neonates and adverse outcomes,

particularly worse neurodevelopmental outcomes.[31-44] Table 3.1 lists 22 publications, since 1995, that sought to determine associations between elevated NRBC counts in various groups of neonates and short- and long-term outcomes.

Summary

Nucleated RBCs are not normally found in the circulating blood except in small numbers at birth and perhaps a day or so thereafter. The absence of NRBCs in the blood is the result of enucleation of orthochromatic erythroblasts within the bone marrow. Any NRBCs that escape the normal enucleation process and enter the circulation are rapidly removed by the spleen.

TABLE 3.1 Outcome-Implications of an Elevated Nucleated Red Blood Cell Count in a Newborn Infant

Year Pub.	First Author	Journal	Country	Study Population	Number Neonates	Findings
1995	Green	Pediatr	Israel	Preterm <32 wk	46 with and 103 without IVH	NRBC >2.0 × 10(9)/L on day 1 had 63% sensitivity and 79% specificity predicting grade III/IV IVH
1999	Buonocore	Am J Ob/Gyn	Italy	Preterm and term neonates	337	Higher NRBC with HIE had develop. delay at 6 mo and 3 yr
1999	Hanlon-Lundberg	Am J Ob/Gyn	USA	Normal vs cord blood pH <7.2	119 with acidemia	Higher NRBC with acidemia
2000	Minior	Fetal Diagn Ther	USA	SGA	73	High NRBC strongest predictor of IVH and death
2001	Axt-Fliedner	J Ultrasound Med	Germany	Fetuses: Doppler systolic diastolic ratios	134	Higher NRBC in growth restricted fetuses
2003	Ghosh	Int J Gynaecol/Ob	India	Term with asphyxia	75	Higher NRBC correlates with asphyxia and poor early outcome
2003	Hamrick	Pediatr Neurol	USA	Term with perinatal depression	33	Higher NRBC in 13 patients did not correlate with MRI or 30-mo neurodevelop. outcomes
2004	Ferns	Indian J Pathol Micro	India	Term, normal vs birth asphyxia	56	Higher NRBC correlated with low Apgar, low cord pH, and poor short-term outcome
2005	Perrone	Arch Dis Child	Italy	Preterm and term	695	Establishing reference interval
2006	Silva	ObGyn		Preterm case control	176	NRBC >18/100 WBC predicted cerebral white matter injury

Continued

TABLE 3.1 Outcome-Implications of an Elevated Nucleated Red Blood Cell Count in a Newborn Infant—cont'd

Year Pub.	First Author	Journal	Country	Study Population	Number Neonates	Findings
2007	Sheffer-Mimouni	J Am Coll Nutr	Israel	Obese mothers	41	Higher NRBC if mother was obese
2011	Christensen	Neonatology	USA	Preterm and Term	40,000	Establishing reference interval
2011	Walsh	Early Hum Dev	Ireland	HIE vs control	44	Higher NRBC and abnormal EEG correlated with poor 2-yr outcome
2012	Gasparovic	Coll Antropol	Croatia	Pereterm with preeclampsia	77	Higher NRBC (>40/100 WBC) correlated with adverse outcome
2013	Goel	J Clin Neonatol	India	Total 100, asphyxiate vs controls	50 in each group	Higher NRBC correlated with lower Apgar, higher HIE stage, and more mortality
2014	Li	Brain Dev	Japan	43 term with HIE	23 with cooling	Higher NRBC in first 3 days increased risk of abnormal MRI and 2-yr outcome
2014	Hebbar	J Pregnancy	India	Preeclampsia	50 with 50 contr	NRBC <13/100 WBC have low risk of adverse outcome
2015	Cremer	Early Hum Dev	Germany	Preterm infants <32 wk and <1500 g	438	NRBC >10/nL of the mean on days 2–5 had an odds ratio for mortality of 7 (95% CI 2–22) for composite adverse outcome
2017	Boskabadi	J Mater Fetal Med	Iran	Neonates with asphyxia followed for 2 yr	63	NRBC >11/100 WBC had 85% sensitivity 90% specific in prediction complications of asphyxia
2019	Poryo	Wein Med Wochenschr	Germany	VLBW	250	High NRBC and high lactate on day 2 were associated with mortality (p<0.001)
2020	Morton	Pediatr Neo	USA	NICU patients who died	45 NICU deaths	Those with any NRBC (>0) had a higher death rate (p<0.001)
2021	Piggott	Cardiol Young	USA	Neonates who underwent cardiac surgery	264	36 died, 32 of whom had an NRBC value >10/100 WBC High NRBC is a biomarker for death after neonatal heart surgery

Abbreviations; *NRBC*, nucleated red blood cells; *IVH*, intra-ventricular hemorrhage; *HIE*, hypoxic-ischemic encephalopathy; *MRI*, magnetic resonance imaging; *WBC*, white blood cells; *EEG*, electroencephalogram

To judge whether the NRBC count of a newborn infant is normal vs. elevated, it is necessary to compare the patient's value with a reference interval chart for gestational age. By convention, NRBC counts that exceed the 95th percentile upper reference interval for gestational age are considered abnormal. NRBC counts are reported as either RBC per microliter of blood (the absolute NRBC count) or NRBC per 100 WBCs. The latter method has greater accuracy.

When an elevated NRBC count is found in a neonate, an explanation should be sought. Chronic fetal hypoxia can generate elevated fetal erythropoietin levels, thereby driving erythropoiesis and generating elevated hemoglobin, hematocrit, reticulocyte, and NRBC values accompanying hyporegenerative neutropenia and/or thrombocytopenia. Acute hypoxia occurring 1 to 4 hours before birth does not seem to result in high NRBC counts. In fact, in rodent and sheep models simulating fetal hypoxia, at least 12 to 24 hours are required after the onset of hypoxia for NRBC to emerge into the blood, with peek elevations 48 to 72 hours after the hypoxic insult. Among neonates with HIE, if an acute intrapartum event necessitated an emergent delivery, the NRBC count is typically normal. Also, in neonates with HIE, a normal NRBC count is modestly predictive of survival and greater odds that they will not be diagnosed with neurodevelopmental impairment at 2 years. We speculate that neonates with HIE who have significantly elevated NRBC counts at birth have experienced hypoxia that occurred earlier or chronically (at least 24 hours or more before birth). One mechanism contributing to elevated NRBC counts after fetal hypoxia is diminished clearance of NRBC from the blood. The delayed NRBC clearance in these patients is presumably the result of injury to or dysfunction of the normal splenic and hepatic NRBC clearance mechanisms, thereby prolonging the NRBC half-life in the blood.

REFERENCES

1. Constantino BT, Cogionis B. Nucleated RBCs—significance in the peripheral blood film. *Lab Med.* 2000;31:223-229.
2. Christensen RD, Henry E, Andres RL, et al. Reference ranges for blood concentrations of nucleated red blood cells in neonates. *Neonatology.* 2011;99:289-294.
3. Quigley HG, Means Jr RT, Glader B. The birth, life, and death of red blood cells: erythropoiesis, the mature red blood cell, and cell destruction. In: Greer JP, Arber DA, Glader B, et al., eds. *Wintrobe's Clinical Hematology.* 13th ed. Philadelphia: Lippincott Williams & Wilkins; 2014:83-124.
4. Mei Y, Liu Y, Ji P. Understanding terminal erythropoiesis: an update on chromatin condensation, enucleation, and reticulocyte maturation. *Blood Rev.* 2021;46:100740.
5. Radosinska J, Vrbjar N. Erythrocyte deformability and Na,K-ATPase activity in various pathophysiological situations and their protection by selected nutritional antioxidants in humans. *Int J Mol Sci.* 2021;22(21):11924.
6. Tsiftsoglou AS. Erythropoietin (EPO) as a key regulator of erythropoiesis, bone remodeling and endothelial transdifferentiation of multipotent mesenchymal stem cells (MSCs): implications in regenerative medicine. *Cells.* 2021;10(8):2140.
7. Christensen RD, Yoder BA, Baer VL, et al. Early-onset neutropenia in small-for-gestational-age infants. *Pediatrics.* 2015;136(5):e1259-e1267.
8. Green DW, Hendon B, Mimouni FB. Nucleated erythrocytes and intraventricular hemorrhage in preterm neonates. *Pediatrics.* 1995;96:475-478.
9. Buonocore G, Perrone S, Gioia D, et al. Nucleated red blood cell count at birth as an index of perinatal brain damage. *Am J Obstet Gynecol.* 1999;181:1500-1505.
10. Hanlon-Lundberg KM, Kirby RS. Nucleated red blood cells as a marker of acidemia in term neonates. *Am J Obstet Gynecol.* 1999;181:196-201.
11. Perrone S, Bracci R, Buonocore G. New biomarkers of fetal-neonatal hypoxic stress. *Acta Paediatr Suppl.* 2002;91:135-138.
12. Ghosh B, Mittal S, Kumar S, et al. Prediction of perinatal asphyxia with nucleated red blood cells in cord blood of newborns. *Int J Gynaecol Obstet.* 2003;81(3):267-271.
13. Ferns SJ, Bhat BV, Basu D. Value of nucleated red blood cells in predicting severity and outcome of perinatal asphyxia. *Indian J Pathol Microbiol.* 2004;47(4)503-504.
14. Goel M, Dwivedi R, Gohiya P, et al. Nucleated red blood cell in cord blood as a marker of perinatal asphyxia. *J Clin Neonatol.* 2013;2(4):179-182.
15. Boskabadi H, Zakerihamidi M, Sadeghian MH, et al. Nucleated red blood cells count as a prognostic biomarker in predicting the complications of asphyxia in neonates. *J Matern Fetal Neonatal Med.* 2017;30(21):2551-2556.
16. Christensen RD, Baer VL, Yaish HM. Thrombocytopenia in late preterm and term neonates after perinatal asphyxia. *Transfusion.* 2015;55(1):187-196.
17. Blackwell SC, Hallak M, Hotra JW, et al. Timing of fetal nucleated red blood cell count elevation in response to acute hypoxia. *Biol Neonate.* 2004;85:217-220.
18. Minior VK, Levine B, Ferber A, et al. Nucleated red blood cells as a marker of acute and chronic fetal hypoxia in a rat model. *Rambam Maimonides Med J.* 2017;28:e0025.
19. Widness JA, Teramo KA, Clemons GK, et al. Temporal response of immunoreactive erythropoietin to acute hypoxemia in fetal sheep. *Pediatr Res.* 1986;20:15-19.
20. Bahr TM, Albertine KH, Christensen RD, et al. Nucleated red blood cell emergence-time in newborn lambs following a dose of darbepoetin alfa. *Cur Pediatr Rev.* 2023;19(4):425-428.
21. Blackwell SC, Refuerzo JS, Wolfe HM, et al. The relationship between nucleated red blood cell counts and early-onset neonatal seizures. *Am J Obstet Gynecol.* 2000;182:1452-1457.
22. Hermansen MC. Potential for brief but severe intrapartum injury among neonates with early-onset seizures and elevated nucleated red blood cell counts. *Am J Obstet Gynecol.* 2001;184(4):782-783.
23. Christensen RD, Lambert DK, Richards DS. Estimating the nucleated red blood cell 'emergence time' in neonates. *J Perinatol.* 2014;34:116-119.
24. Bahr TM, Henry E, O'Brien EA, et al. Nucleated red blood cell counts of neonates born emergently one to four hours after a maternal cardiac arrest. *Neonatology.* 2022;119:255-259.
25. Bahr TM, Ohls RK, Baserga MC, et al. Implications of an elevated nucleated red blood cell count in neonates with moderate to severe hypoxic-Ischemic encephalopathy. *J Pediatr.* 2022;246:12-18.
26. Wojan F, Stray-Gundersen S, Nagel MJ, et al. Short exposure to intermittent hypoxia increases erythropoietin levels in healthy individuals. *J Appl Physiol.* 2021;130(6):1955-1960.
27. Pedersen SJV, Chok R, McKillop S, et al. Peripheral nucleated red blood cells and mortality in critically ill children. *J Pediatr Hematol Oncol.* 2022;44(3):79-83. doi:10.1097/MPH.0000000000002294.
28. Ballantine JD, Kwon S, Liem RI. Nucleated red blood cells in children with sickle cell disease hospitalized for pain. *J Pediatr Hematol Oncol.* 2019;41(8):e487-e492. doi:10.1097/MPH.0000000000001467.
29. Steinberg MH, Gatling RR, Tavassoli M. Evidence of hyposplenism in the presence of splenomegaly. *Scand J Haematol.* 1983;31(5):437-439. doi:10.1111/j.1600-0609.1983.tb01539.x.
30. Schaer C, Schmugge M, Frey B. Prognostic value of nucleated red blood cells in critically ill children. *Swiss Med Wkly.* 2014;144:w13944. doi:10.4414/smw.2014.13944.

31. Axt-Fliedner R, Wrobel M, Hendrik HJ, et al. Nucleated red blood cell count and doppler ultrasound in low- and high-risk pregnancies. *Clin Exp Obstet Gynecol*. 2000;27(2):85-88.

32. Hamrick SE, Miller SP, Newton NR, et al. Nucleated red blood cell counts: not associated with brain injury or outcome. *Pediatr Neurol*. 2003;29(4):278-283.

33. Perrone S, Vezzosi P, Longini M, et al. Nucleated red blood cell count in term and preterm newborns: reference values at birth. *Arch Dis Child Fetal Neonatal Ed*. 2005;90(2):F174-F175.

34. Silva AM, Smith RN, Lehmann CU, et al. Neonatal nucleated red blood cells and the prediction of cerebral white matter injury in preterm infants. *Obstet Gynecol*. 2006;107(3):550-556.

35. Sheffer-Mimouni G, Mimouni FB, Dollberg S, et al. Neonatal nucleated red blood cells in infants of overweight and obese mothers. *J Am Coll Nutr*. 2007;26(3):259-263.

36. Walsh BH, Boylan GB, Murray DM. Nucleated red blood cells and early EEG: predicting Sarnat stage and two year outcome. *Early Hum Dev*. 2011;87(5):335-339.

37. Gasparović VE, Ahmetasević SG, Colić A. Nucleated red blood cells count as first prognostic marker for adverse neonatal outcome in severe preeclamptic pregnancies. *Coll Antropol*. 2012; 36(3):853-857.

38. Li J, Kobata K, Kamei Y, et al. Nucleated red blood cell counts: an early predictor of brain injury and 2-year outcome in neonates with hypoxic-ischemic encephalopathy in the era of cooling-based treatment. *Brain Dev*. 2014;36(6):472-478.

39. Hebbar S, Misha M, Rai L. Significance of maternal and cord blood nucleated red blood cell count in pregnancies complicated by preeclampsia. *J Pregnancy*. 2014:496416.

40. Cremer M, Roll S, Gräf C, et al. Nucleated red blood cells as marker for an increased risk of unfavorable outcome and mortality in very low birth weight infants. *Early Hum Dev*. 2015; 91(10):559-563.

41. Boskabadi H, Zakerihamidi M, Sadeghian MH, et al. Nucleated red blood cells count as a prognostic biomarker in predicting the complications of asphyxia in neonates. *J Matern Fetal Neonatal Med*. 2017;30(21):2551-2556.

42. Poryo M, Wissing A, Aygün A, et al. Reference values for nucleated red blood cells and serum lactate in very and extremely low birth weight infants in the first week of life. *Early Hum Dev*. 2017;105:49-55.

43. Morton SU, Brettin K, Feldman HA, et al. Association of nucleated red blood cell count with mortality among neonatal intensive care unit patients. *Pediatr Neonatol*. 2020;61(6): 592-597.

44. Piggott KD, Norlin C, Laviolette C, et al. Nucleated red blood cells as a biomarker for mortality in infants and neonates requiring veno-arterial extracorporeal membrane oxygenation for cardiac disease. *Perfusion*. 2021:2676591211050607.

Chapter 4

Age-Appropriate Biology of Neonatal Neutrophils

Shelley M. Lawrence, MD, MS

Chapter Outline

Introduction

Unraveling the complexities of intrinsic mechanisms behind the normal transition of the suppressed in utero neutrophil into the fully operational postpartum cell has been a goal of neutrophil biologists for nearly a century. Even though neonatal neutrophils have been historically described as functionally deficient when compared with adult cells, these phenotypic and functional disparities have been evolutionarily perfected over centuries and are essential to the divergent environments and pathogenic challenges to which they are exposed. Compared to the oxygen concentration of 21% in the earth's atmosphere, the intrauterine environment is exceedingly hypoxic, with measured oxygen concentrations in the range of 3% to 5%.[1] Because of this low oxygen content, cellular suppressive mechanisms that stabilize or counter hypoxia-inducible factor-1α (HIF-1α) are vital to prevent the expression HIF-1α proinflammatory genes. After parturition and in the immediate postnatal period, the neonate will also be newly exposed to trillions of microbes that will become essential constituents of their microbiome and for which immune tolerance is essential to prevent an acute and robust inflammatory response.

Like other major organs, the immune system matures during fetal development with well-described cellular transformations originating from the earliest hematopoietic precursors in the yolk sac and progressing to the well-developed myeloid progenitor cells in the bone marrow. The survival of extremely preterm infants exposes the severity of these immaturity-related impairments that places them at high risk for infection and sepsis-related mortality. In this chapter we explore differences between neonatal and adult neutrophils, describe neutrophil maturation throughout pregnancy, and highlight variances in neonatal neutrophil proficiency by gestational age and how these differences may impact long-term outcomes following infection or sepsis.

Development

Fetal hematopoiesis originates in the extraembryonic yolk sac around the third week of embryogenesis, where a transient population of primeval myeloid, megakaryocyte, and erythroid cells is formed.[2,3] Around weeks 7 to 8 of gestation, however, genuine, self-renewing hematopoietic stem cells (HSCs) are derived from specialized intraembryonic endothelial cells located in the ventral wall of the descending aorta.[4-6] These primitive HSCs will seed the thymus, liver, and spleen, where hematopoiesis will continue until the seventh month of gestation.[2,7] After this time, the bone marrow will become the primary source of red cells, white cells, and platelets.[8,9]

Primitive neutrophil precursors initially appear in the human clavicular marrow between 10 and 11 weeks of fetal development and are detected in the peripheral vasculature by the end of the first trimester.[10,11] Mature neutrophils can be identified by 14 to 16 weeks postconception and are formed by HSCs positioned in specialized niches in the trabecular regions near the endosteum of the long bones, where they reside near osteoblasts.[12] Once formed, neutrophils will exit the bone marrow into the bloodstream by traversing through the cell bodies of the bone marrow endothelium rather than through the cell junctions, by a process known as transcellular migration.[13,14]

Neutrophils reside in three distinct groups, or pools, known as the proliferative (bone marrow storage and release), circulating (bloodstream), and marginating pools. These pools are maintained by a delicate physiologic balance that is closely regulated by the individual's state of health and the maturational stage of the cell. Neutrophil homeostasis is also directly regulated by the controlled production of granulocyte–colony-stimulating factor (G-CSF), granulocyte macrophage–CSF (GM-CSF), interleukin-19 (IL-19), CXCL1, CCL2, and CXCL10 by nearby conventional dendritic cells.[15,16]

Within the bone marrow, neutrophil development is defined by granule formation within the maturing cell in a process known as neutrophil granulopoiesis. Neutrophil granulopoiesis and maturation are stimulated by IL-19 produced predominantly by osteoclasts, which activates IL-19 receptor (IL-20Rβ)/Stat3 signaling in neutrophil progenitors to promote their expansion and facilitate their differentiation.[16] Beginning between the myelocyte and promyelocyte stages of development, granulopoiesis proceeds over the subsequent 4 to 6 days to yield mature, segmented neutrophils (Fig. 4.1).[17] The formation of neutrophil granules is a continuous process by which granule proteins are packaged as they are produced in the process called "targeting by timing." In general, azurophilic granules are synthesized in promyelocytes, specific granule proteins in myelocytes, and gelatinase granule proteins in metamyelocytes and band cells, after which granule formation concludes and secretory vesicles form.[6,17,18] Because the formation of neutrophil granules occurs in a continuum, granule proteins may be found in more than one granule type. Direct sorting, shuttling, and packaging of granule proteins are important for proper neutrophil granule formation, with adaptor protein complexes (APs) and the monomeric Golgi-localized γ-adaptin ear homology ARF (GGA) binding protein playing key roles in this process.[19,20]

Exocytosis of neutrophil granules occurs in the reverse order of their formation and in a hierarchic fashion based on the magnitude of the stimulus and the function of their contents (see Fig. 4.1).[17,21] Thus, minimal stimulation will trigger the extrusion of secretory vesicles first. Although secretory vesicles are not considered genuine neutrophil granules, they are important reservoirs of membrane-associated receptors that allow the neutrophil to establish firm contact with activated vascular endothelium and transmigrate into inflamed tissues.[6] Next to degranulate are gelatinase granules, containing matrix-degrading enzymes (gelatinases) and membrane receptors, that are necessary for extravasation into inflamed tissues during early inflammatory processes. Specific granules follow and contain potent antimicrobial substances, which can be extruded either into phagosomes, that provide lethal enclosures for intracellular pathogen killing and clearance, or extracellularly. Last to degranulate are azurophilic granules, which are unique in that they are tightly controlled and can only be activated by potent stimuli. Once mobilized, these granules extrude highly toxic acidic hydrolases and microbicidal proteins into phagolysosomes. These structures provide specialized intracellular containment vacuoles that protect the surrounding cells and tissues from injury, which would occur if these noxious substances were to be expelled extracellularly.

PROLIFERATIVE NEUTROPHIL POOL

A delicate balance between granulopoiesis, bone marrow storage and release, intravascular margination, and transmigration into peripheral tissues is required to maintain neutrophil homeostasis.[15,22] Mitotic neutrophil precursors that comprise the proliferative pool are important in maintaining and replenishing neutrophil numbers, including myeloblasts, promyelocytes, and myelocytes.[23,24]

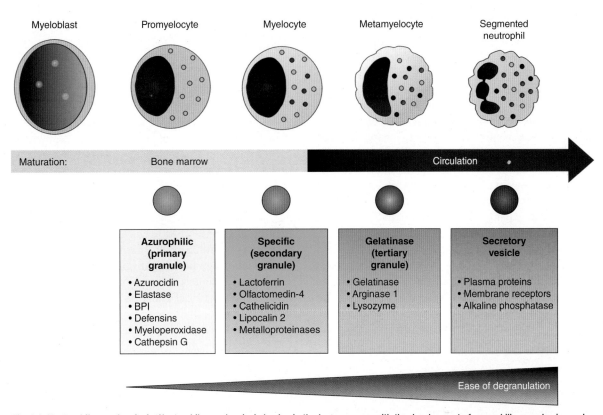

Fig. 4.1 Neutrophil granulopoiesis. Neutrophil granulopoiesis begins in the bone marrow with the development of azurophilic granules in myeloblasts/promyelocytes and concludes after the creation of secretory vesicles in mature, segmented cells. Neutrophil maturation is defined by nuclear segmentation and the sequential formation of three different granules and secretory vesicles. Degranulation occurs in reverse order of granule formation. Thus, secretory vesicles are the first to be mobilized after minimal neutrophil stimulation. These vesicles contain membrane-associated receptors that are essential for chemotactic-directed migration and the establishment of firm contact with activated vascular endothelium. Azurophilic granules are the last to be mobilized and contain toxic microbicidal proteins that are crucial for killing pathogenic microorganisms.

In steady-state conditions, human adults produce nearly 100 billion neutrophils every day. These cells[25,26] are generally short-lived cells with a half-life of ~19 hours.[27] In contrast, term neonates have greatly diminished neutrophil proliferative pools, estimated to contain only 10% adult values.[28] While adults produce between 4 and 5 $\times 10^9$ neutrophils/kg body weight per day, term newborns generate nearly a quarter[28] and preterm infants only 20% of adult values.[29] Moreover, the proliferative pool in a developing fetus or postpartum neonate experiences significant cell turnover, with more than two thirds of these cells residing in an active cell cycle.[10,30]

Proliferative Pool and the Microbiome

The coevolution of mammals and their microbiota has led to direct regulation of the host neutrophil proliferative pool by microbial-derived mediators. In steady-state granulopoiesis, tonic microbial signaling leads to activation of the host systemic innate immune system via Toll-like receptor 4 (TLR4), a member of the highly conserved family of pattern recognition receptors that recognizes and binds to gram-negative lipopolysaccharide, pathogen-associated molecular patterns (PAMPs), and endogenous molecules generated as a result of tissue injury.[31] This relationship is well demonstrated in adult mice, where the complexity of the intestinal microbiome directly controls the size of bone marrow neutrophil mitotic progenitors that function to maintain vigilance against potential pathogens.[31]

In contrast to adults, the immune naïve fetus represents a unique challenge. In the course of natural parturition, newborns are exposed to and colonized by a vast number of microorganisms that comprise the maternal vaginal and rectal microbiota. Because these microbes harbor a variety of foreign nucleic acids, proteins, and antigens, neutrophil tolerance is imperative during the transition to extrauterine life to prevent robust systemic proinflammatory reactions during the establishment of the newborn's microbiota. Interventions that impede the natural development of the newborn's microbiota, such as cesarean delivery or exposure to intrapartum and/or postpartum antibiotics, may place the infant at an elevated risk for necrotizing enterocolitis, late-onset sepsis, prolonged length of stay, or even death.[32-34]

To further explore the association of the microbiome and neutrophils in neonates, Deshmukh et al.[35] used a murine model to demonstrate that induction of IL-17 by the pup's intestinal microbiota resulted in activation of intestinal group 3 innate lymphoid cells. These lymphoid cells subsequently increased their production of G-CSF to enhance the proliferation of neutrophil mitotic precursors in a TLR4- and MyD88-dependent manner. This continuous, very low-level TLR signaling (below the threshold required for induction of adaptive immune responses) by microbial antigens and TLR ligands facilitates neutrophil homeostasis under steady-state conditions.[31] Conversely, invading pathogens elicit an upregulation of TLR induction through detection of PAMPs, causing a rise of proinflammatory cytokines, including IL-1β, tumor necrosis factor (TNF)-α, GM-CSF, and G-CSF.[36,37] This surge of inflammatory mediators triggers emergency granulopoiesis, leading to an acute and drastic increase in the number of bloodstream neutrophils that are available to combat the ensuing infection. This acute proliferation of neutrophils can be attenuated in germ-free mice, where studies have shown severely delayed pathogen clearance and neutrophil recruitment following a challenge with apathogenic bacteria.[31] Therefore maintenance of neutrophil homeostasis, proper cell functioning, and robust neutrophil proliferative during emergency granulopoiesis are all directly dependent upon the establishment of a healthy and robust microbiome after birth.

Hypoproductive Neutropenia in the Neonate

During the very early phases of deep tissue or bloodstream infections or inflammation, quiescent neutrophil progenitors are activated and their number in circulation rises rapidly from the depletion of bone marrow reserves of mature and nearly mature cells.[38]

This triggers the release of a large quantity of immature granulocytes into the bloodstream in a process often referred to as a "left shift". The left shift can be detected by clinical hematology analyzers and is routinely used to assess a person's probability of serious infection and/or sepsis.[39]

Human adults maintain a large reserve pool, estimated to contain more than 20 times the number of neutrophils found in circulation. These cells can be quickly mobilized during times of sepsis to rapidly boost neutrophil numbers.[7,10,25,40,41] In contrast, very low birth weight infants (or those <1500 g at birth) are more likely to develop neutropenia (or an absolute neutrophil count <1000 cells/μL), when challenged by infectious pathogens due to their inability to generate or recruit significant neutrophil numbers. The development of neutropenia can be devastating in neonates, as it substantially increases a neonate's risk for sepsis-related morbidity and mortality.[7,10,41]

Neonates who are born small for gestational age (SGA; or birth weight <10th percentile) also experience a high rate of neutropenia compared to non-SGA infants, with an incidence of 6% vs. 1%, respectively. SGA-associated neutropenia usually persists for the first week of life and is accompanied by thrombocytopenia in more than 60% of neonates.[42] Because the severity of neutropenia is directly correlated with the number of nucleated red blood cells, in utero growth restriction rather than maternal conditions resulting in placental deficiencies, such as preeclampsia or other hypertensive disorders, is thought to be the primary cause.[42] Previous conclusions regarding direct relationships between neutropenia and preeclampsia,[43] or related placental deficiencies, have been disproven using regression models that suggest no higher incidence of low neutrophil counts over and above that calculated for SGA alone.[42,44]

For reasons that remain unclear, SGA infants have an increased probability of being diagnosed with late-onset sepsis and a fourfold elevated risk of developing necrotizing enterocolitis.[42] The primary mechanism underlying neutropenia in SGA infants is diminished neutrophil production, rather than excessive margination or accelerated neutrophil destruction, because a normal immature to total neutrophil ratio is maintained.[42] Experimental models have shown diminished neutrophil production from pluripotent hematopoietic progenitors and reduced concentrations of granulocyte-macrophage progenitors, resulting in (1) downregulation of neutrophil transcription and growth factors due to elevated levels of erythropoietin and enhanced reticulocytosis[45] and (2) insufficient production of G-CSF. However, a placental inhibitor of neutrophil production that has yet to be identified cannot be ruled out as a potential cause for SGA-associated neutropenia.[42]

The highest frequency of neutropenia without an identified cause is observed in extremely low birth weight infants (those born <1000 g).[46] In this patient population, neutropenia is usually not associated with sepsis,[47] and those with and without neutropenia experience similar mortality rates.[46] Fortunately, neutrophil numbers in preterm and term infants will rise over the first few weeks of life to achieve adult values around 1 month of age, irrespective of gestational age or intrauterine growth.[29]

Therapies targeted at increasing neutrophil numbers, including recombinant G-CSF (rG-CSF) and GM-CSF (rGM-CSF), have been trialed in clinical studies with disappointing results, even though study sizes have been small. While the bloodstream concentration of neutrophils increased following the administration of either drug, mortality in preterm infants with proven or suspected sepsis, who also received concurrent antibiotics, was no different than controls 14 days from the beginning of the intervention.[48,49] In particular, the PROGRAMS trial investigated the specific use of rGM-CSF in the first 5 days of life in SGA infants because of its collective ability not only to increase neutrophil numbers but also its proficiency to generate a TH1 immune response and activate monocytes and neutrophils to improve bactericidal activity. This study, however, also failed to show improved sepsis-free survival to day 14 from trial entry compared to the control group.[50]

Further subgroup analysis of all rG-CSF and rGM-CSF data by the Cochrane Group identified 97 preterm infants from three different studies who received either drug with systemic infection and neutropenia at the time of study enrollment and demonstrated marked reduction in mortality by day 14 (risk ratio 0.34 [95% confidence interval (CI) 0.12–0.92]; number needed to treat 6 [95% CI 3–33]).[49] Their findings suggest that additional, appropriately powered studies should be undertaken to determine the efficacy of these drugs in this defined patient population.[51] Alternative therapies,

such as low dose IL-19, demonstrated efficacy at reversing neutropenia in rodent models related to chemotherapy, irradiation, and induction by chloramphenicol exposure, but human trials are currently lacking.[16]

Defects in neutrophil production can also lead to life-threatening severe congenital neutropenia (SCN), or Kostmann syndrome, which presents clinically with recurrent invasive fungal and bacterial infections.[52,53] SCN is also associated with a predisposition for myelodysplastic syndrome and acute myeloid leukemia, with a rate of malignant transformation exceeding 20% in those affected.[52,53] Secondary mutations in genes encoding the neutrophil primary granule protein elastase account for more than half of all SNC cases.[54] Genetic defects generally lead to neutrophil elastase misfolding, resulting in intracellular accumulation and mislocalization of the modified protein that causes endoplasmic reticulum stress and induction of apoptosis through activation of the unfolded-protein response mechanism.[54] Many causes of SNC originate in the earliest phases of granulocyte monocyte progenitor commitment to neutrophil differentiation, or at the myeloblast-to-promyelocyte maturational stage.[55]

CIRCULATING AND MARGINATING NEUTROPHIL POOLS

Once released from the proliferative pool, maturing neutrophils (including metamyelocytes, bands, and segmented cells) are equally distributed between those free flowing in the bloodstream (circulating pool) and those that cannot be readily retrieved by routine blood sampling (marginating pool).[56] First observed in the 1960s, marginating neutrophils were discovered following autologous transfusion of ex vivo radiolabeled neutrophils in healthy adult volunteers.[57] After the transfusion, nearly half of these cells disappeared from circulation but could be readily recovered following adrenalin dosing or strenuous exercise.[57] Although the lungs and pulmonary vasculature are considered the primary sources of marginating neutrophils, the liver, spleen, and bone marrow have also been shown to harbor a large number of these cells.[58]

The importance of continued neutrophil maturation outside of the bone marrow has only recently been elucidated. Investigations suggest that while the establishment of the cytotoxic capacity of neutrophils occurs during bone marrow granulopoiesis, the signaling components that facilitate antimicrobial defensive mechanisms are primarily transcribed in the periphery, or at later stages of neutrophil maturation. This developmental continuum, or neutrotime, may function to finetune the neutrophil's protective mechanisms after environmental exposures in real time.[59]

Following birth, marginating neutrophils may be recruited into the bloodstream due to the surge of stress-related birth hormones, including cortisol, epinephrine, and norepinephrine, although the exact mechanisms have not been well defined. This rapid accumulation of circulating neutrophils during the first 6 to 24 hours of life in term infants results in neutrophil numbers never again encountered in one's lifetime while healthy.[60] In preterm infants 28 weeks or more gestational age, neutrophil levels peak earlier (~6–12 hours of life), rising to levels around 25,000 to 28,000 cells/μL. Those less than 28 weeks of gestational age experience a more gradual but dramatic increase in cell numbers, with peak levels reaching up to 40,000 cells/μL around 24 hours of life.[60] Irrespective of gestational age at birth, all newborns will subsequently undergo a gradual decline in neutrophil numbers over the next 72 hours, with neutrophil composition and counts closely approximating that of adults by the third day of life.[60]

After birth, neonates also have an abundance of bloodstream immature granulocytes (promyelocytes, myelocytes, and metamyelocytes) when compared to adults (12% vs. 5%, respectively).[6,61] These early neutrophil precursors generally lack gelatinase granules and secretory vesicles, which may hinder early proinflammatory responses and increase the newborn's susceptibility to infection by hindering the cell's ability to transmigrate into inflamed tissues.[61] Alternatively, the higher quantity of immature granulocytes may simultaneously guard against inappropriate inflammatory responses during the critical period of establishing its microbiome. Further investigations are necessary to establish the significance of these findings.

Functional Characteristics of Neonatal Neutrophils

Historically, neonatal neutrophils have been described as dysfunctional when compared to adult cells due to shortages of important cell membrane receptors, reduced intracellular signaling pathways, and impaired cellular functions, which coalesce to heighten a newborn's susceptibility to infection and septic shock (Fig. 4.2). When compared to adult cells, however, unstimulated cord blood neutrophils from term, healthy infants have increased levels of proinflammatory cytokines, including IFN-γ, IL-1ß, and TNF-α,[62] and exhibit prolonged survival capacity due to a reduced capacity to undergo programmed apoptosis,[63] irrespective of labor exposure. Following stimulation by TNF-α and LPS, neonatal neutrophils also upregulate the expression of proinflammatory IL-1ß compared to adult cells.[64] Even though neonatal neutrophils appear primed and ready for combat against threatening pathogens, heightened neutrophil inflammatory responses are often coupled to powerful inhibitory mechanisms (see later).

Recognition of PAMPs by Toll-like receptors induces the innate immune system to generate proinflammatory cytokines, type I interferon, and other immune mediators that typically favor differentiation and activation of TH1 cells that are vital in protecting against intracellular viral and bacterial infections. In neonates, however, a greater concentration of TH2-polarizing cytokines, including IL-6 and IL-10, are produced following TLR 1-9 activation. Better adapted to defend against parasitic infections, TH2-mediated immune responses are deficient against bacterial and viral infections, leaving newborns more vulnerable to sepsis-related morbidity and mortality. Moreover, TH2-mediated immune responses greatly increase the neonate's future risk of developing atrophy, allergy, and asthma.[65-67]

Reduced intracellular mediators of the TLR signaling pathway and/or higher concentrations of plasma adenosine may explain the dampened responsiveness observed with neonatal neutrophils in relation to TH1-mediated activation.[66] Research suggests that adenosine enhances the production of TH2-polarizing cytokines, including IL-6, by binding G protein–coupled A3 adenosine receptors (A3ARs) and increasing intracellular cAMP levels. While this reaction may hinder neutrophil migration to sites of inflammation[66] and increase a newborn's susceptibility to intracellular pathogens, it may also enable colonization of commensal microorganisms after birth by prohibiting excessive inflammation.

Group B *Streptococcus* (GBS) remains a leading cause of neonatal early-onset sepsis (EOS) in term neonates and can elicit variable immunologic responses in the

Neutrophil Development in the Fetus

Preterm infants

1. Neutrophil production primarily from the **liver**
2. ↑↑ Immature granulocytes in circulation
3. ↑↑ Neutrophils in circulation in the first 24 hours of life
4. ↓↓ Storage pool and cell mass per gram BW
5. ↓ Chemotaxis
6. ↓↓ Rolling and firm adhesion
7. ↓↓ Transmigration
8. ↓↓ Phagocytosis
9. ↓ Apoptosis

Term infants

1. Neutrophil production primarily from the **bone marrow**
2. ↑ Immature granulocytes in circulation
3. ↑ Neutrophils in circulation in the first 24 hours of life
4. ↓ Storage pool and cell mass per gram BW
5. ↓ Chemotaxis
6. ↓ Rolling and firm adhesion
7. ↓ Transmigration
8. ↓ Phagocytosis
9. ↓ Apoptosis

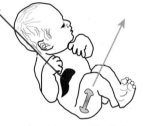

Fig. 4.2 Differences between preterm and term neonatal neutrophils. Preterm neutrophils are primarily derived from myeloid precursors located in the fetal liver. At around 7 months of gestation, neutrophil production transitions to the bone marrow. Preterm neonates have a higher percentage of immature granulocytes circulating in the bloodstream, which have notable deficiencies in chemotaxis, rolling and adhesion to vascular endothelium, transmigration, and phagocytosis when compared to term and adult neutrophils. Moreover, preterm infants will achieve the highest concentration of neutrophils in circulation within the first 24 hours of life. While preterm infants ≥28 weeks of gestational age will experience peak neutrophil levels around 6 to 12 hours of life (at 25–28,000 cells/µL), those born <28 weeks of gestational age experience a more gradual but dramatic increase in cell numbers, with peak levels reaching up to 40,000 cells/µL around 24 hours of life. *BW,* Body weight. (Lawrence SM, Corriden R, Nizet V. Age-Appropriate Functions and Dysfunctions of the Neonatal Neutrophil. *Front Pediatr.* 2017 Feb 28;5:23. doi: 10.3389/fped.2017.00023. PMID: 28293548; PMCID: PMC5329040.)

newborn. While GBS hemolysin can activate pro-IL-1ß processing and IL-1ß release by neonatal neutrophils to increase their recruitment to inflamed or infected tissues,[68] molecular mimicry by GBS capsular sialic acid and ß protein can dampen innate immune responses by binding to inhibitory sialic acid-binding immunoglobulin-like lectin receptors (Siglecs) on neutrophils. This binding triggers SHP-2 phosphatase-dependent signaling, which dampens neutrophil activation and phagocytic killing.[69,70] In murine pups, GBS also induces the production of IL-10 compared to adult animals, which impedes neutrophil recruitment to sites of inflammation and impedes bacterial clearance. This response can be attenuated in TLR2 deficient pups, however, where improved GBS phagocytosis by neonatal neutrophils hinders bacterial dissemination.[71]

When challenged with peptidoglycan, a major cell component of gram-positive bacteria, neonatal neutrophils exhibited an exaggerated proinflammatory response due to upregulation of CD11b, TNF-α, and IL-8 expression. Peptidoglycan exposure improved their chemotactic capabilities and generation of reactive oxygen species (ROS) through activation of the heat shock proteins HSPA1A and OLR1.[72] Conversely, complement-mediated phagocytosis of gram-negative bacteria is lower in neonatal neutrophils (especially preterm infants) compared with adults due to lower concentrations of the cell membrane and cytoplasmic receptor CR3 (CD11b/CD18, $\alpha_M\beta_2$, MAC-1), which binds lipopolysaccharide and is a critical pathogen recognition receptor for gram-negative bacteria. Following neutrophil stimulation, neonatal levels of CR3 remained lower than adult cells, resulting in impaired activation and diminished recruitment to and accumulation at the site of inflammation.[73]

Neonatal neutrophils also demonstrate delayed apoptosis. Overexpression of IL-1ß and IL-8 and activation of nuclear factor kappa B has been shown to upregulate antiapoptotic genes.[74] Reduced cellular expression of Siglec-9 and its downstream signaling protein SHP-1, an inhibitory tyrosine phosphate, also promote neonatal neutrophil survival by delaying programmed cell death via apoptosis.[75] While prolonging cell survival may enhance bacterial clearance, it can also boost local proinflammatory responses that cause tissue injury and contribute to adverse neonatal outcomes.[76] Pathogen-induced programmed cell death via apoptosis with subsequent clearance by tissue macrophages and monocytes is essential for the resolution of inflammation and promotion of tissue repair. The consequences of delayed neutrophil apoptosis and turnover are demonstrated by Grigg et al.,[77] who showed a direct correlation with higher rates of chronic lung disease and pulmonary injury.

MICROBICIDAL PROTEINS AND ACTIVITY

As previously discussed, degranulation of neutrophil granules occurs in reverse order of their formation, so that azurophilic (or primary) granules are the last and most difficult to retrieve. Studies have shown that degranulation capabilities are the same between term neonatal and adult neutrophils, while those from preterm infants have substantial impairments. Specifically, neutrophils from preterm infants have deficient degranulation of specific (secondary) and azurophilic granule proteins, including bactericidal/permeability-increasing protein (BPI), elastase, and lactoferrin.[78,79]

Unstimulated neutrophils from adults and term, healthy newborns contain similar concentrations of the azurophilic granule proteins defensin and myeloperoxidase, while BPI is reduced threefold[80] (Table 4.1). Intriguingly, recent findings demonstrate neutrophils from human and murine males exhibit higher protein expression of azurophilic granule components compared to females, contributing to accumulating evidence of sex dimorphic mammalian biology.[81] BPI is an important neutrophil protein, as it enhances the phagocytosis of gram-negative bacterium by acting as

TABLE 4.1   Granule Proteins in Neonatal Compared to Adult Neutrophils

Variable	Preterm	Term	Comment
Degranulation Capabilities	Decreased	Normal	Only known for BPI, elastase, and lactoferrin[78, 79,]
Respiratory Burst	Decreased	Increased	[129, 132-134]
Granule Protein Levels			
Myeloperoxidase	Normal	Normal	[80]
Defensins	Unknown	Normal	[80]
BPI	Decreased	Decreased	[79, 80]
Lactoferrin	Decreased	Decreased	[87]
OLFM4	Increased	Increased	[62]
Rolling and Firm Adhesion			
CR3	Decreased	Decreased	[40, 103]
LFA-1 Levels	Normal	Normal	[40, 73, 92]
L-Selectin	Decreased	Decreased	[40, 92, 103-105]
Phagocytosis	Decreased	Normal	Reduced in neonates with sepsis or noninfective clinical stress for some organisms[151]
CR1	Decreased	Normal	[152, 153]
Fcγ	Normal	Normal	[40]
FcγRII	Decreased	Normal	[112, 154]
FcγIII	Decreased	Normal	Adult levels in preterm infants reached by two weeks of age [112]
Galectin-3	Decreased	Decreased/ Normal	[120-122]

BPI, Bactericidal/permeability-increasing protein; *OLFM4,* olfactomedin 4.

an opsonin.[80,82] BPI also has a strong affinity for the lipid A portion of LPS, the endotoxin of gram-negative bacteria, and can function as a neutralizing agent against its proinflammatory properties.[80,83] Therefore, preterm infants who are deficient in BPI mobilization are at an increased risk of becoming septic with gram-negative bacteria, such as *Escherichia coli*, the leading cause of EOS. Using the potent neutrophil stimulation agent phorbol myristate acetate, Nupponen et al.[79] demonstrated that term and adult neutrophils produced similar concentrations of BPI, while preterm neonatal cells continued to experience diminished production. Plasma levels of BPI, however, can surge in term infants with EOS to achieve levels comparable to those of adults with bacteremia[84] or pneumonia[79,85] and older children with sepsis syndrome.[86] Thus, neutrophil mobilization of BPI demonstrates an age-dependent maturational effect.

Concentrations of the specific granule protein lactoferrin were also found to be about half of adult values in term neonatal neutrophils, while preterm infants had even lower quantities.[87] Lactoferrin binds free iron and is directly bacteriostatic and bactericidal against gram-positive and -negative bacteria, viruses, and fungi.[88] Olfactomedin-4 (OLFM4), another specific granule protein, has potent antiinflammatory properties and can attenuate neutrophil bacterial killing and host innate immunity against both gram-positive and -negative bacteria.[89] At baseline, OLFM4 expression is greatly upregulated in unstimulated cord blood neutrophils from healthy term newborns compared to adult cells,[62] but levels can rapidly surge even higher in septic neonates.[90] OLFM4 expression is associated with decreased concentrations of IL-1ß, IL-6, G-CSF, and GM-CSF. Additionally, OLFM4 can restrict neutrophil cathepsin c–mediated protease activity and Nod-like receptor-mediated NF-κB activation. Collectively, these OLFM4 attributes prohibit antimicrobial killing and substantially increase sepsis-related mortality.[89]

CHEMOTAXIS AND MIGRATION

As the "police force" of the immune system, neutrophils comprise nearly 60% of leukocytes in humans, and the majority of myeloid granulopoiesis are dedicated to their production.[27] Neutrophils are alerted to tissue inflammation in the earliest stages of infection by chemoattractants, derived from either the pathogen (i.e., fMLP, LPS) and/or host (i.e., cytokines, cytokines, or leukotrienes), that are subsequently released into the bloodstream. These agents activate quiescent neutrophils and create a biochemical gradient that is sensed by specialized G protein–coupled receptors, located on the neutrophil cell membrane. Induction of G protein–coupled receptors activates intracellular signaling cascades, leading to cell polarization, cytoskeletal rearrangement, and adhesion molecule clustering that enable the stimulated neutrophil to hone in on and migrate toward inflamed tissue in a process known as chemotaxis.[91,92]

Chemotactic abilities are similar between neonatal and adult neutrophils, irrespective of gestational age,[56,93] but neonatal cells have reduced chemoattractant responsiveness.[94-96] Even though the number and affinity of the cell-surface receptors are similar, neonatal neutrophil deficiencies are attributed to decreased intracellular calcium mobilization that causes aberrations in chemoattractant-induced signaling[97] and impaired microfilamentous cytoskeletal organization capabilities from delays in F-actin induction.[98]

After birth, IGs comprise a higher percentage of circulating neutrophils, and these cells are inept at chemotaxis compared to more developmentally mature cells.[62,99] By 4 weeks of age, however, neutrophils from term infants typically achieve similar chemotactic abilities as adult cells. Conversely, deficiencies persisted in almost half of preterm infants at 42 weeks corrected gestations age,[95,96] indicating the developmental program of neutrophil maturation is not corrected following birth and exposure to extrauterine environmental factors. Infant health can also affect chemotaxis, with improvements observed in neonates who are ventilated for severe respiratory distress syndrome (but otherwise healthy)[96] and those with superficial infections[100] compared to stable preterm and term infants.[96] Septic infants with gram-negative bacteremia, however, had poorly chemotactic neutrophils,[93,100] as did neonates exposed to maternal magnesium sulfate with impairments directly correlated to maternal serum magnesium levels.[101]

Once the activated neutrophil arrives at the inflamed site, extravasation into the tissue is necessary and requires four steps: (1) capture and rolling, (2) firm adhesion, (3) crawling, and (4) diapedesis/transmigration.

To initiate the contact between the neutrophil and vascular endothelium, interaction with L-selectin on the neutrophil and P- or E-selectin on the endothelium is necessary during capture and rolling. Once contact is established, chemokines located on the inflamed endothelium bind to distinct chemokine receptors on the neutrophil cell surface, eliciting a conformational change of neutrophil with the shedding of L-selectin,[102] induction of β2 integrin expression (including LFA-1 or lymphocyte function associated antigen-1), and activation of CR3, by inside-out signaling.[103]

L-selecting levels are decreased, and shedding is impaired in neonatal neutrophils, which may hinder slow rolling and adhesion maneuvers.[104] L-selectin first appears on fetal neutrophils around 21 weeks of gestation,[40,105] and its concentration on the cell surface rises in an age-dependent manner.[40,103] Despite improved levels with advancing fetal maturational age, the overall quantity and ease of L-selectin release remain well below that of adult cells at term gestation, with considerable deficits observed in neonates less than 30 weeks of gestational age.[40,92,103] Once L-selectin is shed from the neutrophil, β2 integrins establish firm adhesion with the endothelium by binding to members of the immunoglobulin superfamily of adhesion molecules, such as ICAM-1 and ICAM-2 (intracellular adhesion molecule 1 and 2), VCAM-1 (vascular cell adhesion molecule-1), and RAGE (receptor for advanced glycation end products).[17,92,106] Interestingly, fetal exposure to antenatal betamethasone may hinder neonatal neutrophil firm adhesion to the vascular endothelium through reduced expression of endothelial adhesion molecules E-selectin, ICAM-1, and VCAM-1.[107] Moreover, the ability of the neonatal vascular endothelium to upregulate its expression of adhesion molecules following LPS exposure is also significantly decreased and inversely related to gestational age.[103,108]

Neonatal neutrophils are also observed to have impaired upregulation of CR3 following chemotactic stimulation, which may impede transmigration into inflamed tissue. Intriguingly, levels of CR3 in midgestational age neonates are similar to those of patients with leukocyte adhesion deficiency type 1 syndrome (LAD-1).[6,40,103] Measurements of cytosolic and cell membrane CR3 stores showed that neonates had only 10% of adult levels at 27 weeks of gestational age,

48% at 36 weeks, and 57 ± 4% at term, with adult levels attained around 11 months of age.[40] In contrast, the appearance of LFA-1 in the neutrophil cell membrane is not dependent on maturation, with equivalent abundance in adults and neonates, irrespective of gestational age.[40,73,92] Therefore, only about half as many term neonatal neutrophils transmigrate through the vascular endothelium in response to infection or inflammation when compared to adult cells.[6,40]

PHAGOCYTOSIS

Once within the inflamed tissue, oxygen deprivation created by the pathologic conditions of the infection drives HIF-dependent activation of prosurvival pathways in the neutrophils[109] to enhance their bactericidal activity.[110] Activated neutrophils then travel along the chemotactic gradient toward the site of microbial invasion until the pathogenic intruder is encountered. Using receptors for complement and the Fc domain of immunoglobulins, including CR1, CR3, FcγRII, and FcγIII, neutrophils will engulf or phagocytose identified pathogens.[6,40] Term neonates and adults have similar numbers of CR1[111] and both Fcγ receptors,[112] while CR3 receptors are reduced as previously discussed.[40] Preterm infants express 80% to 88% of adult levels of FcγRII but only 50% of FcγIII at birth but will rapidly attain adult FcγIII levels by 2 weeks of life. Together these four receptors primarily mediate the binding, ingestion, and killing of bacteria.[29]

Neutrophils from term, healthy neonates and adults have similar efficiency in the opsonization and ingestion of gram-positive and -negative bacteria,[113] while neutrophils from preterm infants demonstrated less competence. Neonates less than 33 weeks gestational age experience slower uptake and ingestion of bacteria, which persists for up to 2 months postnatal age despite no apparent maturational defect.[114] One reason for this deficiency may be lower levels of circulating opsonization factors, particularly maternal immunoglobulins, which are actively transported across the placenta during the last trimester of pregnancy. Administration of intravenous immunoglobulins (IVIG) to preterm infants less than 32 weeks gestational age normalized the phagocytic capacity of these neutrophils but failed to reduce either (1) mortality during the hospital stay or (2) death or major disability at 2 years of age in infants with suspected or proven sepsis in a large cohort of neonates.[115,116]

Neonates, especially those born extremely premature or exposed to prolonged courses of antibiotics, are at an increased risk of acquiring invasive fungemia. As discussed previously, deficiencies of opsonization factors observed in preterm infants decrease the ability of neutrophils to phagocytose *Candida albicans*,[78,117] yet both neonatal and adult neutrophils were equally unable to phagocytose unopsonized *C. albicans* yeast but equally capable of phagocytosing unopsonized *C. parapsilosis*.[118] Likewise, the oxidative burst was equally robust when challenged with *C. albicans* hyphae in all groups but nonexistent against *C. parapsilosis* and attenuated against *C. albicans* yeast forms.[6,118] Therefore, the ability of neutrophils to phagocytose *Candida* not only depends on the size and form of the pathogen (i.e., hyphae or yeast) but also on the species.[6,118,119]

Another neutrophil cell membrane receptor that is critical in the phagocytosis of *Candida* species is galectin-3, an S-type lectin receptor with proinflammatory autocrine/paracrine effects.[119,120] Galectin-3 can distinguish between pathogenic and nonpathogenic fungi by recognizing and binding to ß-(1-2) oligomannan on their cell surface.[119] Galectin-3 may also function to enhance ROS production, promote neutrophil degranulation, and impede apoptosis.[120] Galectin-3 can also bind to the neutrophil cell membrane following its extracellular release by activated or damaged neutrophils resulting in the colligation of CD66a and CD66b, which functions to improve the cell's phagocytic capabilities.[120] There is conflicting data regarding serum and plasma levels of galectin-3 in term neonates compared to adults, although serum levels in preterm infants may be lower than their term counterparts and increase throughout gestation.[119,121] Galectin-3 levels may also be higher in neonates delivered vaginally compared to cesarean without labor. Research suggests labor exposure may function to prime neonatal neutrophils and render them more responsive to challenges with gram-negative bacteria[122] and/or fungi.[119,121]

RESPIRATORY BURST

Once engulfed by the neutrophil, microbes are trapped within phagosomes that fuse with azurophilic and specific granules to form phagolysosomes, which are specialized containment units designed to confine the oxidative and highly toxic reactions needed to destroy bacteria within the cell, while protecting the host tissue against harmful metabolites.[123,124] The formation of phagolysosomes is associated with a sharp rise in hexose monophosphate shunt metabolism of glucose and, in turn, a proportional increase in molecular oxygen consumption and is referred to as the respiratory burst.[123] Nicotinamide adenine dinucelotide phosphate (NADPH) oxidase, which is localized on the phagolysosome membrane, is activated by phagocytosis and is essential in driving the respiratory burst through the reduction of oxygen (O_2) to yield hydroxydioxylic acid (HO_2) and hydrogen peroxide (H_2O_2).[123,125] Inactivating mutations of NADPH oxidase result in chronic granulomatous disease (CGD), which is characterized by recurrent bacterial and fungal infections. CGD is also associated with the formation of granulomas, which are caused by the neutrophils' inability to completely kill and eliminate pathogens.[126]

HO_2 and H_2O_2 cause substantial acidification of the phagolysosome but are weakly bactericidal.[127] The addition of myeloperoxidase from azurophilic granules, however, catalyzes oxidation reactions between H_2O_2 and chloride (Cl^-) to form hypochlorous acid ($HOCl$),[128] hydroxyl radicals ($\cdot OH$), and chloramines, all of which are potent oxidants[129] that further contribute to the microbicidal capabilities of neutrophils.[127] The resulting reactions between the oxygenation radicals and engulfed microbes produce electronically excited products that cause light emission in the visible spectrum, known as chemiluminescence.[130]

The generation of O_2^- can be detected using the nitroblue tetrazolium test,[131] which remains negative (clear) in patients with NADPH oxidase deficiencies (i.e., CGD), but produces a positive (or blue) reaction in neutrophils that function normally. Neonatal neutrophils from healthy newborns induce an intensely positive reaction that corresponds to enhanced oxygen consumption in the initial phase of the respiratory burst and normal or elevated production of H_2O_2,[132] whereas neutrophils from neonates with perinatal distress[133] or stressed preterm and term infants[129] demonstrated respiratory burst suppression with decreased bactericidal activity against both gram-positive and -negative bacteria. Deficient respiratory burst reactions normalized to adult cellular function in preterm infants by 2 months of age, but they remained depressed in chronically ill infants receiving intensive care.[134]

NEUTROPHIL EXTRACELLULAR TRAPS

Neutrophils can also entrap and kill pathogens by extruding their chromatin material, loaded with antimicrobial molecules, extracellularly in a process known as neutrophil extracellular trap (NET) formation. In general, NETs are composed of sticky chromatin, which is laden with citrullinated histones, elastase, myeloperoxidase, lactoferrin, and defensins and function to entrap and kill a variety of bacteria, fungi, and protozoa.[135] NETs can be produced by neutrophils via two distinct pathways: (1) initiation in response to LPS, TNF-α, or IL-8[136,137] that requires activation of NADPH-oxidase,[138] ROS production,[139] and induction of the RIPK3-MLKL cascade[140,141]; and (b) a ROS-independent pathway that follows activation by either the complement system,[142] TLR2, and/or fibronectin.[140] Neonatal neutrophils, irrespective of gestational age, fail to form NETs via the ROS-dependent fashion even though they can generate sufficient endogenous ROS and have NADPH activity equivalent to adult cells.[143] The inability to form NETs in this fashion was shown by Yost et al.[144] to be caused by NET-inhibitory factor (nNIF), which appears to be unique to neonatal neutrophils and functions as an important regulator of fetal and neonatal inflammation. Others have shown preterm, term, and adult neutrophils possess a similar ability to produce NETs following exposure to fibronectin together with either purified β-glucan or *C. albicans* hyphae in a ROS-independent manner.[145] None of the neutrophils, however, formed NETs when exposed to fibronectin or β-glucan independently.[145]

Conclusion

Our knowledge of neutrophil biology has expanded substantially over the last half century with advancements in laboratory techniques and scientific methodologies. Neutrophils are no longer regarded as short-lived, indiscriminate phagocytes of the immune system but as essential cells that are vital for proper adaptive immune responses, resolution of proinflammatory reactions, and tissue repair and regeneration. While we have historically characterized neonatal neutrophils as being dysfunctional when compared to adult cells, we now understand that phenotypic and functional

variances are necessary. These cells have adapted and evolved to protect the developing fetus from maternal immunity, while also enduring extremely hypoxic in utero environmental conditions without triggering HIF-1α-mediated proinflammatory responses.[146] The establishment of the naïve newborn's microbiome in the immediate postpartum period also necessitates neutrophil suppression, even if the inability to mount a sufficient proinflammatory response may be detrimental to the neonate if exposed to pathogenic microorganisms.

Infectious disease is the second leading cause of neonatal mortality worldwide, preceded only by complications related to preterm birth.[147] Nature does not intend for the survival of most preterm infants outside the womb without the additional support of complex medical interventions and technologies. As with other organ systems, the immune system is significantly affected by preterm birth. Not only are adaptive immune responses generally absent, but components of innate immunity may also be lacking. For example, the vernix is absent prior to 28 weeks of gestation and the protective skin layer, known as the stratum covrneum, does not develop until the third trimester of pregnancy.[66,92,148] Postnatal neutrophil deficits are, therefore, exacerbated in the most immature neonates, resulting in a 10-fold greater risk for early infection compared to term infants and 30% mortality rate in those infected.[149,150] As neonatologists continue to strive to push the limits of viability to even younger gestational ages, understanding the complexities of neutrophil biology during fetal development and the neonatal period must be a high priority to improve survival and long-term neurodevelopmental outcomes associated with infectious diseases and neonatal sepsis.

REFERENCES

1. Maltepe E, Saugstad OD. Oxygen in health and disease: regulation of oxygen homeostasis—clinical implications. *Pediatr Res.* 2009;65(3):261-268. doi:10.1203/PDR.0b013e31818fc83f.
2. Tavian M, Péault B. Embryonic development of the human hematopoietic system. *Int J Dev Biol.* 2005;49(2-3):243-250. doi:10.1387/ijdb.041957mt.
3. Tober J, Koniski A, McGrath KE, et al. The megakaryocyte lineage originates from hemangioblast precursors and is an integral component both of primitive and of definitive hematopoiesis. *Blood.* 2007;109(4):1433-1441. doi:10.1182/blood-2006-06-031898.
4. Bertrand JY, Chi NC, Santoso B, et al. Haematopoietic stem cells derive directly from aortic endothelium during development. *Nature.* 2010;464(7285):108-111. doi:10.1038/nature08738.

5. Kissa K, Herbomel P. Blood stem cells emerge from aortic endothelium by a novel type of cell transition. *Nature.* 2010; 464(7285):112-115. doi:10.1038/nature08761.

6. Lawrence SM, Corriden R, Nizet V. Age-appropriate functions and dysfunctions of the neonatal neutrophil. *Front Pediatr.* 2017;5:23. doi:10.3389/fped.2017.00023.

7. Luis TC, Killmann NM, Staal FJ. Signal transduction pathways regulating hematopoietic stem cell biology: introduction to a series of Spotlight Reviews. *Leukemia.* 2012;26(1):86-90. doi:10.1038/leu.2011.260.

8. Baron MH, Isern J, Fraser ST. The embryonic origins of erythropoiesis in mammals. *Blood.* 2012;119(21):4828-4837. doi:10.1182/blood-2012-01-153486.

9. Palis J, Yoder MC. Yolk-sac hematopoiesis: the first blood cells of mouse and man. *Exp Hematol.* 2001;29(8):927-936. doi:10.1016/s0301-472x(01)00669-5.

10. Christensen RD, Rothstein G. Pre- and postnatal development of granulocytic stem cells in the rat. *Pediatr Res.* 1984;18(7):599-602. doi:10.1203/00006450-198407000-00006.

11. Slayton WB, Li Y, Calhoun DA, et al. The first-appearance of neutrophils in the human fetal bone marrow cavity. *Early Hum Dev.* 1998;53(2):129-144. doi:10.1016/s0378-3782(98)00049-8.

12. Zhang J, Niu C, Ye L, et al. Identification of the haematopoietic stem cell niche and control of the niche size. *Nature.* 2003;425(6960):836-841. doi:10.1038/nature02041.

13. Burdon PC, Martin C, Rankin SM. Migration across the sinusoidal endothelium regulates neutrophil mobilization in response to ELR + CXC chemokines. *Br J Haematol.* 2008;142(1):100-108. doi:10.1111/j.1365-2141.2008.07018.x.

14. Summers C, Rankin SM, Condliffe AM, et al. Neutrophil kinetics in health and disease. *Trends Immunol.* 2010;31(8):318-324. doi:10.1016/j.it.2010.05.006.

15. Jiao J, Dragomir AC, Kocabayoglu P, et al. Central role of conventional dendritic cells in regulation of bone marrow release and survival of neutrophils. *J Immunol.* 2014;192(7):3374-3382. doi:10.4049/jimmunol.1300237.

16. Xiao M, Zhang W, Liu W, et al. Osteocytes regulate neutrophil development through IL-19: a potent cytokine for neutropenia treatment. *Blood.* 2021;137(25):3533-3547. doi:10.1182/blood.2020007731.

17. Faurschou M, Borregaard N. Neutrophil granules and secretory vesicles in inflammation. *Microbes Infect.* 2003;5(14):1317-1327. doi:10.1016/j.micinf.2003.09.008.

18. Borregaard N, Sørensen OE, Theilgaard-Mönch K. Neutrophil granules: a library of innate immunity proteins. *Trends Immunol.* 2007;28(8):340-345. doi:10.1016/j.it.2007.06.002.

19. Pham CT. Neutrophil serine proteases: specific regulators of inflammation. *Nat Rev Immunol.* 2006;6(7):541-550. doi:10.1038/nri1841.

20. Sheshachalam A, Srivastava N, Mitchell T, et al. Granule protein processing and regulated secretion in neutrophils. *Front Immunol.* 2014;5:448. doi:10.3389/fimmu.2014.00448.

21. Kennedy AD, DeLeo FR. Neutrophil apoptosis and the resolution of infection. *Immunol Res.* 2009;43(1-3):25-61. doi:10.1007/s12026-008-8049-6.

22. Lawrence SM, Nizet V. Neutrophil granulopoiesis and homeostasis. In: Polin R, Abman S, Rowitch D, et al, eds. *Fetal and Neonatal Physiology.* 6th ed. Philadelphia: Elsevier; 2021.

23. Boll IT, Fuchs G. A kinetic model of granulocytopoiesis. *Exp Cell Res.* 1970;61(1):147-152. doi:10.1016/0014-4827(70)90268-5.

24. Tak T, Tesselaar K, Pillay J, et al. What's your age again? Determination of human neutrophil half-lives revisited. *J Leukoc Biol.* 2013;94(4):595-601. doi:10.1189/jlb.1112571.

25. Donohue DM, Reiff RH, Hanson ML, et al. Quantitative measurement of the erythrocytic and granulocytic cells of the marrow and blood. *J Clin Invest.* 1958;37(11):1571-1576. doi:10.1172/jci103750.

26. Strydom N, Rankin SM. Regulation of circulating neutrophil numbers under homeostasis and in disease. *J Innate Immun.* 2013;5(4):304-314. doi:10.1159/000350282.

27. Lahoz-Beneytez J, Elemans M, Zhang Y, et al. Human neutrophil kinetics: modeling of stable isotope labeling data supports short blood neutrophil half-lives. *Blood.* 2016;127(26):3431-3438. doi:10.1182/blood-2016-03-700336.

28. Erdman SH, Christensen RD, Bradley PP, et al. Supply and release of storage neutrophils. A developmental study. *Biol Neonate.* 1982;41(3-4):132-137. doi:10.1159/000241541.

29. Carr R, Huizinga TW. Low soluble FcRIII receptor demonstrates reduced neutrophil reserves in preterm neonates. *Arch Dis Child Fetal Neonatal Ed.* 2000;83(2):F160. doi:10.1136/fn.83.2.f160.

30. Edwards SW. *Biochemistry and Physiology of the Neutrophil.* 1st ed. New York: Cambridge University Press Publishing; 1994.

31. Balmer ML, Schürch CM, Saito Y, et al. Microbiota-derived compounds drive steady-state granulopoiesis via MyD88/TICAM signaling. *J Immunol.* 2014;193(10):5273-5283. doi:10.4049/jimmunol.1400762.

32. Bizzarro MJ, Dembry LM, Baltimore RS, et al. Changing patterns in neonatal *Escherichia coli* sepsis and ampicillin resistance in the era of intrapartum antibiotic prophylaxis. *Pediatrics.* 2008;121(4):689-696. doi:10.1542/peds.2007-2171.

33. Cotten CM, Taylor S, Stoll B, et al. Prolonged duration of initial empirical antibiotic treatment is associated with increased rates of necrotizing enterocolitis and death for extremely low birth weight infants. *Pediatrics.* 2009;123(1):58-66. doi:10.1542/peds.2007-3423.

34. Greenwood C, Morrow AL, Lagomarcino AJ, et al. Early empiric antibiotic use in preterm infants is associated with lower bacterial diversity and higher relative abundance of *Enterobacter. J Pediatr.* 2014;165(1):23-29. doi:10.1016/j.jpeds.2014.01.010.

35. Deshmukh HS, Liu Y, Menkiti OR, et al. The microbiota regulates neutrophil homeostasis and host resistance to *Escherichia coli* K1 sepsis in neonatal mice. *Nat Med.* 2014;20(5):524-530. doi:10.1038/nm.3542.

36. Bugl S, Wirths S, Radsak MP, et al. Steady-state neutrophil homeostasis is dependent on TLR4/TRIF signaling. *Blood.* 2013;121(5):723-733. doi:10.1182/blood-2012-05-429589.

37. Hirai H, Zhang P, Dayaram T, et al. C/EBPβ is required for 'emergency' granulopoiesis. *Nat Immunol.* 2006;7(7):732-739. doi:10.1038/ni1354.

38. Weinschenk NP, Farina A, Bianchi DW. Premature infants respond to early-onset and late-onset sepsis with leukocyte activation. *J Pediatr.* 2000;137(3):345-350. doi:10.1067/mpd.2000.107846.

39. Christensen RD, Rothstein G. Exhaustion of mature marrow neutrophils in neonates with sepsis. *J Pediatr.* 1980;96(2):316-318. doi:10.1016/s0022-3476(80)80837-7.

40. Carr R. Neutrophil production and function in newborn infants. *Br J Haematol.* 2000;110(1):18-28. doi:10.1046/j.1365-2141.2000.01992.x.

41. Christensen RD, Harper TE, Rothstein G. Granulocyte-macrophage progenitor cells in term and preterm neonates. *J Pediatr.* 1986;109(6):1047-1051. doi:10.1016/s0022-3476(86)80297-9.

42. Christensen RD, Yoder BA, Baer VL, et al. Early-onset neutropenia in small-for-gestational-age infants. *Pediatrics.* 2015;136(5): e1259-e1267. doi:10.1542/peds.2015-1638.

43. Koenig JM, Christensen RD. Incidence, neutrophil kinetics, and natural history of neonatal neutropenia associated with

maternal hypertension. *N Engl J Med.* 1989;321(9):557-562. doi:10.1056/nejm198908313210901.

44. Wirbelauer J, Thomas W, Rieger L, et al. Intrauterine growth retardation in preterm infants ≤32 weeks of gestation is associated with low white blood cell counts. *Am J Perinatol.* 2010;27(10):819-824. doi:10.1055/s-0030-1254547.

45. Christensen RD, Koenig JM, Viskochil DH, et al. Down-modulation of neutrophil production by erythropoietin in human hematopoietic clones. *Blood.* 1989;74(2):817-822.

46. Christensen RD, Henry E, Wiedmeier SE, et al. Low blood neutrophil concentrations among extremely low birth weight neonates: data from a multihospital health-care system. *J Perinatol.* 2006;26(11):682-687. doi:10.1038/sj.jp.7211603.

47. Teng RJ, Wu TJ, Garrison RD, et al. Early neutropenia is not associated with an increased rate of nosocomial infection in very low-birth-weight infants. *J Perinatol.* 2009;29(3):219-224. doi:10.1038/jp.2008.202.

48. Aktaş D, Demirel B, Gürsoy T, et al. A randomized case-controlled study of recombinant human granulocyte colony stimulating factor for the treatment of sepsis in preterm neutropenic infants. *Pediatr Neonatol.* 2015;56(3):171-175. doi:10.1016/j.pedneo.2014.06.007.

49. Carr R, Modi N, Doré C. G-CSF and GM-CSF for treating or preventing neonatal infections. *Cochrane Database Syst Rev.* 2003;3:CD003066. doi:10.1002/14651858.Cd003066.

50. Carr R, Brocklehurst P, Doré CJ, et al. Granulocyte-macrophage colony stimulating factor administered as prophylaxis for reduction of sepsis in extremely preterm, small for gestational age neonates (the PROGRAMS trial): a single-blind, multicentre, randomised controlled trial. *Lancet.* 2009;373(9659):226-233. doi:10.1016/s0140-6736(09)60071-4.

51. Chaudhuri J, Mitra S, Mukhopadhyay D, et al. Granulocyte colony-stimulating factor for preterms with sepsis and neutropenia: a randomized controlled trial. *J Clin Neonatol.* 2012;1(4):202-206. doi:10.4103/2249-4847.105993.

52. Dale DC, Link DC. The many causes of severe congenital neutropenia. *N Engl J Med.* 2009;360(1):3-5. doi:10.1056/NEJMp0806821.

53. Klimenkova O, Ellerbeck W, Klimiankou M, et al. A lack of secretory leukocyte protease inhibitor (SLPI) causes defects in granulocytic differentiation. *Blood.* 2014;123(8):1239-1249. doi:10.1182/blood-2013-06-508887.

54. Grenda DS, Murakami M, Ghatak J, et al. Mutations of the ELA2 gene found in patients with severe congenital neutropenia induce the unfolded protein response and cellular apoptosis. *Blood.* 2007;110(13):4179-4187. doi:10.1182/blood-2006-11-057299.

55. Hoogendijk AJ, Pourfarzad F, Aarts CEM, et al. Dynamic transcriptome-proteome correlation networks reveal human myeloid differentiation and neutrophil-specific programming. *Cell Rep.* 2019;29(8):2505-2519.e4. doi:10.1016/j.celrep.2019.10.082.

56. Saverymuttu SH, Peters AM, Keshavarzian A, et al. The kinetics of 111indium distribution following injection of 111indium labelled autologous granulocytes in man. *Br J Haematol.* 1985;61(4):675-685. doi:10.1111/j.1365-2141.1985.tb02882.x.

57. Mauer AM, Athens JW, Ashenbrucker H, et al. Leukokinetic studies. II. A method for labeling granulocytes *in vitro* with radioactive diisopropylfluorophosphate (DFP). *J Clin Invest.* 1960;39(9):1481-1486. doi:10.1172/jci104167.

58. Athens JW, Haab OP, Raab SO, et al. Leukokinetic studies. IV. The total blood, circulating and marginal granulocyte pools and the granulocyte turnover rate in normal subjects. *J Clin Invest.* 1961;40(6):989-995. doi:10.1172/jci104338.

59. Chevre R, Soehnlein O. Neutrophil life in three acts: a production by different stage directors. *Nat Immunol.* 2021;22(9):1072-1074. doi:10.1038/s41590-021-00997-z.

60. Schmutz N, Henry E, Jopling J, et al. Expected ranges for blood neutrophil concentrations of neonates: the Manroe and Mouzinho charts revisited. *J Perinatol.* 2008;28(4):275-281. doi:10.1038/sj.jp.7211916.

61. Lawrence SM, Eckert J, Makoni M, et al. Is the use of complete blood counts with manual differentials an antiquated method of determining neutrophil composition in newborns? *Ann Clin Lab Sci.* 2015;45(4):403-413.

62. Makoni M, Eckert J, Anne Pereira H, et al. Alterations in neonatal neutrophil function attributable to increased immature forms. *Early Hum Dev.* 2016;103:1-7. doi:10.1016/j.earlhumdev.2016.05.016.

63. Kobayashi SD, Voyich JM, Whitney AR, et al. Spontaneous neutrophil apoptosis and regulation of cell survival by granulocyte macrophage-colony stimulating factor. *J Leukoc Biol.* 2005;78(6):1408-1418. doi:10.1189/jlb.0605289.

64. Contrino J, Krause PJ, Slover N, et al. Elevated interleukin-1 expression in human neonatal neutrophils. *Pediatr Res.* 1993;34(3):249-252. doi:10.1203/00006450-199309000-00002.

65. Angelone DF, Wessels MR, Coughlin M, et al. Innate immunity of the human newborn is polarized toward a high ratio of IL-6/TNF-alpha production *in vitro* and *in vivo. Pediatr Res.* 2006;60(2):205-209. doi:10.1203/01.pdr.0000228319.10481.ea.

66. Wynn JL, Levy O. Role of innate host defenses in susceptibility to early-onset neonatal sepsis. *Clin Perinatol.* 2010;37(2):307-337. doi:10.1016/j.clp.2010.04.001.

67. Philbin VJ, Levy O. Developmental biology of the innate immune response: implications for neonatal and infant vaccine development. *Pediatr Res.* 2009;65(5 Pt 2):98r-105r. doi:10.1203/PDR.0b013e31819f195d.

68. Mohammadi N, Midiri A, Mancuso G, et al. Neutrophils directly recognize group B Streptococci and contribute to interleukin-1β production during infection. *PLoS ONE.* 2016;11(8):e0160249. doi:10.1371/journal.pone.0160249.

69. Ali SR, Fong JJ, Carlin AF, et al. Siglec-5 and Siglec-14 are polymorphic paired receptors that modulate neutrophil and amnion signaling responses to group B Streptococcus. *J Exp Med.* 2014;211(6):1231-1242. doi:10.1084/jem.20131853.

70. Carlin AF, Uchiyama S, Chang YC, et al. Molecular mimicry of host sialylated glycans allows a bacterial pathogen to engage neutrophil Siglec-9 and dampen the innate immune response. *Blood.* 2009;113(14):3333-3336. doi:10.1182/blood-2008-11-187302.

71. Andrade EB, Alves J, Madureira P, et al. TLR2-induced IL-10 production impairs neutrophil recruitment to infected tissues during neonatal bacterial sepsis. *J Immunol.* 2013;191(9):4759-4768. doi:10.4049/jimmunol.1301752.

72. Fong ON, Chan KY, Leung KT, et al. Expression profile of cord blood neutrophils and dysregulation of HSPA1A and OLR1 upon challenge by bacterial peptidoglycan. *J Leukoc Biol.* 2014;95(1):169-178. doi:10.1189/jlb.0413219.

73. McEvoy LT, Zakem-Cloud H, Tosi MF. Total cell content of CR3 (CD11b/CD18) and LFA-1 (CD11a/CD18) in neonatal neutrophils: relationship to gestational age. *Blood.* 1996;87(9):3929-3933.

74. Allgaier B, Shi M, Luo D, et al. Spontaneous and Fas-mediated apoptosis are diminished in umbilical cord blood neutrophils

compared with adult neutrophils. *J Leukoc Biol.* 1998;64(3): 331-336. doi:10.1002/jlb.64.3.331.

75. Rashmi R, Bode BP, Panesar N, et al. Siglec-9 and SHP-1 are differentially expressed in neonatal and adult neutrophils. *Pediatr Res.* 2009;66(3):266-271. doi:10.1203/PDR.0b013e3181b1bc19.

76. Kotecha S, Mildner RJ, Prince LR, et al. The role of neutrophil apoptosis in the resolution of acute lung injury in newborn infants. *Thorax.* 2003;58(11):961-967. doi:10.1136/thorax.58.11.961.

77. Grigg JM, Savill JS, Sarraf C, et al. Neutrophil apoptosis and clearance from neonatal lungs. *Lancet.* 1991;338(8769):720-722. doi:10.1016/0140-6736(91)91443-x.

78. Bektas S, Goetze B, Speer CP. Decreased adherence, chemotaxis and phagocytic activities of neutrophils from preterm neonates. *Acta Paediatr Scand.* 1990;79(11):1031-1038. doi:10.1111/j.1651-2227.1990.tb11379.x.

79. Nupponen I, Turunen R, Nevalainen T, et al. Extracellular release of bactericidal/permeability-increasing protein in newborn infants. *Pediatr Res.* 2002;51(6):670-674. doi:10.1203/00006450-200206000-00002.

80. Levy O, Martin S, Eichenwald E, et al. Impaired innate immunity in the newborn: newborn neutrophils are deficient in bactericidal/permeability-increasing protein. *Pediatrics.* 1999;104(6):1327-1333. doi:10.1542/peds.104.6.1327.

81. Lu RJ, Taylor S, Contrepois K, et al. Multi-omic profiling of primary mouse neutrophils predicts a pattern of sex and age-related functional regulation. *Nat Aging.* 2021;1(8):715-733. doi:10.1038/s43587-021-00086-8.

82. Iovine NM, Elsbach P, Weiss J. An opsonic function of the neutrophil bactericidal/permeability-increasing protein depends on both its N- and C-terminal domains. *Proc Natl Acad Sci U S A.* 1997;94(20):10973-10978. doi:10.1073/pnas.94.20.10973.

83. Elsbach P. The bactericidal/permeability-increasing protein (BPI) in antibacterial host defense. *J Leukoc Biol.* 1998;64(1):14-18. doi:10.1002/jlb.64.1.14.

84. Froon AH, Dentener MA, Greve JW, et al. Lipopolysaccharide toxicity-regulating proteins in bacteremia. *J Infect Dis.* 1995;171(5):1250-1257. doi:10.1093/infdis/171.5.1250.

85. Froon AH, Bonten MJ, Gaillard CA, et al. Prediction of clinical severity and outcome of ventilator-associated pneumonia. Comparison of simplified acute physiology score with systemic inflammatory mediators. *Am J Respir Crit Care Med.* 1998;158(4):1026-1031. doi:10.1164/ajrccm.158.4.9801013.

86. Wong HR, Doughty LA, Wedel N, et al. Plasma bactericidal/permeability-increasing protein concentrations in critically ill children with the sepsis syndrome. *Pediatr Infect Dis J.* 1995;14(12):1087-1091. doi:10.1097/00006454-199512000-00011.

87. Ambruso DR, Bentwood B, Henson PM, et al. Oxidative metabolism of cord blood neutrophils: relationship to content and degranulation of cytoplasmic granules. *Pediatr Res.* 1984;18(11):1148-1153. doi:10.1203/00006450-198411000-00019.

88. Valenti P, Antonini G. Lactoferrin: an important host defence against microbial and viral attack. *Cell Mol Life Sci.* 2005;62(22):2576-2587. doi:10.1007/s00018-005-5372-0.

89. Liu W, Yan M, Sugui JA, et al. Olfm4 deletion enhances defense against *Staphylococcus aureus* in chronic granulomatous disease. *J Clin Invest.* 2013;123(9):3751-3755. doi:10.1172/jci68453.

90. Wynn JL, Guthrie SO, Wong HR, et al. Postnatal age is a critical determinant of the neonatal host response to sepsis. *Mol Med.* 2015;21(1):496-504. doi:10.2119/molmed.2015.00064.

91. Corriden R, Chen Y, Inoue Y, et al. Ecto-nucleoside triphosphate diphosphohydrolase 1 (E-NTPDase1/CD39) regulates neutrophil chemotaxis by hydrolyzing released ATP to adenosine. *J Biol Chem.* 2008;283(42):28480-28486. doi:10.1074/jbc.M800039200.

92. Nussbaum C, Sperandio M. Innate immune cell recruitment in the fetus and neonate. *J Reprod Immunol.* 2011;90(1):74-81. doi:10.1016/j.jri.2011.01.022.

93. Krause PJ, Herson VC, Boutin-Lebowitz J, et al. Polymorphonuclear leukocyte adherence and chemotaxis in stressed and healthy neonates. *Pediatr Res.* 1986;20(4):296-300. doi:10.1203/00006450-198604000-00004.

94. Fox SE, Lu W, Maheshwari A, et al. The effects and comparative differences of neutrophil specific chemokines on neutrophil chemotaxis of the neonate. *Cytokine.* 2005;29(3):135-140. doi:10.1016/j.cyto.2004.10.007.

95. Sacchi F, Rondini G, Mingrat G, et al. Different maturation of neutrophil chemotaxis in term and preterm newborn infants. *J Pediatr.* 1982;101(2):273-274. doi:10.1016/s0022-3476(82)80139-x.

96. Carr R, Pumford D, Davies JM. Neutrophil chemotaxis and adhesion in preterm babies. *Arch Dis Child.* 1992;67(7 Spec No):813-817. doi:10.1136/adc.67.7_spec_no.813.

97. Weinberger B, Laskin DL, Mariano TM, et al. Mechanisms underlying reduced responsiveness of neonatal neutrophils to distinct chemoattractants. *J Leukoc Biol.* 2001;70(6):969-976.

98. Hilmo A, Howard TH. F-actin content of neonate and adult neutrophils. *Blood.* 1987;69(3):945-949.

99. Boner A, Zeligs BJ, Bellanti JA. Chemotactic responses of various differentiational stages of neutrophils from human cord and adult blood. *Infect Immun.* 1982;35(3):921-928. doi:10.1128/iai.35.3.921-928.1982.

100. Laurenti F, Ferro R, Marzetti G, et al. Neutrophil chemotaxis in preterm infants with infections. *J Pediatr.* 1980;96(3 Pt 1):468-470. doi:10.1016/s0022-3476(80)80700-1.

101. Mehta R, Petrova A. Intrapartum magnesium sulfate exposure attenuates neutrophil function in preterm neonates. *Biol Neonate.* 2006;89(2):99-103. doi:10.1159/000088560.

102. Kansas GS. Selectins and their ligands: current concepts and controversies. *Blood.* 1996;88(9):3259-3287.

103. Nussbaum C, Gloning A, Pruenster M, et al. Neutrophil and endothelial adhesive function during human fetal ontogeny. *J Leukoc Biol.* 2013;93(2):175-184. doi:10.1189/jlb.0912468.

104. Anderson DC, Abbassi O, Kishimoto TK, et al. Diminished lectin-, epidermal growth factor-, complement binding domain-cell adhesion molecule-1 on neonatal neutrophils underlies their impaired CD18-independent adhesion to endothelial cells *in vitro. J Immunol.* 1991;146(10):3372-3379.

105. Rebuck N, Gibson A, Finn A. Neutrophil adhesion molecules in term and premature infants: normal or enhanced leucocyte integrins but defective L-selectin expression and shedding. *Clin Exp Immunol.* 1995;101(1):183-189. doi:10.1111/j.1365-2249.1995.tb02296.x.

106. Borregaard N, Cowland JB. Granules of the human neutrophilic polymorphonuclear leukocyte. *Blood.* 1997;89(10):3503-3521.

107. Fuenfer MM, Herson VC, Raye JR, et al. The effect of betamethasone on neonatal neutrophil chemotaxis. *Pediatr Res.* 1987;22(2):150-153. doi:10.1203/00006450-198708000-00009.

108. Lorant DE, Li W, Tabatabaei N, et al. P-selectin expression by endothelial cells is decreased in neonatal rats and human premature infants. *Blood.* 1999;94(2):600-609.

109. Peyssonnaux C, Datta V, Cramer T, et al. HIF-1alpha expression regulates the bactericidal capacity of phagocytes. *J Clin Invest.* 2005;115(7):1806-1815. doi:10.1172/jci23865.

110. Nordenfelt P, Tapper H. Phagosome dynamics during phagocytosis by neutrophils. *J Leukoc Biol.* 2011;90(2):271-284. doi:10.1189/jlb.0810457.

111. Anderson DC, Freeman KL, Heerdt B, et al. Abnormal stimulated adherence of neonatal granulocytes: impaired induction of surface Mac-1 by chemotactic factors or secretagogues. *Blood.* 1987;70(3):740-750.

112. Carr R, Davies JM. Abnormal FcRIII expression by neutrophils from very preterm neonates. *Blood.* 1990;76(3):607-611.

113. Falconer AE, Carr R, Edwards SW. Impaired neutrophil phagocytosis in preterm neonates: lack of correlation with expression of immunoglobulin or complement receptors. *Biol Neonate.* 1995;68(4):264-269. doi:10.1159/000244245.

114. Källman J, Schollin J, Schalèn C, et al. Impaired phagocytosis and opsonisation towards group B streptococci in preterm neonates. *Arch Dis Child Fetal Neonatal Ed.* 1998;78(1):F46-F50. doi:10.1136/fn.78.1.f46.

115. INIS Collaborative Group, Brocklehurst P, Farrell B, et al. Treatment of neonatal sepsis with intravenous immune globulin. *N Engl J Med.* 2011;365(13):1201-1211. doi:10.1056/NEJMoa1100441.

116. Ohlsson A, Lacy JB. Intravenous immunoglobulin for suspected or proven infection in neonates. *Cochrane Database Syst Rev.* 2015;3:CD001239. doi:10.1002/14651858.CD001239.pub5.

117. Xanthou M, Valassi-Adam E, Kintsonidou E, et al. Phagocytosis and killing ability of *Candida albicans* by blood leucocytes of healthy term and preterm babies. *Arch Dis Child.* 1975;50(1):72-75. doi:10.1136/adc.50.1.72.

118. Destin KG, Linden JR, Laforce-Nesbitt SS, et al. Oxidative burst and phagocytosis of neonatal neutrophils confronting *Candida albicans* and *Candida parapsilosis.* *Early Hum Dev.* 2009;85(8):531-535. doi:10.1016/j.earlhumdev.2009.05.011.

119. Linden JR, De Paepe ME, Laforce-Nesbitt SS, et al. Galectin-3 plays an important role in protection against disseminated candidiasis. *Med Mycol.* 2013;51(6):641-651. doi:10.3109/13693786.2013.770607.

120. Linden JR, Kunkel D, Laforce-Nesbitt SS, et al. The role of galectin-3 in phagocytosis of *Candida albicans* and *Candida parapsilosis* by human neutrophils. *Cell Microbiol.* 2013;15(7):1127-1142. doi:10.1111/cmi.12103.

121. Sundqvist M, Osla V, Jacobsson B, et al. Cord blood neutrophils display a galectin-3 responsive phenotype accentuated by vaginal delivery. *BMC Pediatr.* 2013;13:128. doi:10.1186/1471-2431-13-128.

122. Fermino ML, Polli CD, Toledo KA, et al. LPS-induced galectin-3 oligomerization results in enhancement of neutrophil activation. *PLoS One.* 2011;6(10):e26004. doi:10.1371/journal.pone.0026004.

123. Allen RC. Neutrophil leukocyte: combustive microbicidal action and chemiluminescence. *J Immunol Res.* 2015;2015:794072. doi:10.1155/2015/794072.

124. Klebanoff SJ, Clark RA. *The Neutrophil: Function and Clinical Disorders.* New York City: North-Holland; 1978.

125. Allen RC. Reduced, radical, and excited state oxygen in leukocyte microbicidal activity. *Front Biol.* 1979;48:197-233.

126. Segal AW. The molecular and cellular pathology of chronic granulomatous disease. *Eur J Clin Invest.* 1988;18(5):433-443. doi:10.1111/j.1365-2362.1988.tb01037.x.

127. Clark RA. Activation of the neutrophil respiratory burst oxidase. *J Infect Dis.* 1999;179(2):S309-S317. doi:10.1086/513849.

128. Allen RC. Halide dependence of the myeloperoxidase-mediated antimicrobial system of the polymorphonuclear leukocyte in the phenomenon of electronic excitation. *Biochem Biophys Res Commun.* 1975;63(3):675-683. doi:10.1016/s0006-291x(75)80437-2.

129. Urlichs F, Speer CP. Neutrophil function in preterm and term infants. *NeoReviews.* 2004;5:e417-e429.

130. Allen RC, Stjernholm RL, Steele RH. Evidence for the generation of an electronic excitation state(s) in human polymorphonuclear leukocytes and its participation in bactericidal activity. *Biochem Biophys Res Commun.* 1972;47(4):679-684. doi:10.1016/0006-291x(72)90545-1.

131. Segal AW. Nitroblue-tetrazolium tests. *Lancet.* 1974;2(7891):1248-1252. doi:10.1016/s0140-6736(74)90758-2.

132. Newburger PE. Superoxide generation by human fetal granulocytes. *Pediatr Res.* 1982;16(5):373-376. doi:10.1203/00006450-198205000-00011.

133. Drossou V, Kanakoudi F, Tzimouli V, et al. Impact of prematurity, stress and sepsis on the neutrophil respiratory burst activity of neonates. *Biol Neonate.* 1997;72(4):201-209. doi:10.1159/000244481.

134. Strunk T, Temming P, Gembruch U, et al. Differential maturation of the innate immune response in human fetuses. *Pediatr Res.* 2004;56(2):219-226. doi:10.1203/01.Pdr.0000132664.66975.79.

135. Brinkmann V, Reichard U, Goosmann C, et al. Neutrophil extracellular traps kill bacteria. *Science.* 2004;303(5663):1532-1535. doi:10.1126/science.1092385.

136. Sørensen OE, Borregaard N. Neutrophil extracellular traps—the dark side of neutrophils. *J Clin Invest.* 2016;126(5):1612-1620. doi:10.1172/jci84538.

137. Remijsen Q, Kuijpers TW, Wirawan E, et al. Dying for a cause: NETosis, mechanisms behind an antimicrobial cell death modality. *Cell Death Differ.* 2011;18(4):581-588. doi:10.1038/cdd.2011.1.

138. Parker H, Dragunow M, Hampton MB, et al. Requirements for NADPH oxidase and myeloperoxidase in neutrophil extracellular trap formation differ depending on the stimulus. *J Leukoc Biol.* 2012;92(4):841-849. doi:10.1189/jlb.1211601.

139. Kirchner T, Möller S, Klinger M, et al. The impact of various reactive oxygen species on the formation of neutrophil extracellular traps. *Mediators Inflamm.* 2012;2012:849136. doi:10.1155/2012/849136.

140. Desai J, Mulay SR, Nakazawa D, et al. Matters of life and death. How neutrophils die or survive along NET release and is "NETosis" = necroptosis? *Cell Mol Life Sci.* 2016;73(11-12):2211-2219. doi:10.1007/s00018-016-2195-0.

141. Fuchs TA, Abed U, Goosmann C, et al. Novel cell death program leads to neutrophil extracellular traps. *J Cell Biol.* 2007;176(2):231-241. doi:10.1083/jcb.200606027.

142. Wang H, Wang C, Zhao MH, et al. Neutrophil extracellular traps can activate alternative complement pathways. *Clin Exp Immunol.* 2015;181(3):518-527. doi:10.1111/cei.12654.

143. Yost CC, Cody MJ, Harris ES, et al. Impaired neutrophil extracellular trap (NET) formation: a novel innate immune deficiency of human neonates. *Blood.* 2009;113(25):6419-6427. doi:10.1182/blood-2008-07-171629.

144. Yost CC, Schwertz H, Cody MJ, et al. Neonatal NET-inhibitory factor and related peptides inhibit neutrophil extracellular trap formation. *J Clin Invest.* 2016;126(10):3783-3798. doi:10.1172/jci83873.

145. Byrd AS, O'Brien XM, Laforce-Nesbitt SS, et al. NETosis in neonates: evidence of a reactive oxygen species-independent pathway in response to fungal challenge. *J Infect Dis.* 2016;213(4):634-639. doi:10.1093/infdis/jiv435.

146. Bhandari T, Nizet V. Hypoxia-inducible factor (HIF) as a pharmacological target for prevention and treatment of infectious diseases. *Infect Dis Ther.* 2014;3(2):159-174. doi:10.1007/s40121-014-0030-1.

147. Mukhopadhyay S, Puopolo KM. Risk assessment in neonatal early onset sepsis. *Semin Perinatol.* 2012;36(6):408-415. doi:10.1053/j.semperi.2012.06.002.

148. Visscher MO, Adam R, Brink S, et al. Newborn infant skin: physiology, development, and care. *Clin Dermatol.* 2015;33(3): 271-280. doi:10.1016/j.clindermatol.2014.12.003.

149. Stoll BJ, Hansen N. Infections in VLBW infants: studies from the NICHD Neonatal Research Network. *Semin Perinatol.* 2003;27(4):293-301. doi:10.1016/s0146-0005(03)00046-6.

150. Stoll BJ, Hansen NI, Higgins RD, et al. Very low birth weight preterm infants with early onset neonatal sepsis: the predominance of gram-negative infections continues in the National Institute of Child Health and Human Development Neonatal Research Network, 2002-2003. *Pediatr Infect Dis J.* 2005;24(7): 635-639. doi:10.1097/01.inf.0000168749.82105.64.

151. Wright Jr WC, Ank BJ, Herbert J, et al. Decreased bactericidal activity of leukocytes of stressed newborn infants. *Pediatrics.* 1975;56(4):579-584.

152. Ambruso DR, Stork LC, Gibson BE, et al. Increased activity of the respiratory burst in cord blood neutrophils: kinetics of the NADPH oxidase enzyme system in subcellular fractions. *Pediatr Res.* 1987;21(2):205-210. doi:10.1203/00006450-19870 2000-00019.

153. Smith JB, Campbell DE, Ludomirsky A, et al. Expression of the complement receptors CR1 and CR3 and the type III Fc gamma receptor on neutrophils from newborn infants and from fetuses with Rh disease. *Pediatr Res.* 1990;28(2):120-126. doi:10.1203/00006450-199008000-00009.

154. Abughali N, Berger M, Tosi MF. Deficient total cell content of CR3 (CD11b) in neonatal neutrophils. *Blood.* 1994;83(4):1086-1092.

Chapter 5

New Erythrocyte Diagnostic Parameters in Neonatal Medicine

Robert D. Christensen, MD, Timothy M. Bahr, MS, MD, and Allison J. Judkins, MD

Chapter Outline

Introduction

In 1929 Wintrobe published a method for measuring the percent of blood comprised of red cells—the hematocrit.[1] Soon thereafter he reported a method for measuring the volume of the average circulating red blood cell (RBC), in femtoliters (fL, 10^{-15} L), as a way to judge whether a patient's RBCs are normal size or smaller or larger than normal.[2] In that publication Wintrobe also reported a way to determine the average hemoglobin content of a RBC, in picograms (pg, 10^{-12} g), as a way to judge whether the amount of hemoglobin within the RBCs is normal. Lastly, he described the concentration of hemoglobin in RBCs (g/dL blood) as the mean corpuscular hemoglobin (MCH) concentration.[2] These basic measurements formulated the basis of his classification of anemias as microcytic, normocytic, or macrocytic and for judging whether erythrocytes were hypochromic.[3] Although the methods for performing these measurements have markedly improved through advancing technology, Wintrobe's classification has remained for the past 90 years the standard approach to anemia evaluation.[4]

Some of the recent additions to the automated complete blood cell count (CBC) reveal yet more useful information about a patient's erythrocytes. These additions include the four parameters discussed in this chapter: specifically the reticulocyte hemoglobin count (RET-He), fragmented red blood cell count (FRC), percentage of microcytic erythrocytes (Micro-R), and percentage of hypochromic erythrocytes (HYPO-He). In most parts of the world these four additional RBC parameters are readily available to clinicians as part of each automated CBC. In the United States the RET-He is similarly available to all who order the test as part of a CBC with no added phlebotomy volume from the patient or laboratory run time. However, in the United States the FRC, Micro-R, and HYPO-He are currently designated as research parameters. They can be obtained on virtually every CBC, but the values are only released from the clinical laboratory under certain regulatory conditions. One reason for this has been the lack of reference ranges for these tests, particularly in neonatal subjects, by which to judge whether the values are low, normal, or elevated.

Our group has sought to remedy this by creating rigorous reference intervals for each of these four new erythrocyte parameters. We have done this with three goals in mind: (1) We hope that the neonatologists in

Europe and Asia who currently have all four of these tests available with each CBC run will take advantage of the reference intervals shown in this chapter and thereby will learn more about each patient's erythrocytes with these tests. (2) We hope that the neonatologists in the Americas will use the RET-He routinely when considering iron sufficiency in their patients and will work with their clinical pathology laboratories to, under proper regulatory guidance, further assess the value of the three other new tests in clinical practice. (3) We hope that this body of work will facilitate the process of eventually having all of these new erythrocyte parameters released by the clinical laboratory to the clinicians as an integral part of every CBC run on a neonate, along with the hemoglobin, hematocrit, RBC indices, and red cell distribution width (RDW), and that so doing will help neonatologists recognize various erythrocyte abnormalities in their patients.

Flow-Cytometric Evaluation as an Integral Part of a Modern CBC

Adding the technology of flow cytometry to automated CBC analysis created the possibility of several new diagnostic parameters. The technology involves the blood sample being diluted and moving through a tube thin enough that the cells pass by one at a time. Characteristics about the cell are measured using lasers and electrical impedance. To focus on specific aspects of the blood, for instance on leukocytes or reticulocytes or nucleated RBCs, the sample is separated into a number of different channels depending somewhat on the model of counter. Such analyzers typically use EDTA (lavender-top) tubes or microtainer tubes. Evolving technology is making it possible for an automated CBC, with expanded parameter reporting, to be done on a blood sample as small as 15 µL (0.015 mL).

Reticulocyte Hemoglobin Content

Advances in flow-cytometric testing of erythrocytes revealed a way to quantify the amount of hemoglobin within reticulocytes. This is important because when iron bioavailability is diminished during early iron deficiency states erythrocyte production begins to make subtle changes, producing RBC of smaller size and with less hemoglobin. Because the typical reticulocyte circulates for only about 1 day, measuring the amount of hemoglobin per reticulocyte could give an account of iron availability for hemoglobin production within the recent few days. Thus at the onset of iron-limited erythropoiesis the RET-He value drops before the mean corpuscular volume (MCV) or MCH fall and before other markers such as zinc protoporphyrin to heme ratio fall. The latter measurement is made on mature RBCs, most of which have been in the circulation, at the time of phlebotomy, for several months. Consequently, early iron deficiency does not increase the zinc protoporphyrin to heme ratio until many weeks of iron deficient erythropoiesis has occurred.[5]

Fig. 5.1 illustrates how the RET-He value is measured. The initial reports of RET-He did not include children or neonates,[5] but studies published over 17 years ago by Ullrich and Brugnara[6] and by Brugnara et al.[7] indicated that the RET-He was an excellent indicator of the iron status of children. They showed that RET-He values obtained from the Sysmex and the Bayer ADVIA analyzers had very good agreement, and that both could identify iron deficiency in children who were on chronic dialysis, with a sensitivity over 93% and a specificity over 83%. Subsequent studies from Spain by Mateos et al. reported that the RET-He was the most accurate marker of iron deficiency in children. From a battery of tests studied, they suggested that the RET-He should be used as a screening tool for the identification of iron deficiency without or with anemia.[8]

Ervasti et al. from Finland were the first to report RET-He values in cord blood of term infants (mean, 35.6 pg, reference range 33.0–38.1 pg).[9] Subsequently Lorenz et al. from Tubingen, Germany, provided the first information of RET-He levels from preterm neonates. They observed that the iron status parameters typically used in adult patients were not suitable to define the iron status of preterm infants. They suggested that RET-He was a superior metric to ferritin, transferrin saturation, and MCV as a marker of iron deficiency in preterm and very low birth weight neonates.[10,11]

Subsequently much has been learned about the importance of RET-He as an early marker of iron deficient erythropoiesis in neonates.[12-22] In 2016 we published

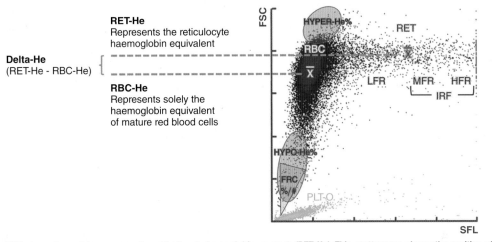

Fig. 5.1 The RET channel, used to measure the reticulocyte hemoglobin content *(RET-He)*. This scattergram shows the position of each cell passing through the detector, according to its size (Y-axis FSC; cell volume) and its RNA content (X-axis SFL; side flow). Gates are set in this channel to quantify the red blood cells *(RBC)*, reticulocytes *(RET)* and platelets *(PLT)* per microliter of blood in the sample. The hemoglobin within the RBC gate is measured as the RBC-He, and the hemoglobin within the reticulocyte gate is measured as the RET-He (the DELTA-He is the difference between the two measurements). (From Sysmex.)

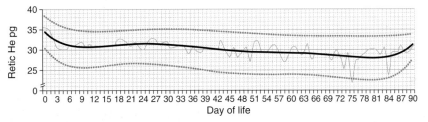

Fig. 5.2 Neonatal reference intervals for RET-He, measured in picograms (pg). The *lower and upper dashed lines* represent the 5th percentile lower reference interval and the 95th percentile upper reference interval over the first 90 days following birth. The *solid line* represents the mean value. (From Christensen RD, Henry E, Bennett ST, et al. Reference intervals for reticulocyte parameters of infants during their first 90 days after birth. *J Perinatol.* 2016;36:61-66.)

the reference interval for RET-He (Fig. 5.2).[23] In 2019 German et al. from Seattle reported a retrospective cohort of neonates cared for at the University of Washington neonatal intensive care unit (NICU) who received a RET-He as part of routine care within the first 120 days after birth. From 249 infants, the measurements at birth were lower in the lowest gestational age neonates, then initially decreased, then slowly increased. They concluded that the slow uptrend with enteral iron supplementation suggested that neonates may be unable to improve their iron sufficiency status adequately or rapidly despite typical iron supplementation.[16]

Serum ferritin is a standard metric for assessing iron sufficiency. We recently reported 190 paired measurements of serum ferritin and RET-He in neonates. We found that 92% of the pairs were concordant; that is, if the tests were abnormal, the two values moved in the same direction. However among the 8% where the two tests were discordant, the discrepancy was almost always a high ferritin and low RET-He in a neonate with evidence of an inflammatory process. In those 8%, other markers of iron deficient erythropoiesis (low MCV, high Micro-R%, low MCH, and high HYPO-He %) indicated that the low RET-He measurement was likely the correct metric, and the high ferritin was the result of inflammation because it is an acute phase reactant, while the RET-He is not.[20-22] Thus advantages of the RET-He include that it takes no more phlebotomy volume than the CBC, which is typically done as part of an evaluation for iron deficiency, that its costs and turnaround time are substantially less than those of a serum ferritin, and its value is not elevated by inflammation.

Fragmented RBC Count

The value of NICU care can be enhanced by discovering new laboratory tests that improve clinical decision making at lower cost, while requiring less phlebotomy blood loss. It is possible that the automated FRC parameter can provide this type of value. Fig. 5.3 shows examples of a major component of the automated FRC enumeration, schistocytes. These RBC fragments are created by microangiopathic damage to circulating erythrocytes. Fig. 5.3A points out a schistocyte on a photomicrograph, and Fig. 5.3B is an electron micrographic example of RBCs in the process of becoming schistocytes by being tethered and torn on fibrin strands in the microvasculature.

Jiang et al. from Japan demonstrated in 2001 that the FRC parameter was useful for diagnosing and following microangiopathic conditions like disseminated intravascular coagulation (DIC), hemolytic uremic syndrome, and transplant associated microangiopathy.[24] With the automated quantification system from Sysmex, they demonstrated that the FRC count correlated very well with manual schistocyte counts. The automated method for quantifying FRC is shown in Fig. 5.4. This parameter can be expressed by the clinical hematology laboratory in two ways: either the fragmented cells as a percentage of total RBC (FRC%) or as an absolute number (FRC/µL blood).

Subsequent to the Jaing report, Banno et al., also from Japan, described the FRC as a valuable index for identifying and determining the severity of thrombotic thrombocytopenic purpura and thrombotic microangiopathy. Their group reported a significant correlation between FRC, reticulocyte count, RDW, fibrinogen degradation products, lactate dehydrogenase, and clinical disease progression.[25] Lesesve et al. from France further validated the utility of the automated FRC parameter using both the Siemens ADVIA series and the Sysmex XE-2100 model, to identify schistocytes, with a negative predictive value for excluding schistocytosis close to 100%.[26-28] Abe et al. from

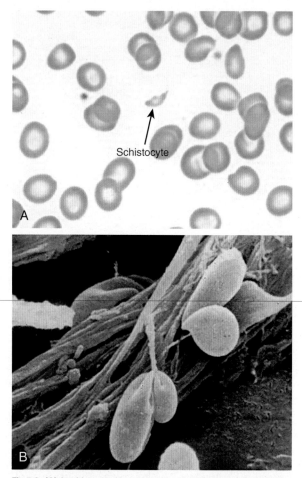

Fig 5.3 (A) A schistocyte is a red blood cell (RBC) fragment, indicating the cell was damaged as it passed through an area of the circulation containing fibrin strands, typically from endothelial cell damage, on which passing RBC can become tethered and torn. **(B)** Electron micrograph showing fibrin strands in the microcirculation on which RBCs have become tethered and may become torn as the blood flow pushes them downstream. If the damaged membrane of a torn RBC reseals, it can thereafter circulate as a schistocyte.

Japan, in a somewhat similar study, reported that the FRC count had 90% sensitivity and 96% specificity for identifying a microangiopathic disorder.[29]

The first study of FRC in neonates, of which we are aware, was from our group in 2019, where we used retrospective data from over 40,000 CBCs of neonates to define a reference interval for this parameter over the first 90 days after birth.[30] Fig. 5.5 shows our histogram of FRC counts of neonates, with a roughly

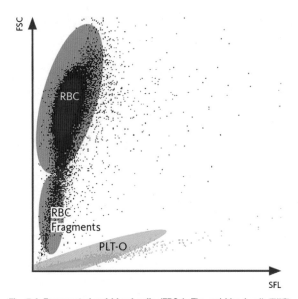

Fig. 5.4 Fragmented red blood cells (FRCs). The red blood cell *(RBC)* fragments in a blood sample, including schistocytes, are measured in the gate immediately smaller than normal RBCs, as shown below. PLT-O is an optical measure of platelets. *SFL* (side fluorescence; the X-axis) is the side-scatter of each cell flowing through the detector and is a surrogate for its RNA content. *FSC* (forward scatter; the Y-axis) is a measure of the size of the cell. FRC can be expressed in two ways: as a percentage of the RBC in the sample (FRC%) or as the absolute number of fragmented red cells per microliter of blood (FRC/µL). (From Sysmex.)

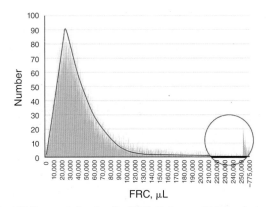

Fig. 5.5 Fragmented red cells (*FRC*/µL) from >40,000 values of newborn infants. The Y-axis shows the number of records at each of the FRC values on the ordinate. The *red line* shows the distribution of values. The *red circle* to the extreme right shows the upper 2.5% of values, comprised of 96 counts. (From Judkins AJ, MacQueen BC, Christensen RD, Henry E, Snow GL, Bennett ST. Automated quantification of fragmented red blood cells: neonatal reference intervals and clinical disorders of neonatal intensive care unit patients with high values. *Neonatology.* 2019;115(1):5-12. doi:10.1159/000491626.)

parametric distribution among the great majority of neonates, ranging from 0 to 100,000 RBC fragments/µL blood; however, the distribution had a long tail to the right, with a cluster of 96 values to the extreme right (counts >210,000/µL). By examining the medical records of these 96 neonates we found that 37% had proven sepsis, 29% had proven DIC, 17% had a chromosomal trisomy or another genetic syndrome, 14% had necrotizing enterocolitis (NEC), and 7% had iron deficiency (defined as a RET-He <25 pg; some had more than one diagnosis).

As part of that report we generated reference FRC intervals for neonates during their first 90 days after birth (Fig. 5.6).[30] Using these reference intervals, we later reported three cases of neonates with coagulopathy where the cause of the bleeding disorder was initially uncertain.[31] In such a neonate, distinguishing DIC from liver disease can require additional testing. We did not have the FRC values of these three patients in real time, but we obtained them subsequently to find that had we known of these values in real time, the underlying pathology would have been clear. Fig. 5.7 illustrates how, in these three neonates with coagulopathy, the FRC/µL measurement differentiates DIC from the coagulopathy of liver disease.

In another study of the potential usefulness of the FRC parameter in neonatology practice, we collected 270 CBCs from 90 neonates suspected of having either sepsis, NEC, or DIC, the three most common microangiopathic conditions of NICU patients.[32] For each CBC we compared routine manual schistocyte enumeration by the clinical laboratory technologist with the automated FRC. When the two counts disagreed, we used a gold standard from a greater than 1000 RBC differential cell count. The clinical laboratory and the automated FRC counts agreed in 63% (95% confidence interval [CI] 55–70%) of the CBCs. Among the 37% where they disagreed, the FRC count was more accurate in 100% (95% CI 88–100%) of the instances. We found that an elevated FRC count was specific for sepsis and was sensitive and specific for NEC and DIC. We concluded that the automated FRC count has distinct advantages over routine manual evaluation for schistocytosis; specifically, the FRC count uses a much larger sample size, has a lower expense, and shows superior accuracy in diagnosing schistocyte-producing conditions in neonates.[32]

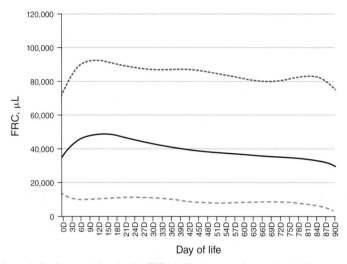

Fig. 5.6 Neonatal reference intervals for fragmented red cells *(FRC)*/µL. The *lower and upper dashed lines* represent the 5th percentile lower reference interval and the 95th percentile upper reference interval during the first 90 days following birth. The *solid line* represents the mean value. (From Judkins AJ, MacQueen BC, Christensen RD, et al. Automated quantification of fragmented red blood cells: neonatal reference intervals and clinical disorders of neonatal intensive care unit patients with high values. *Neonatology.* 2019;115:5-12.)

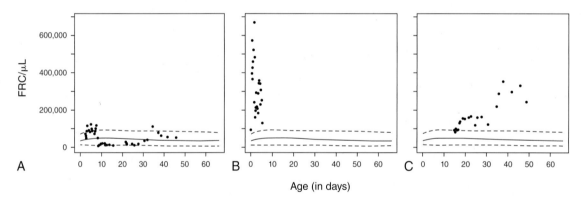

Fig. 5.7 Illustration of how, in a neonate with coagulopathy, the fragmented red cells *(FRC)*/µL measurement differentiates disseminated intravascular coagulation (DIC) from the coagulopathy of liver disease. **A–C,** Serial FRC measurements from an individual neonate with coagulopathy and an uncertain diagnosis. The *dots,* each representing a FRC measurement, are plotted overlaying the reference interval chart. **A,** Normal FRC counts; patient eventually diagnosed with the coagulopathy of liver disease (gestational alloimmune liver disease). **B,** Very elevated FRC counts; patient eventually diagnosed with DIC. **C,** Rising FRC counts; patient eventually diagnosed with hemolytic uremic syndrome associated with *E. coli* 0157:H7 shiga-toxin. We speculate that if we would have had access to the FRC count in real time, we might have made the correct diagnosis much more rapidly than we did. (From Bahr TM, Judkins AJ, Baer VL, et al. The fragmented red cell count can support the diagnosis of a microangiopathic neonatal condition. *J Perinatol.* 2020;40:354-355).

Proportion of Erythrocytes that are Microcytic or Hypochromic

The Micro-R is a unique means of quantifying RBC microcytosis. It is defined by the manufacturer of the analyzer as the percent of RBCs that have a MCV below 60 fL. Fig. 5.8 illustrates how the automated Micro-R measurement is made.

The MCV is the average size of all erythrocytes in a blood sample, whereas the Micro-R specifically quantifies the population of very small RBCs in that sample. Thus a patient with some large RBCs (perhaps from

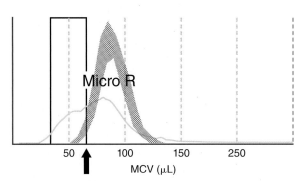

Fig. 5.8 Quantifying erythrocyte microcytosis using the Micro-R. The X-axis is mean corpuscular volume (MCV), in microliters, as a measure of the size of the individual red blood cells (RBCs) flowing through the detector. The Y-axis is a count of the individual RBCs flowing through the detector. The *arrow* indicates a MCV of 60 fL and the *black-outlined box* shows the window defining the proportion of RBC with an MCV <60 fL, which by convention is taken as the "Micro-R". The *darker blue histogram* shows the reference interval for MCV in a healthy population, and the *light blue line* shows the histogram of a patient who has erythrocyte microcytosis, which curve is shifted to the left of the reference interval curve. (From Sysmex.)

reticulocytosis) who also has a population of small RBCs (perhaps from early iron-limited erythropoiesis) might have a normal MCV because the larger and smaller cells are averaged to generate the MCV. However, a neonate with early iron-limited erythropoiesis will be recognized by an elevated Micro-R even if the MCV is normal.

The MCV reference interval for adults is 80 to 96 fL.[3,4] In neonates the normal range for MCV depends on the gestational and postnatal age of the patient. For instance, in term infants at birth it is 100 to 116 fL, and the intervals are yet higher at younger gestational ages.[33] In healthy adults the Micro-R is typically less

than 1%,[34-37] meaning that fewer than 1% of the RBC are less than 60 fL. (The Micro-R reference interval for neonates is shown in Fig. 5.10A, later.) Most neonates over their first 90 days will have a Micro-R of less than 3% of their RBC, while the upper reference interval can be as high 7%. Thus neonates, despite having a much higher MCV than adults, have a higher Micro-R than adults, meaning neonates normally have a higher population of microcytes than do adults.[38]

The HYPO-He is a unique metric to quantify hypo-hemoglobinized RBCs and is defined as the percent of RBC that have a MCH below 17 pg. Fig. 5.9 illustrates

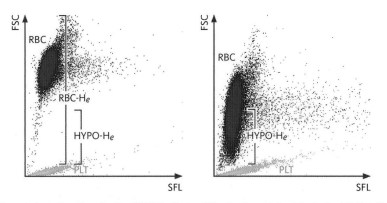

Fig. 5.9 Quantifying erythrocyte hypochromia using the HYPO-He. Each cell flowing through the detector is plotted on the RET scattergram based on its fluorescence intensity, as shown on the X-axis (*SFL* = side fluorescence) and its high-angle forward scattered light signal shown on the Y-axis (*FSC* = forward scatter). Thus the Y-axis shows RBC size, and the X axis shows RBC cellular content (principally hemoglobin). The *left panel* shows a blood sample from a healthy individual, with a HYPO-He of <1%. The *right panel* shows a sample from a patient with a very high proportion of RBC with a MCH <17 pg. In this example the HYPO-He is 60%. *PLT,* Platelet; *MCH,* mean corpuscular hemoglobin; *RBC,* red blood cells. (From Sysmex.)

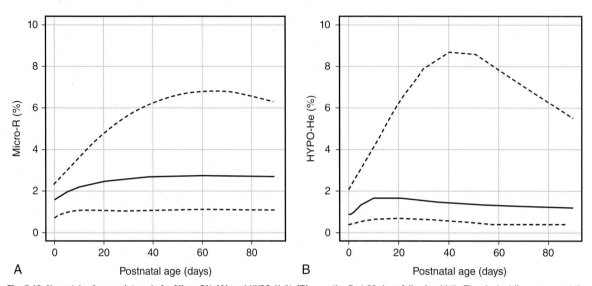

Fig. 5.10 Neonatal reference intervals for Micro-R% **(A)** and HYPO-He% **(B)** over the first 90 days following birth. The *dashed lines* represent the lower and upper reference intervals, and the *solid line* represents the mean value. (From Bahr TM, Christensen TR, Henry E, et al. Neonatal reference intervals for the complete blood count parameters MicroR and HYPO-He: sensitivity beyond the red cell indices for identifying microcytic and hypochromic disorders. *J Pediatr.* 2021;239:95-100.e2. Available at: https://doi.org/10.1016/j.jpeds.2021.08.002.)

how the automated HYPO-He measurement is made. The MCH reference interval for adults is 26 to 32 pg,[4,5] and the HYPO-He in healthy adults is typically less than 1%.[34-37] In neonates the MCH reference interval, like the MCV, is dependent on gestational and postnatal age and is considerably higher than in adults.[33] As shown in Fig. 5.10B, most neonates have a HYPO-He less than 2%, but the upper reference interval is as high as 8.5% peaking 35 to 50 days after birth.[38]

Elevations in the proportions of microcytic and hypochromic erythrocytes are characteristics of iron-limited erythropoiesis. However, these two parameters are also elevated in neonates with alpha thalassemia trait or hemoglobin H disease, where the Micro-R can be quite high, while the HYPO-He is also elevated but typically less so.[38,39] In a limited number of neonates with hereditary spherocytosis, we found the Micro-R is high, but the HYPO-He is normal to low because they have a population of microspherocytes, which are small but hyperdense.

Summary

A CBC is one of the most frequently ordered laboratory tests in neonates, particularly those cared for in a NICU.

Anemia is common among NICU patients and can have a variety of causes. Treatment of the anemia is more evidence based when its cause is known. Iron deficiency, occult blood loss, phlebotomy losses, and hemolysis can all be contributing to anemia in a neonate.

In evaluating a neonate whether or not they are anemic the RET-He has advantages over the serum ferritin level in identifying a lack of bioavailable iron. Although the serum ferritin may be a more popular test to assess iron status, it requires an additional phlebotomy, with more blood withdrawn. Moreover, a serum ferritin might have a false-positive result, being normal or high during neonatal inflammatory conditions.

In a neonate with coagulopathy, an elevated FRC count can point the differential diagnosis toward a microangiopathic disorder, while a normal FRC count in such a neonate tends to exclude DIC from the differential, making the coagulopathy of liver disease much more likely.

An elevated Micro-R in company with an elevated HYPO-He is more sensitive that a low MCV and/or a low MCH in diagnosing neonatal iron limited erythro poiesis. Table 5.1 illustrates the typical changes in RET-He, FRC, Micro-R, and HYPO-He accompanying various neonatal erythrocyte disorders.

TABLE 5.1 Changes in the Erythrocytic Parameters, RET-He, FRC, Micro-R, and HYPO-He, in Various Pathologic Conditions Affecting NICU Patients

Pathologic Condition	RET-He	FRC	Micro-R	HYPO-He
Iron limited erythropoiesis	↓	Normal to ↑	↑	↑
Iron deficiency anemia	↓↓	↑ to ↑↑	↑↑	↑↑
Necrotizing enterocolitis	Normal	↑↑	Normal	Normal
Sepsis	Normal	↑↑	Normal	Normal
Coagulopathy of DIC	Normal	↑ to ↑↑	Normal	Normal
Coagulopathy of liver disease	Normal	Normal	Normal	Normal
Alpha thalassemia trait or Hgb H disease	Normal	↑ to ↑↑	↑↑	↑
Hereditary spherocytosis	Normal	↑	↑↑	Normal

FRC, fragmented red cells; *HYPO-He,* hypochromic population; *Micro-R,* microcytic population; *RET-He,* reticulocyte hemoglobin.

REFERENCES

1. Wintrobe MM. A simple and accurate hematocrit. *J Lab Clin Med.* 1929;15:287-289.
2. Wintrobe MM. The volume and hemoglobin content of the red blood corpuscle. *Am J Med Sci.* 1929;177:513-523.
3. Wintrobe MM. Classification of the anemias on the basis of differences in the size and hemoglobin content of the red corpuscles. *Proc Soc Exp Biol Med.* 1930;27:1071-1072.
4. Smock KJ. Examination of the blood and bone marrow. In: Greer JP, Arber DA, Appelbaum FR, et al., eds. *Wintrobe's Clinical Hematology.* 14th ed. Philadelphia: Wolters Kluwer; 2019:2-3.
5. Mast AE, Blinder MA, Lu Q, et al. Clinical utility of the reticulocyte hemoglobin content in the diagnosis of iron deficiency. *Blood.* 2002;99:1489-1491
6. Ullrich C, Wu A, Armsby C, et al. Screening healthy infants for iron deficiency using reticulocyte hemoglobin content. *JAMA.* 2005;294(8):924-930.
7. Brugnara C, Schiller B, Moran J. Reticulocyte hemoglobin equivalent (Ret He) and assessment of iron-deficient states. *Clin Lab Haematol.* 2006;28(5):303-308.
8. Mateos ME, De-la-Cruz J, López-Laso E, et al. Reticulocyte hemoglobin content for the diagnosis of iron deficiency. *J Pediatr Hematol Oncol.* 2008;30(7):539-542.
9. Ervasti M, Kotisaari S, Sankilampi U, et al. The relationship between red blood cell and reticulocyte indices and serum markers of iron status in the cord blood of newborns. *Clin Chem Lab Med.* 2007;45(8):1000-1003.
10. Lorenz L, Peter A, Poets CF, et al. A review of cord blood concentrations of iron status parameters to define reference ranges for preterm infants. *Neonatology.* 2013;104(3):194-202.
11. Lorenz L, Arand J, Büchner K, et al. Reticulocyte haemoglobin content as a marker of iron deficiency. *Arch Dis Child Fetal Neonatal Ed.* 2015;100(3):F198-F202.
12. Al-Ghananim RT, Nalbant D, Schmidt RL, et al. Reticulocyte hemoglobin content during the first month of life in critically ill very low birth weight neonates differs from term infants, children, and adults. *J Clin Lab Anal.* 2016;30(4):326-334.
13. Lorenz L, Peter A, Arand J, et al. Reticulocyte haemoglobin content declines more markedly in preterm than in term

infants in the first days after birth. *Neonatology.* 2017;112(3). 246-250.
14. Ennis KM, Dahl LV, Rao RB, et al. Reticulocyte hemoglobin content as an early predictive biomarker of brain iron deficiency. *Pediatr Res.* 2018;84(5):765-769.
15. Gelaw Y, Woldu B, Melku M. The role of reticulocyte hemoglobin content for diagnosis of iron deficiency and iron deficiency anemia, and monitoring of iron therapy: a literature review. *Clin Lab.* 2019;65(12).
16. German K, Vu PT, Irvine JD, et al. Trends in reticulocyte hemoglobin equivalent values in critically ill neonates, stratified by gestational age. *J Perinatol.* 2019;39(9):1268-1274.
17. Dzirba TA, Moss MF, Dionisio LM. Assessment of reticulocyte hemoglobin content in infants in intensive care units. *Int J Lab Hematol.* 2020;42(4):e180-e184.
18. Bahr TM, Lozano-Chinga M, Agarwal AM, et al. Dizygotic twins with prolonged jaundice and microcytic, hypochromic, hemolytic anemia with pyropoikilocytosis. *Blood Cells Mol Dis.* 2020;85:102462.
19. Amin K, Bansal M, Varley N, et al. Reticulocyte hemoglobin content as a function of iron stores at 35-36 weeks post menstrual age in very premature infants. *J Matern Fetal Neonatal Med.* 2021; 34(19):3214-3219.
20. Bahr TM, Baer VL, Ohls RK, et al. Reconciling markedly discordant values of serum ferritin versus reticulocyte hemoglobin content. *J Perinatol.* 2021;41(3):619-626.
21. Bahr TM, Carr NR, Christensen TR, et al. Early iron supplementation and iron sufficiency at one month of age in NICU patients at-risk for iron deficiency. *Blood Cells Mol Dis.* 2021; 90:102575.
22. Gerday E, Brereton JB, Bahr TM, et al. Urinary ferritin; a potential noninvasive way to screen NICU patients for iron deficiency. *J Perinatol.* 2021;41(6):1419-1425.
23. Christensen RD, Henry E, Bennett ST, et al. Reference intervals for reticulocyte parameters of infants during their first 90 days after birth. *J Perinatol.* 2016;36(1):61-66.
24. Jiang M, Saigo K, Kumagai S, et al. Quantification of red blood cell fragmentation by automated haematology analyser XE-2100. *Clin Lab Haematol.* 2001;23:167-172.

25. Banno S, Ito Y, Tanaka C, et al. Quantification of red blood cell fragmentation by the automated hematology analyzer XE-2100 in patients with living donor liver transplantation. *Clin Lab Haematol.* 2005;27:292-296.

26. Lesesve JF, Salignac S, Lecompte T, et al. Automated measurement of schistocytes after bone marrow transplantation. *Bone Marrow Transpl.* 2004;34:357-362.

27. Lesesve JF, Asnafi V, Braun F, et al. Fragmented red blood cells automated measurement is a useful parameter to exclude schistocytes on the blood film. *Int J Lab Hematol.* 2012;34(6):566-576.

28. Lesesve JF, Speyer E, Perol JP. Fragmented red cells reference range for the Sysmex XN®-series of automated blood cell counters. *Int J Lab Hematol.* 2015;37(5):583-587.

29. Abe Y, Wada H, Yamada E, et al. The effectiveness of measuring for fragmented red cells using an automated hematology analyzer in patients with thrombotic microangiopathy. *Clin Appl Thromb Hemost.* 2009;15:257-262.

30. Judkins AJ, MacQueen BC, Christensen RD, et al. Automated quantification of fragmented red blood cells: neonatal reference intervals and clinical disorders of neonatal intensive care unit patients with high values. *Neonatology.* 2019;115(1):5-12.

31. Bahr TM, Judkins AJ, Baer VL, et al. The fragmented red cell count can support the diagnosis of a microangiopathic neonatal condition. *J Perinatol.* 2020;40(2):354-355.

32. Bahr TM, Judkins AJ, Christensen RD, et al. Neonates with suspected microangiopathic disorders: performance of standard manual schistocyte enumeration vs. the automated fragmented red cell count. *J Perinatol.* 2019;39(11):1555-1561.

33. Christensen RD, Jopling J, Henry E, et al. The erythrocyte indices of neonates, defined using data from over 12,000 patients in a multihospital health care system. *J Perinatol.* 2008;28:24-28.

34. d'Onofrio G, Zini G, Ricerca BM, et al. Automated measurement of red blood cell microcytosis and hypochromia in iron deficiency and beta-thalassemia trait. *Arch Pathol Lab Med.* 1992;116(1):84-89.

35. Maconi M, Cavalca L, Danise P, et al. Erythrocyte and reticulocyte indices in iron deficiency in chronic kidney disease: comparison of two methods. *Scand J Clin Lab Invest.* 2009;69(3):365-370.

36. Urrechaga E, Borque L, Escanero JF. Percentage of hypochromic erythrocytes as a potential marker of iron availability. *Clin Chem Lab Med.* 2011;50:685-687.

37. Archer NM, Brugnara C. Diagnosis of iron-deficient states. *Crit Rev Clin Lab Sci.* 2015;52(5):256-272.

38. Bahr TM, Christensen TR, Henry E, et al. Neonatal reference intervals for the complete blood count parameters Micro-R and HYPO-He: sensitivity beyond the red cell indices for identifying microcytic and hypochromic disorders. *J Pediatr.* 2021;239: 95-100.e2.

39. Bahr TM, Knudsen MC, Lozano-Chinga M, et al. Infantile pyknocytosis: end-tidal CO, %Micro-R measurements, next-generation sequencing, and transfusion avoidance with darbepoetin. *Biomed Hub.* 2020;5(3):227-234.

Chapter 6

Neonatal Iron Homeostasis

Kendell R. German, MD and Sandra E. Juul, MD, PhD

Chapter Outline

Introduction

Iron is critical for various tissues throughout the body, including red blood cells and the brain. While iron can be stored, it cannot be synthesized de novo in the body and therefore is an essential micronutrient that must be provided in the diet. An important feature of iron is that it is not actively excreted from the body, so regulation of total body iron occurs at the level of dietary absorption. Based on the need to ensure adequate iron intake to meet the body's demands coupled with the importance of avoiding iron overload, iron uptake is typically closely regulated to ensure iron homeostasis is optimized. Iron acquisition begins prior to birth, with active iron transfer from the mother to fetus.[1] These accumulated fetal iron stores are used as the primary iron source for the first 4 to 6 months after term birth, when dietary iron intake usually increases.[2] Dietary absorption of iron is also tightly regulated, although the timing of development of this homeostatic mechanism is not known.

There are various conditions under which iron homeostasis may be disrupted. Despite the body's tight regulatory mechanisms, iron deficiency is prevalent worldwide, affecting 1.6 to 2 billion individuals.[3,4] In 2002 the World Health Organization estimated that anemia resulting from iron deficiency was one of the 10 most important factors contributing to the global burden of diseases, with children and pregnant women at particularly high risk.[3] Although individuals from low- and middle-resource countries are at highest risk, it is not well recognized that pregnant women and children in high-resource countries, such as the United States, are also at high risk. For example, Auerbach et al. screened a cohort of 102 consecutive, nonselected, nonanemic pregnant women in the United States and found that 42% were iron deficient.[5]

When an infant's iron balance is disrupted, it is the role of the clinician to identify this disruption and provide needed supplementation, guided by iron status parameters. Failure to recognize and treat either iron deficiency or overload can have long-term consequences that persist throughout an individual's life. These effects may be hematologic in nature with extreme iron deficiency resulting in anemia, or they may be developmental, with iron deficiency leading to long-term neurodevelopmental impacts. Because of the potential adverse long-term consequences, ensuring optimal iron status is an essential part of neurodevelopmental care of at-risk infants.[6]

In Utero Iron Accretion

Breast milk is low in iron; therefore an infant's iron needs during the first 4 to 6 months of life are typically supported by stores accrued during the third trimester of pregnancy, until iron-rich sources of supplementary foods are introduced in a child's diet.[7] A young infant's iron balance appears to be highly dependent on iron loading during pregnancy.[8,9] Because this period is critical to ensuring adequate iron stores for the first several months of a healthy child's life, several mechanisms are in place to ensure adequate placental iron transfer from mother to fetus.

Although the exact mechanism by which iron crosses the placenta is not known, several iron transporters that are critical to postnatal iron transfer are recognized to play a role in this process in utero. Iron transfer occurs to a certain extent throughout pregnancy, but the majority occurs in the third trimester.[10] This is one reason why preterm infants are at added risk for iron deficiency postnatally. The transfer of iron across the placenta is an active process carried out primarily by the syncytiotrophoblasts.[1] In the primate placenta, maternal blood bathes fetal tissue, thus diminishing the distance that iron must travel to pass from mother to fetus. Iron is transported in the circulation bound to a protein called transferrin. Maternal transferrin-bound iron is actively transported across the placenta via transferrin receptor 1.[1] While transferrin receptor 1 is ubiquitous in cells throughout the body (except in mature erythrocytes), there is a particularly high concentration of this receptor on placental syncytiotrophoblasts, thus facilitating fetal iron acquisition.[1] Iron enters syncytiotrophoblast cells via transferrin receptor 1, then is exported to the fetal side by ferroportin. The presence of ferroportin on cell surfaces, which affects the ability of cells to absorb and release iron, is regulated by hepcidin. Hepcidin is a negative regulator of iron, as will be discussed subsequently, and thus elevated hepcidin levels lead to decreased ferroportin within cell membranes and therefore decreased iron absorption and availability. To promote fetal iron transfer, maternal hepcidin values are particularly low during pregnancy.[11]

The transfer of iron from mother to fetus is a tightly regulated process as both iron deficiency and overload during pregnancy are associated with adverse effects. The iron requirements for a woman during pregnancy are estimated to be 1 g over the duration of pregnancy. This includes expansion of the maternal red cell mass with expansion of the blood volume during pregnancy,[11] placental needs (90 mg), and fetal transfer (270 mg iron).[10,12] Additionally, the fetus has significant iron demands throughout pregnancy but particularly during the period of rapid brain growth and expansion of the fetal red cell mass in the third trimester. Fetal iron transfer is prioritized over maternal needs when mothers have mild iron deficiency; however, more severe deficiency states cannot be overcome.[11] Thus severe maternal iron deficiency puts both the mother and developing fetus at risk for adverse effects of iron deficiency. This is of significant concern as pregnant women represent one of the groups at highest risk for iron deficiency. The incidence of iron deficiency during gestation ranges from approximately 45% in well-resourced countries to up to 80% in low-income countries.[5,11] This has significant health implications for mother and fetus. Maternal iron deficiency has been associated with adverse perinatal outcomes including in utero growth restriction, preterm birth, low birth weight, peripartum hemorrhage, and even increased maternal mortality.[11,13,14] Maternal conditions that decrease fetal iron transfer include maternal obesity, diabetes, and preeclampsia. Maternal alcohol use and smoking are also associated with decreased maternal-to-fetus iron transfer.[11] It is unclear whether this disruption in placental iron transfer is caused by impaired placental function or an inappropriate elevation of the proinflammatory hormone hepcidin in mothers with these conditions.[15]

Adverse long-term outcomes are possible in infants born with inadequate prenatal iron transfer. The fetal origins hypothesis links in utero exposures and environment to adult-onset disease.[16,17] Fetal nutritional disruptions, including iron deficiency, have been associated with an increased incidence of abnormal brain structure and development as well as neuropsychiatric disruptions later in adulthood.[18-20] This likely reflects the importance of iron in brain development. In addition to its erythropoietic effects, iron plays key roles in energy production in the brain, synaptogenesis, dendritic pruning, and neurotransmitter production.[21-27] The hippocampus appears to be particularly sensitive to iron deficiency during pregnancy and early infancy.[11,28] This is perhaps due to its high energy demand and rapid growth during pregnancy and the first 2 years of life. Consequently, iron deficiency during fetal life can have adverse effects on hippocampal development leading to long-term disruptions in neurodevelopmental conditions predominantly controlled by the hippocampus, including recognition memory.[29] In addition to hippocampal function in particular, iron deficiency can impact the fetal brain more globally. This is likely due to a combination of brain-specific functions of iron as well as the high oxygen consumption of the brain during fetal life, for which iron is a critical component. The brain uses approximately 60% of total fetal oxygen availability, emphasizing the importance of optimized oxygen delivery in the maternoplacental unit.[30]

While much of the research examining fetal iron deficiency is focused on the impacts on the fetal brain, emerging research is showing additional long-term impacts of fetal iron deficiency. For example, Gambling et al. showed in an animal model that iron deficiency during fetal life was associated with long-term elevated blood pressure in offspring.[31]

Fetal iron deficiency is associated with adverse outcomes, but iron overload also appears to be associated with adverse outcomes, emphasizing the importance of tight iron regulation. Chang et al. showed an increased risk of low birth weight and prematurity with an elevated hematocrit in a population of adolescent women, highlighting the U-shaped relationship between high and low iron status in the perinatal period.[32,33] Additionally, several studies have suggested an association between impaired glucose regulation in iron-replete pregnant women treated with iron.[34-36] As we will summarize, this U-shape relationship persists in infancy, childhood, and adulthood, highlighting the critical nature of iron homeostasis and targeting supplementation to those with iron deficiency.

Iron Regulation in Neonates

Both iron deficiency and overload can have detrimental effects.[32] Because of the importance of ensuring iron homeostasis, regulation mechanisms are in place. Notably, iron cannot be easily excreted from the body once absorbed, therefore much of the regulation process for iron takes place in the gut lumen, at the site of iron absorption. As shown in Fig. 6.1, ingested ferric iron (Fe^{3+}) is reduced to ferrous iron (Fe^{2+}) in the gut lumen by ferric reductase. Fe^{2+} is absorbed into the intestinal epithelial cell from the gut lumen via divalent metal transporter-1. Human lactoferrin, from breast milk, is absorbed along with its bound iron by a specific receptor. Iron then binds to ferritin intracellularly. Iron exits the epithelial cell on the basolateral surface via ferroportin-1. Fe^{2+} is oxidized to Fe^{3+} by hephaestin as it exits the cell. Iron binds transferrin as it exits the cell and is transported through the circulation as transferrin-bound Fe^{2+}.[37]

This process is under tight regulatory control by hepcidin. Hepcidin is a polypeptide hormone primarily produced in the liver. It has been clearly shown to serve as the primary regulator of iron in older children and adults,[38,39] and there are emerging studies suggesting that its regulatory mechanisms are intact in neonates.[40-44] Hepcidin acts as a negative regulator of iron absorption and availability (see Fig. 6.1). It causes the internalization and degradation of the ferroportin transmembrane channel.[39] Ferroportin is the primary channel through which iron exits cells in the intestinal and in storage cells for iron such as macrophages. Therefore internalization of ferroportin in

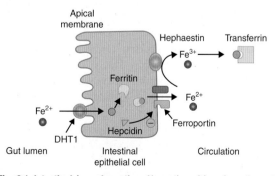

Fig. 6.1 Intestinal iron absorption. Absorption of iron from the gut lumen through the intestinal epithelial cell to the circulation.

intestinal epithelium causes iron to be trapped in the epithelial cell. It is then lost in feces as the epithelial cell is naturally sloughed over time. In storage cells such as macrophages, hepcidin leads to sequestration of iron within these cells. Therefore the net effect of an increase in hepcidin is decreased iron absorption and availability.[39,45]

The production of hepcidin varies based on both the body's total body iron status and other clinical conditions such as infection and, more broadly, inflammation.[38] Additionally, erythroferrone, which promotes erythropoiesis, leads to a downregulation of hepcidin, thus making iron available for red blood cell production.[46] When an individual's iron needs exceed the availability of iron within the body, hepcidin production decreases, leading to increased absorption of iron. This is the case in pregnancy, when iron demands of the increasing maternal red cell mass, the placenta, and the fetus rapidly increase from a woman's baseline iron demands. During a healthy pregnancy, hepcidin values therefore decrease to allow increased iron absorption from the gut to accommodate this increased demand.[11]

Some bacteria, most notably gram-negative bacteria, have been found to be siderophilic (i.e., require iron for normal function and replication). As an evolutionary adaptation, humans have evolved to increase their hepcidin production with infection and inflammation.[47] This leads to decreased iron absorption as well as sequestration of iron within storage cells such as macrophages and hepatocytes. This leads to less free iron available for bacterial replication. While this certainly has historic benefits, the more widespread upregulation of hepcidin with any form of inflammation, including inflammation of chronic disease, has detrimental effects. Chronic inflammatory conditions, such as inflammatory bowel disease, have been linked to inappropriate upregulation in hepcidin resulting in functional iron deficiency.[38] This is one of the theorized mechanisms behind mothers with obesity, a potentially proinflammatory condition, having infants at higher risk of iron deficiency.[15,48]

As noted previously, several regulatory mechanisms are in place to ensure adequate fetal iron accretion during pregnancy. In healthy, term infants, iron stores accrued during fetal life provide an adequate iron source to support a period of low iron intake from breast milk (though what iron is present is highly bioavailable due to lactoferrin) during the first 4 to 6 months of age, after which complimentary foods are typically introduced. In fact, neonatal iron status in healthy term infants is highly dependent on this loading, and infants born with low stores are unlikely to catch up without supplementation.

Preterm infants and term infants born with inadequate prenatal stores due to placental dysfunction or other causes are at risk for iron deficiency. When supplemental iron is offered, it does appear that neonates can regulate their iron status through mechanisms that approach adult mechanisms, though results are somewhat conflicting in this population. Bahr et al. found that hepcidin levels were lower in neonates at risk for iron deficiency, including preterm infants,[40] and studies by our group and others have shown hepcidin values to correlate with iron treatment and markers of iron status, including ferritin.[41,42,44] Similar to older children and adults, hepcidin values in neonates have been shown to increase with inflammation and sepsis, suggesting that infants may also be able to regulate hepcidin to sequester iron from siderophilic bacteria.[44,49,50] However, not all studies support the idea that neonates can regulate their iron status. Yapakçi et al.[51] showed no difference in hepcidin values following transfusion, though an increase was seen by Lorenz et al.[43] Domellöf et al. examined iron uptake via iron-isotopes.[52] They found no difference in iron absorption rates in iron supplemented vs. unsupplemented infants at 6 months of age, but did see a difference at 9 months. They concluded that younger infants may not have the ability to regulate absorption based on need, though as this study was conducted in a population with presumed low incidence of iron deficiency, this may have confounded their results as many infants at 6 months may have remained iron sufficient through prenatal stores.

In sum, the available evidence suggests that iron is tightly regulated in children and adults through the actions of hepcidin, erythropoietin, and erythroferrone to avoid both overload and deficiency. While these mechanisms may be less robust in neonates, there is evidence that even preterm neonates have some regulatory control over their iron status through the action of these regulatory hormones.

Measures of Iron Status

A number of regulatory hormones and proteins are involved in iron regulation as noted previously, and many of these can be used to assess iron status. These measures can be more challenging to interpret in neonates due to the normal hematologic changes of infancy; therefore age-specific norms must be used to interpret these measures appropriately.

HEMOGLOBIN AND HEMATOCRIT

Hemoglobin and/or hematocrit are by far the most commonly used measures to assess iron deficiency worldwide. These measures are inexpensive, widely available, and require little blood, all strong advantages. The majority of iron in the body is used for erythropoiesis. Consequently, severe iron deficiency results in iron deficiency anemia. The American Academy of Pediatrics (AAP) recommends universal screening for anemia via hemoglobin measurement (with a primary goal of identifying iron deficiency anemia) at 1 year of age,[53] whereas the US Preventive Services Task Force (USPSTF) finds insufficient evidence to support universal screening.[54] We believe these recommendations should be updated, as iron deficiency anemia is a late finding of severe iron deficiency, and preterm infants, even those who received iron supplementation during hospitalization, have a high prevalence of iron deficiency as early as 4 months posthopitalization.

Hemoglobin is a nonspecific marker of iron deficiency and therefore carries several disadvantages as a sole marker of iron deficiency, particularly in the neonatal population. First, animal models have demonstrated that iron is prioritized for erythropoiesis over other iron demands in the body, including brain iron needs.[55] As a result, infants may experience iron deficiency at the tissue level prior to the onset of anemia. Various animal model and human studies have shown that brain maldevelopment may occur prior to the onset of anemia in iron deficient infants.[56-59] Therefore anemia is a late marker of iron deficiency, and infants may have irreversible developmental impacts prior to the onset of anemia, making reliance on hemoglobin and hematocrit as sole markers of iron status in at-risk neonates highly problematic.

A second disadvantage, which is shared by most markers of iron status in neonates, is that hematologic

parameters undergo normal variation with advancing gestational and chronologic age due to physiologic anemia and the transition from primarily fetal hemoglobin-containing red blood cells to adult hemoglobin-containing red blood cells.[60] It is therefore important that age-specific norms be used to assess anemia in the neonatal population. Similarly, the presence of microcytosis is common in iron deficiency anemia in older children and adults. However, due to the high proportion of immature red blood cells in neonates, the mean corpuscular volume in neonates is typically higher in infants, which could mask underlying iron deficiency anemia if using pediatric or adult normative ranges.[61]

Finally, while the majority of anemia in the adult population can be attributed to iron deficiency, iron deficiency is not the sole cause of anemia, particularly in neonates.[56] Despite their recommendation to screen toddlers for anemia using hemoglobin measurements, the AAP acknowledges that not all anemia is caused by iron deficiency and that many toddlers with iron deficiency may not be anemic.[53] Blood disorders such as hemoglobinopathies, phlebotomy, infections such as malaria, toxin exposure such as lead, and other nutritional deficiencies may all cause anemia.[3] This leads to the possibility of iron overload if anemic infants are inappropriately diagnosed with iron deficiency when, in fact, their low hemoglobin and hematocrit values are caused by an alternative etiology.

In summary, due to the detrimental effects of preanemic iron deficiency, we argue that hemoglobin and hematocrit are not good measures of iron status, particularly in at-risk neonates. Alternative measures, including those listed subsequently, should be used to evaluate iron status in the neonatal population and guide any needed supplementation.

FERRITIN

Ferritin is a commonly used maker of iron status. Ferritin serves as the storage form of iron within the body. Low ferritin values reliably indicate iron deficiency. However, ferritin is an acute phase reactant and therefore can be elevated in the setting of infection and inflammation.[62,63] Given a relatively high rate of inflammation in critically ill neonates, this can often result in falsely elevated ferritin values, leading to underdiagnosis of iron deficiency. In a retrospective cohort of preterm neonates who received both ferritin and zinc protoporphyrin-to-heme (ZnPPH) ratio values as measures of iron status, our group found poor correlation between the highest ferritin value measured during a child's hospitalization and neurodevelopmental outcomes, with improved correlation with ZnPPH values, potentially due to falsely elevated ferritin values reflecting inflammation rather than iron sufficiency.[64] The AAP acknowledges this challenge in their recommendations and thus advise concurrent assessment of ferritin and C-reactive protein for diagnosis of iron deficiency in toddlers with anemia, or the use of reticulocyte hemoglobin (RET-He), which is not significantly affected by inflammation.[53]

ZINC PROTOPORPHYRIN-TO-HEME RATIO

In the production of hemoglobin, either iron or zinc can be incorporated into the protoporphyrin ring resulting in zinc protoporphyrin instead of heme.[65] When less iron is available, the proportion of zinc incorporated increases, thus raising the ZnPPH value. Therefore high ZnPPH values correlate with iron deficiency.[66,67] ZnPPH has been validated to assess iron status in neonates as well as children and adults.[65,67-71] ZnPPH carries the advantage of being less affected by inflammation than ferritin[63,69] and is low cost but can be affected by lead intoxication.[72] It is also unclear how quickly ZnPPH values respond to changes in iron status. ZnPPH values measure the ZnPPH content of the red blood cell pool as a whole; given the average life cycle of red blood cells in neonates of approximately 80 days, it is possible that ZnPPH values may lag behind changes in iron status. However, Labbe et al. suggests that given that ZnPPH is measured by fluorescence, minute changes in ZnPPH content of newly nascent cells may impact the overall ZnPPH values, implying more immediate responsiveness.[71,73]

RETICULOCYTE HEMOGLOBIN

RET-He refers to the hemoglobin content of a reticulocyte, measured in picograms (pg). It is analogous to the mean corpuscular hemoglobin, also measured in pg. As it reflects iron-containing hemoglobin content in newly formed cells, it has been hypothesized to be an acute marker of iron status. In animal models, it was shown to predate tissue-level iron deficiency, a strong potential benefit; these findings are being confirmed in neonatal clinical trials.[74] An additional advantage is that RET-He can be measured concurrently with a complete blood cell count (CBC) and reticulocyte count on most CBC analyzers, making this a very cost-effective measure that requires limited phlebotomy.[75] Several studies have identified normal ranges for RET-He in the neonatal population; however, values that correlate with optimal tissue iron status as suggested by short- and long-term neurodevelopmental changes have yet to be established.[76-79]

TOTAL IRON BINDING CAPACITY AND PERCENT TRANSFERRIN SATURATION

Iron is typically transported in the circulation bound to transferrin. The total iron binding capacity (TIBC) refers to the amount of possible iron binding sites in the total transferrin pool, thus representing both transferrin-bound iron and unsaturated transferrin. The proportion of transferrin that is saturated with iron (i.e., saturated transferrin divided by the TIBC) yields the percent transferrin saturation. A low transferrin saturation and high TIBC typically reflect iron deficiency.[80]

MEASURES UNDER INVESTIGATION

There are several novel markers under investigation that carry important advantages over currently available measures. MicroR and Hypo-HE can potentially be measured with some CBC analyzers such as the Sysmex analyzer (though currently are not reported clinically). MicroR pertains to a measure of microcytosis, reflecting the percentage of cells falling below the 5th percentile mean corpuscular volume, and Hypo-HE measures hypohemoglobinized red blood cells, reflecting the percentage of cells falling below the 5th percentile mean corpuscular hemoglobin. Both measures may be disrupted with preanemic iron deficiency.[81]

Excitingly, several studies are exploring the use of urinary markers of iron sufficiency, including urine ferritin and hepcidin.[41,44,82,83] Once validated, these have the potential to allow monitoring of iron status to adjust iron supplementation while preventing phlebotomy, which worsens iron status and puts infants at risk for other adverse events, including need for transfusion.

Iron and Brain Development

While the majority of iron in the body is used for erythropoiesis, iron is critical for a variety of tissues throughout the body, including the brain.[29] Specifically, iron is required in the brain for synaptogenesis, dendritic growth, myelination, neurotransmitter production, the development of normal structure, and energy metabolism.[59,84,85] Animal models have shown that iron is prioritized for red blood cell production over brain tissue needs, meaning that the brain may become iron deficient prior to the onset of anemia (known as preanemic iron deficiency or tissue-level iron deficiency).[55] Animal models, including rodents and nonhuman primates, have identified that the brain disruptions seen with iron deficiency are specifically attributable to iron deficiency, rather than anemia and impaired oxygen delivery, through isolating anemia and iron deficiency via knock-out rodent models and through evaluation of preanemic iron deficiency.[57-59,85] Also of note, there appear to be critical windows of brain development during the perinatal and early childhood period, when iron deficiency leads to disruptions in brain structure and function, which are not reversible with later supplementation,[59,84] emphasizing the need to establish optimal iron status during these vulnerable periods. The effects of iron deficiency during the perinatal and neonatal period have been associated with short-, medium-, and long-term developmental impacts.

Although iron is required throughout the brain, susceptibility periods and the timing of brain iron needs differ over time in different areas of the brain.[86] The hippocampus, which is undergoing rapid growth and development in the late prepartum and neonatal/toddler period, appears to be particularly susceptible to brain iron deficiency.[26,28,87-89] Iron deficiency has been shown to cause less complex dendritic arborization in the rat brain hippocampus and permanent disruptions in the metabolic profile.[88,89] The hippocampus is particularly involved in recognition memory, which may explain why this area of development may be significantly affected in iron deficient infants.

There are two primary hypotheses to explain why iron deficiency in the peripartum/neonatal period might not be reversible with later supplementation. Some researchers believe that there is a critical window in brain development where alterations in substrate availability (such as iron) lead to maldevelopment in these regions and thus brain structure, which is permanently changed.[28,89,90] Alternatively (and perhaps concurrently), iron deficiency may alter the regulation of genes involved in brain function, such as synaptic plasticity, leading to epigenetic changes that persist throughout an individual's lifetime.[26,91] In either instance, the potential irreversibility of iron deficiency alterations points to the importance of optimizing iron status in the perinatal, neonatal, and toddler period.

Disruptions in neurodevelopment with iron deficiency have been seen in the short, medium, and long term. In the neonatal period, iron deficiency can be seen with changes in neuronal conduction speed, temperament changes, and differences in neonatal reflexes.[92-96] Perinatal deficiency, even if corrected in early childhood, can lead to developmental differences that persist into childhood, adolescence, and even adulthood. At early childhood and school age, children with a history of iron deficiency are shown to have lower language skills, higher inattention scores, disruptions in sleep patterns, impaired recognition memory, disrupted motor development, slower processing speed, and social interaction differences.[97-100] Older children and adults have worse executive function.[101] Lozoff et al. have also found that adults with a history of iron deficiency in infancy have lower educational attainment in adulthood, which they hypothesize may be related to the impacts of iron deficiency in childhood adversely affecting their school experience.[102] While adverse effects can be seen with iron deficiency, long-term adverse effects are also associated with ubiquitous iron supplementation in children and infants who are not iron deficient, highlighting the importance of targeted supplementation.[103,104]

Iron Supplementation

Because of the risks of anemia and disruptions in brain development, various regulatory bodies recommend that infants and toddlers at risk for iron deficiency be screened for deficiency and supplemented as needed. However, the timing of supplementation, the duration, and the amount are unclear.[105]

The AAP and the European Society of Pediatric Gastroenterology, Hepatology, and Nutrition (ESPHAN) recommend that preterm infants receive 2 to 3 mg/kg/day of enteral iron supplementation between infancy and the introduction of complimentary iron-containing foods.[53,106] This may be provided either as supplements or in iron-fortified formula for infants who are formula fed. More recent studies have suggested that 2 to 3 mg/kg/day may be inadequate to achieve optimal iron status in high-risk infants, such as those born extremely preterm, with positive associations seen between iron dose and neurodevelopmental outcome with regimens up to 12 mg/kg/day.[64,107] A strong disadvantage of these studies is that they are retrospective in nature; hopefully future prospective trials, such as a randomized clinical trial being run by Kahn (NCT04691843) aimed at comparing iron supplementation up to 12 mg/kg/day vs. standard of care and its effects on neurodevelopment in early childhood, will shed further light on this important question.

While enteral supplements are typically well tolerated in the neonatal population[108] (as opposed to in adults who commonly report gastrointestinal upset with iron supplementation), some iron deficient infants may potentially require parenteral iron, either due to NPO status or inadequate enteral absorption. Historically, intravenous iron was typically administered as an iron salt, such as iron sucrose. These formulations provide readily available iron, but high doses may put infants at risk for nontransferrin bound iron, which is a prooxidant, meaning that they must be administered in small and frequent doses.[109] More recently, slow-release iron preparations have gained popularity for treatment of iron deficiency during pregnancy.[110,111] While understudied in the neonatal population, these formulations may provide the opportunity to supplement infants who either cannot tolerate enteral supplements or who are unresponsive to enteral supplements, potentially due to upregulation of hepcidin in the setting of chronic inflammation.

While the benefits of providing adequate supplementation to iron deficient neonates are clear, over-supplementation of iron sufficient infants may also be detrimental. We therefore propose that iron indices should be monitored in infants receiving iron supplements, particularly those above 2 mg/kg/day, to ensure appropriate levels. Also, measures to improve fetal iron loading and decrease iron loss are of upmost importance, including optimizing maternal iron status during pregnancy, delayed cord clamping, and minimizing phlebotomy, all of which are practices that improve fetal and neonatal iron status without the risk of adverse outcomes.[112]

Iron Overload

While iron deficiency is associated with adverse effects, so too is iron overload.[113] Dewey et al. and Brannon et al. describe iron status in neonates as a U-shaped curve with the best outcomes seen in infants who have appropriate iron levels, and worse outcomes in those with iron that is either too high or too low.[32,114] Free iron is a prooxidant, and ferroptosis has been implicated in neonatal brain injury.[115] Also, iron supplements have been associated with higher rates of morbidity and mortality in areas with high rates of certain infections such as malaria.[116,117] Unmonitored iron supplementation should be avoided as iron supplementation of iron sufficient infants has been associated with a variety of adverse effects, including the disruption of absorption of other nutrients and decreased linear growth.[118-120] In pregnant women, iron supplementation of iron sufficient women has been associated with impaired glucose regulation.[34-36] Because of the risks attributable to iron supplementation of iron sufficient infants, the USPSTF finds inconclusive evidence to recommend routine supplementation of iron.[121]

In addition to adverse effects associated with systemic iron overload, unabsorbed enteral iron has been shown to disrupt the gut microbiome.[113] For example, an iron-rich gut environment has been associated with a higher prevalence of pathogenic bacteria and increased pathogenicity of bacteria (such as adhesion to the gut epithelium).[122,123] Therefore high enteral supplements, even if not absorbed, should be avoided. Fig. 6.2 depicts factors that either increase iron status or worsen iron status.

Transfusions and Iron

A large proportion of iron in the body is bound to hemoglobin in red blood cells, with 3.47 mg iron present per gram of hemoglobin. Therefore transfusions represent a measurable source of iron in neonates, many of whom receive red blood cell transfusions.[124] This is particularly true in infants who receive multiple transfusions for hemolytic diseases such as Rh incompatibility, ABO incompatibility, and disseminated intravascular coagulation, where the iron from hemolysed red blood cells remains in the body and is recycled. However, for many preterm

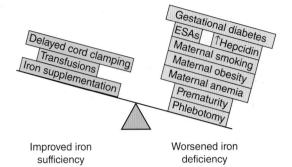

Fig. 6.2 Iron balance in neonates. Factors on the left represent neonatal and maternal factors that increase iron status. Factors on the *left* represent factors that decrease iron status. *ESAs,* Erythropoietic-stimulating agents.

infants, transfusions are given for anemia secondary to repeat phlebotomy and anemia of prematurity. For example, Puia-Dumitrescu et al. showed that average blood loss due to phlebotomy in a cohort of extremely low birth weight infants born between 23 0/7 weeks and 29 6/7 weeks of gestation was 83 mL, with the mean number of transfusions approximately matching this at 8.[125] In these cases, iron in the transfusion basically replaces the iron lost via phlebotomy and therefore does not add to the baseline iron load. In these circumstances, preterm infants may still require iron supplementation to meet the needs of their neonatal iron deficiency.

Erythropoiesis-Stimulating Agents

Erythropoietin (Epo) is a glycoprotein produced in the liver during fetal life, then by the kidneys starting around term gestation. Epo acts to stimulate red blood cell production.[126] Recombinant human Epo (rHEpo) can be given exogenously to stimulate erythropoiesis. Given that low Epo levels are an important cause of anemia of prematurity, with downregulation of Epo in the relative hyperoxic ex utero environment, rhEpo or Darbepoetin (Darbe), an Epo analog with a longer half-life, are commonly used for treatment of anemia in preterm infants. Treatment with erythropoiesis-stimulating agents (ESAs) have been shown to decrease the incidence and volume of red blood cell transfusions in this population.[127] While this is a strong advantage given the potential adverse effects

associated with transfusion, the upregulation of erythropoiesis associated with ESA use does indicate an increase in iron utilization for incorporation into heme. Consequently higher iron doses are commonly needed to accommodate this need in preterm infants treated with ESAs. For example, the Preterm Erythropoietin Neuroprotection Trial (PENUT) recommended that infants receive supplements with iron at a dose of 6 to 12 mg/kg/day based on iron measures. They found that infants treated with Epo received more iron than placebo-treated infants (275.1 mg/kg vs. 207.2 mg/kg cumulative enteral iron at 12 weeks of age) and yet had worse iron sufficiency, suggesting that higher iron doses were needed in those treated with Epo to maintain sufficiency.[127,128] ESA use should be considered in preterm infants to minimize transfusion need as well as potential promotion of positive nonhematologic effects.[129] Iron status should be closely monitored in these infants to avoid worsening deficiency.

Conclusions

Normal iron balance during the neonatal period has positive hematologic and neurodevelopmental effects. While neonates have regulatory mechanisms in place to ensure optimal iron status under typical conditions, infants with critical illness, such as preterm neonates, are at increased risk for disruptions in neonatal iron homeostasis, which may have long-term consequences. Close regulation of iron parameters is needed to guide iron supplementation to minimize the risk of both iron deficiency and overload. Further prospective studies are vitally needed to identify optimal target iron biomarkers that best correlate with long-term outcomes.

REFERENCES

1. Cao C, Fleming MD. The placenta: the forgotten essential organ of iron transport. *Nutr Rev.* 2016;74(7):421-431.
2. Hermoso M, Tabacchi G, Iglesia-Altaba I, et al. The nutritional requirements of infants. Towards EU alignment of reference values: the EURRECA network. *Matern Child Nutr.* 2010;6: 55-83.
3. McLean E, Cogswell M, Egli I, et al. Worldwide prevalence of anaemia, WHO Vitamin and Mineral Nutrition Information System, 1993–2005. *Public Health Nutr.* 2009;12(4):444-454.
4. Benoist BD, McLean E, Egli I, et al. *Worldwide Prevalence of Anaemia 1993-2005: WHO Global Database on Anemia.* Geneva: World Health Organization; 2008.

5. Auerbach M, Abernathy J, Juul S, et al. Prevalence of iron deficiency in first trimester, nonanemic pregnant women. *J Matern Fetal Neonat Med*. 2021;34(6):1002-1005.

6. Kling PJ. Iron nutrition, erythrocytes, and erythropoietin in the NICU: erythropoietic and neuroprotective effects. *Neoreviews*. 2020;21(2):e80-e88.

7. Yang Z, Lönnerdal B, Adu-Afarwuah S, et al. Prevalence and predictors of iron deficiency in fully breastfed infants at 6 mo of age: comparison of data from 6 studies. *Am J Clin Nutr*. 2009; 89(5):1433-1440.

8. Shao J, Lou J, Rao R, et al. Maternal serum ferritin concentration is positively associated with newborn iron stores in women with low ferritin status in late pregnancy. *J Nutr*. 2012;142:2004-2009.

9. Georgieff MK, Wewerka SW, Nelson CA, et al. Iron status at 9 months of infants with low iron stores at birth. *J Pediatr*. 2002; 141(3):405-409.

10. Widdowson EM, Spray CM. Chemical development in utero. *Arch Dis Child*. 1951;26(127):205-214.

11. Georgieff MK. Iron deficiency in pregnancy. *Am J Obstet Gynecol*. 2020;223(4):516-524.

12. Bothwell TH. Iron requirements in pregnancy and strategies to meet them. *Am J Clin Nutr*. 2000;72:257S-264S.

13. Auerbach M, James SE, Nicoletti M, et al. Results of the first American prospective study of intravenous iron in oral iron-intolerant iron-deficient gravidas. *Am J Med*. 2017;130(12): 1402-1407.

14. Breymann C, Auerbach M. Iron deficiency in gynecology and obstetrics: clinical implications and management. *Hematol Am Soc Hematol Ed Progr*. 2017;2017(1):152-159.

15. Flores-Quijano ME, Montalvo-Velarde I, Vital-Reyes VS, et al. Longitudinal analysis of the interaction between obesity and pregnancy on iron homeostasis: role of hepcidin. *Arch Med Res*. 2016;47(7):550-556.

16. Langley-Evans SC. Developmental programming of health and disease. *Proc Nutr Soc*. 2006;65(1):97-105.

17. Barker DJ, Gluckman PD, Godfrey KM, et al. Fetal nutrition and cardiovascular disease in adult life. *Lancet*. 1993;341(8850): 938-941.

18. Monk C, Georgieff MK, Xu D, et al. Maternal prenatal iron status and tissue organization in the neonatal brain. *Pediatr Res*. 2016;79(3):482-488.

19. Schmidt RJ, Tancredi DJ, Krakowiak P, et al. Maternal intake of supplemental iron and risk of autism spectrum disorder. *Am J Epidemiol*. 2014;180(9):890-900.

20. Insel BJ, Schaefer CA, McKeague IW, et al. Maternal iron deficiency and the risk of schizophrenia in offspring. *Arch Gen Psychiatr*. 2008;65(10):1136-1144.

21. Youdim MB, Yehuda S. The neurochemical basis of cognitive deficits induced by brain iron deficiency: involvement of dopamine-opiate system. *Cell Molecul Biol*. 2000;46(3):491-500.

22. Bastian TW, Hohenberg WCV, Mickelson DJ, et al. Iron deficiency impairs developing hippocampal neuron gene expression, energy metabolism, and dendrite complexity. *Dev Neurosci*. 2016;38(4):264-276.

23. Yu GS, Steinkirchner TM, Rao GA, et al. Effect of prenatal iron deficiency on myelination in rat pups. *Am J Pathol*. 1986;125(3): 620-624.

24. Ortiz E, Pasquini JM, Thompson K, et al. Effect of manipulation of iron storage, transport, or availability on myelin composition and brain iron content in three different animal models. *J Neurosci Res*. 2004;77(5):681-689.

25. Tran P, SJ Fretham, ES Carlson, et al. Long-term reduction of hippocampal brain-derived neurotrophic factor activity after fetal-neonatal iron deficiency in adult rats. *Pediatr Res*. 2009; 65(5):493-498.

26. Carlson ES, Stead JDH, Neal CR, et al. Perinatal iron deficiency results in altered developmental expression of genes mediating energy metabolism and neuronal morphogenesis in hippocampus. *Hippocampus*. 2007;17(8):679-691.

27. Barks AK, Liu SX, Georgieff MK, et al. Early-life iron deficiency anemia programs the hippocampal epigenomic landscape. *Nutrients*. 2021;13(11):3857.

28. Fretham SJ, Carlson ES, Wobken J, et al. Temporal manipulation of transferrin-receptor-1-dependent iron uptake identifies a sensitive period in mouse hippocampal neurodevelopment. *Hippocampus*. 2012;22(8):1691-1702.

29. Lozoff B, Georgieff M. Iron deficiency and brain development. *Sem Pediatr Neurol*. 2006;13:158-165.

30. Kuzawa CW. Adipose tissue in human infancy and childhood: an evolutionary perspective. *Am J Phys Anthropol*. 1998;41: 177-209.

31. Gambling L, Dunford S, Wallace DI, et al. Iron deficiency during pregnancy affects postnatal blood pressure in the rat. *J Physiol*. 2003;552:603-610.

32. Dewey KG, Oaks BM. U-shaped curve for risk associated with maternal hemoglobin, iron status, or iron supplementation. *Am J Clin Nutr*. 2017;106:1694S-1702S.

33. Chang SC, O'Brien KO, Nathanson MS, et al. Hemoglobin concentrations influence birth outcomes in pregnant African-American adolescents. *J Nutr*. 2003;133(7):2348-2355.

34. Zhang C, Rawal S. Dietary iron intake, iron status, and gestational diabetes. *Am J Clin Nutr*. 2017;106:1672S-1680S.

35. Kataria Y, Wu Y, Horskjær PH, et al. Iron status and gestational diabetes-a meta-analysis. *Nutrients*. 2018;10(5):621.

36. Bowers KA, Olsen SF, Bao W, et al. Plasma concentrations of ferritin in early pregnancy are associated with risk of gestational diabetes mellitus in women in the Danish National Birth Cohort. *J Nutr*. 2016;146(9):1756-1761.

37. Lönnerdal B, Kelleher SL. Iron metabolism in infants and children. *Food Nutr Bull*. 2007;28:S491-S499.

38. Lopez A, Cacoub P, Macdougall IC, et al. Iron deficiency anaemia. *Lancet*. 2016;387(10021):907-916.

39. Nemeth E, Tuttle MS, Pwelson J, et al. Hepcidin regulates cellular iron efflux by binding to ferroportin and inducing its internalization. *Science*. 2004;306:2090-2093.

40. Bahr TM, Ward DM, Jia X, et al. Is the erythropoietin-erythroferrone-hepcidin axis intact in human neonates? *Blood Cells Molec Dis*. 2021;88:102536.

41. German KR, Comstock BA, Parikh P, et al. Do extremely low gestational age neonates regulate iron absorption via hepcidin? *J Pediatr*. 2022;241:62-67.e1.

42. Berglund S, Lönnerdal B, Westrup B, et al. Effects of iron supplementation on serum hepcidin and serum erythropoietin in low-birth-weight infants. *Am J Clin Nutr*. 2011;94(6): 1553-1561.

43. Lorenz L, Müller KF, Poets CF, et al. Short-term effects of blood transfusions on hepcidin in preterm infants. *Neonatology*. 2015;108(3):205-210.

44. Müller KF, Poets CF, Westerman M, et al. Hepcidin concentrations in serum and urine correlate with iron homeostasis in preterm infants. *J Pediatr*. 2012;160(6):949-953.

45. Coffey R, Ganz T. Iron homeostasis: an anthropocentric perspective. *J Biol Chem*. 2017;292(31):12727-12734.

46. Kautz L, Jung G, Valore EV, et al. Identification of erythroferrone as an erythroid regulator of iron metabolism. *Nat Genet.* 2014;46(7):678-684.

47. Stefanova D, Raychev A, Arezes J, et al. Endogenous hepcidin and its agonist mediate resistance to selected infections by clearing non-transferrin-bound iron. *Blood.* 2017;130(3):245-257.

48. Flores-Quijano ME, Vega-Sánchez R, Tolentino-Dolores MC, et al. Obesity is associated with changes in iron nutrition status and its homeostatic regulation in pregnancy. *Nutrients.* 2019;11(3):693.

49. Tabbah SM, Buhimschi CS, Rodewald-Millen K, et al. Hepcidin, an iron regulatory hormone of innate immunity, is differentially expressed in premature fetuses with early-onset neonatal sepsis. *Am J Perinatol.* 2018;35(9):865-872.

50. Wu TW, Kusano R, Ma Y, et al. The utility of serum hepcidin as a biomarker for late-onset neonatal sepsis. *J Pediatr.* 2013;162(1):67-71.

51. Yapakçi EA, Gökmen Z, Tarcan A, et al. Erythrocyte transfusions and serum prohepcidin levels in premature newborns with anemia of prematurity. *J Pediatr Hematol Oncol.* 2009;31(11):840-842.

52. Domellöf M, Lönnerdal B, Abrams SA, et al. Iron absorption in breast-fed infants: effects of age, iron status, iron supplements, and complementary foods. *Am J Clin Nutr.* 2002;76(1):198-204.

53. Baker RD, Greer FR, Committee on Nutrition American Academy of Pediatrics. Diagnosis and prevention of iron deficiency and iron-deficiency anemia in infants and young children (0-3 years of age). *Pediatrics.* 2010;126(5):1040-1050.

54. Force USPST. *Iron Deficiency Anemia in Young Children: Screening.* 2015. Available at: https://www.uspreventiveservicestaskforce.org/uspstf/recommendation/iron-deficiency-anemia-in-young-children-screening.

55. Zamora T, Guiang SF III, Widness JA, et al. Iron is prioritized to red blood cells over the brain in phlebotomized anemic newborn lambs. *Pediatr Res.* 2016;79(6):922-928.

56. Lozoff B, Clark KM, Jing Y, et al. Dose-response relationships between iron deficiency with or without anemia and infant social-emotional behavior. *J Pediatr.* 2008;152(5):696-702.

57. Pisansky MT, Wickham RJ, Su J, et al. Iron deficiency with or without anemia impairs prepulse inhibition of the startle reflex. *Hippocampus.* 2013;23(10):952-962.

58. Rao R, Ennis K, Lubach GR, et al. Metabolomic analysis of CSF indicates brain metabolic impairment precedes hematological indices of anemia in the iron-deficient infant monkey. *Nutr Neurosci.* 2018;21(1):40-48.

59. Vlasova RM, Wang Q, Willette A, et al. Infantile iron deficiency affects brain development in monkeys even after treatment of anemia. *Front Human Neurosci.* 2021;15:624107.

60. Christensen RD, Jopling J, Henry E, et al. The erythrocyte indices of neonates, defined using data from over 12,000 patients in a multihospital health care system. *J Perinatol.* 2008;28(1):24-28.

61. Christensen R, Yaish H, Henry E, et al. Red blood cell distribution width: reference intervals for neonates. *J Matern Fetal Neonatal Med.* 2015;28(8):883-888.

62. Suchdev PS, Williams AM, Mei Z, et al. Assessment of iron status in settings of inflammation: challenges and potential approaches. *Am J Clin Nutr.* 2017;106:1626S-1633S.

63. German K, Vu PT, Grelli KN, et al. Zinc protoporphyrin-to-heme ratio and ferritin as measures of iron sufficiency in the neonatal intensive care unit. *J Pediatr.* 2018;194:47-53.

64. German KR, Vu PT, Neches S, et al. Comparison of two markers of iron sufficiency and neurodevelopmental outcomes. *Early Hum Dev.* 2021;158:105395.

65. Magge H, Sprinz P, Adams WG, et al. Zinc protoporphyrin and iron deficiency screening trends and therapeutic response in an urban pediatric center. *JAMA Pediatr.* 2013;167(4):361-367.

66. Juul SE, Zerzan JC, Strandjord TP, et al. Zinc protoporphyrin/heme as an indicator of iron status in NICU patients. *J Pediatr.* 2003;142(3):273-278.

67. Labbé RF, Vreman HJ, Stevenson DK. Zinc protoporphyrin: a metabolite with a mission. *Clin Chem.* 1999;45(12):2060-2072.

68. Cheng CF, Zerzan JC, Johnson DB, et al. Zinc protoporphyrin-to-heme ratios in high-risk and preterm infants. *J Pediatr.* 2012;161(1):81-87.e1.

69. Crowell R, Ferris AM, Wood RJ, et al. Comparative effectiveness of zinc protoporphyrin and hemoglobin concentrations in identifying iron deficiency in a group of low-income, preschool-aged children: practical implications of recent illness. *Pediatrics.* 2006;118(1):224-232.

70. Rettmer RL, Carlson TH, Origenes ML, et al. Zinc protoporphyrin/heme ratio for diagnosis of preanemic iron deficiency. *Pediatrics.* 1999;104(3):e37.

71. Yip R, Schwartz S, Deinard MD. Screening for iron deficiency with the erythrocyte protoporphyrin test. *Pediatrics.* 1983;72:214-219.

72. Lamola AA, Yamane T. Zinc protoporphyrin in the erythrocytes of patients with lead intoxication and iron deficiency anemia. *Science.* 1974;186(4167):936-938.

73. Labbé RF, Dewanji A. Iron assessment tests: transferrin receptor vis-à-vis zinc protoporphyrin. *Clin Biochem.* 2004;37(3):165-174.

74. Ennis K, Dahl L, Rao R, et al. Reticulocyte hemoglobin content as an early predictive biomarker of brain iron deficiency. *Pediatr Res.* 2018;84(5):765-769.

75. Canals C, Remacha AF, Sardá MP, et al. Clinical utility of the new Sysmex XE 2100 parameter - reticulocyte hemoglobin equivalent - in the diagnosis of anemia. *Haematologica.* 2005;90(8):1133-1134.

76. Christensen RD, Henry E, Bennett ST, et al. Reference intervals for reticulocyte parameters of infants during their first 90 days after birth. *J Perinatol.* 2016;36(1):61-66.

77. German K, Vu PT, Irvine JD, et al. Trends in reticulocyte hemoglobin quivalent values in critically ill neonates, stratified by gestational age. *J Perinatol.* 2019;39:1268-1274.

78. Al-Ghananim RT, Nalbant D, Schmidt RL, et al. Reticulocyte hemoglobin content during the first month of life in critically ill very low birth weight neonates differs from term infants, children, and adults. *J Clin Lab Anal.* 2016;30(4):326-334.

79. Lorenz L, Arand J, Springer F, et al. Reference ranges of reticulocyte haemoglobin content in preterm and term infants: a retrospective analysis. *Neonatology.* 2017;111(3):189-194.

80. Soldin OP, Bierbower LH, Choi JJ, et al. Serum iron, ferritin, transferrin, total iron binding capacity, hs-CRP, LDL cholesterol and magnesium in children; new reference intervals using the Dade Dimension Clinical Chemistry System. *Clin Chim Acta.* 2004;342(1-2):211-217.

81. Bahr T, Christensen T, Henry E, et al. Neonatal reference intervals for the complete blood count parameters MicroR and HYPO-He: sensitivity beyond the red cell indices for identifying microcytic and hypochromic disorders. *J Pediatr.* 2021;239:95-100.e2.

82. Bahr TM, Christensen RD, Ward DM, et al. Ferritin in serum and urine: a pilot study. *Blood Cells Mol Dis.* 2019;76:59-62.

83. Gerday E, Brereton JB, Bahr TM, et al. Urinary ferritin; a potential noninvasive way to screen NICU patients for iron deficiency. *J Perinatol.* 2021;41(6):1419-1425.

84. Kwik-Uribe CL, Gietzen D, German JB, et al. Chronic marginal iron intakes during early development in mice result in persistent changes in dopamine metabolism and myelin composition. *J Nutr.* 2000;130(11):2821-2830.

85. Rao R, Ennis K, Oz G, et al. Metabolomic analysis of cerebrospinal fluid indicates iron deficiency compromises cerebral energy metabolism in the infant monkey. *Neurochem Res.* 2013;38(3):573-580.

86. Piñero DJ, Li NQ, Connor JR, et al. Variations in dietary iron alter brain iron metabolism in developing rats. *J Nutr.* 2000; 130(2):254-263.

87. Georgieff MK. The role of iron in neurodevelopment: fetal iron deficiency and the developing hippocampus. *Biochem Soc Trans.* 2008;36:1267-1271.

88. Rao R, Tkac I, Townsend EL, et al. Perinatal iron deficiency alters the neurochemical profile of the developing rat hippocampus. *J Nutr.* 2003;133(10):3215-3221.

89. Brunette KE, Tran PV, Wobken JD, et al. Gestational and neonatal iron deficiency alters apical dendrite structure of CA1 pyramidal neurons in adult rat hippocampus. *Dev Neurosci.* 2010;32(3):238-248.

90. Jorgenson LA, Wobken JD, Georgieff MK. Perinatal iron deficiency alters apical dendritic growth in hippocampall CA1 pyramidal neurons. *Dev Neurosci.* 2003;25:412-420.

91. Clardy SL, Wang X, Zhao W, et al. Acute and chronic effects of developmental iron deficiency on mRNA expression patterns in the brain. *J Neural Trans Suppl.* 2006;71:173-196.

92. Amin SB, Orlando M, Eddins A, et al. In utero iron status and auditory neural maturation in premature infants as evaluated by auditory brainstem response. *J Pediatr.* 2010;156:377-381.

93. Berglund SK, Westrup B, Haraldsson E, et al. Effects of iron supplementation on auditory brainstem response in marginally LBW infants. *Pediatr Res.* 2011;70(6):601-606.

94. Algarín C, Peirano P, Garrido M, et al. Iron deficiency anemia in infancy: long-lasting effects on auditory and visual system functioning. *Pediatr Res.* 2003;53(2):217-223.

95. Wachs TD, Pollitt E, Cueto S, et al. Relation of neonatal iron status to individual variability in neonatal temperament. *Dev Psychobiol.* 2005;46(2):141-153.

96. Armony-Sivan R, Eidelman AI, Lanir A, et al. Iron status and neurobehavioral development of premature infants. *J Perinatol.* 2004;24(12):757-762.

97. Tamura T, Goldenberg RL, Hou J, et al. Cord serum ferritin concentrations and mental and psychomotor development of children at five years of age. *J Pediatr.* 2002;140:165-170.

98. Peirano PD, Algarín CR, Garrido MI, et al. Iron deficiency anemia in infancy is associated with altered temporal organization of sleep states in childhood. *Pediatr Res.* 2007;62(6):715-719.

99. Geng F, Mai X, Zhan J, et al. Impact of fetal-neonatal iron deficiency on recognition memory at 2 months of age. *J Pediatr.* 2015;167(6):1226-1232.

100. Lozoff B, Andraca ID, Castillo M, et al. Behavioral and developmental effects of preventing iron-deficiency anemia in healthy full-term infants. *Pediatrics.* 2003;112(4):846-854.

101. Lozoff B, Jimenez E, Hagen J, et al. Poorer behavioral and developmental outcome more than 10 years after treatment for iron deficiency in infancy. *Pediatrics.* 2000;105(4):E51.

102. East P, Doom JR, Blanco E, et al. Iron deficiency in infancy and neurocognitive and educational outcomes in young adulthood. *Dev Psychol.* 2021;57(6):962-975.

103. East P, Doom J, Blanco E, et al. Young adult outcomes associated with lower cognitive functioning in childhood related to iron-fortified formula in infancy. *Nutr Neurosci.* 2020:1-10.

104. Gahagan S, Delker E, Blanco E, et al. Randomized controlled trial of iron-fortified versus low-iron infant formula: developmental outcomes at 16 years. *J Pediatr.* 2019;212:124-130.

105. Björmsjö M, Hernell O, Lönnerdal B, et al. Reducing iron content in infant formula from 8 to 2 mg/L does not increase the risk of iron deficiency at 4 or 6 months of age: a randomized controlled trial. *Nutrients.* 2020;13(1):3.

106. Lapillonne A, Bronsky J, Campoy C, et al. Feeding the late and moderately preterm infant: a position paper of the European Society for Paediatric Gastroenterology, Hepatology and Nutrition Committee on Nutrition. *J Pediatr Gastroenterol Nutr.* 2019;69(2):259-270.

107. German KR, Vu PT, Comstock BA, et al. Enteral iron supplementation in infants born extremely preterm and its positive correlation with neurodevelopment; post hoc analysis of the Preterm Erythropoietin Neuroprotection Trial randomized controlled trial. *J Pediatr.* 2021;238:102-109.e8.

108. Ziegler EE, Nelson SE, Jeter JM. Iron supplementation of breastfed infants from an early age. *Am J Clin Nutr.* 2009; 89(2):525-532.

109. Auerbach M, Macdougall I. The available intravenous iron formulations: history, efficacy, and toxicology. *Hemodial Int.* 2017;21:SS83-SS92.

110. Rogozi-ska E, Daru J, Nicolaides M, et al. Iron preparations for women of reproductive age with iron deficiency anaemia in pregnancy (FRIDA): a systematic review and network meta-analysis. *Lancet Haematol.* 2021;8(7):e503-e512.

111. Khalafallah AA, Hyppa A, Chuang A, et al. A prospective randomised controlled trial of a single intravenous infusion of ferric carboxymaltose vs single intravenous iron polymaltose or daily oral ferrous sulphate in the treatment of iron deficiency anaemia in pregnancy. *Sem Hematol.* 2018;55(4):223-234.

112. Grajeda R, Pérez-Escamilla R, Dewey KG. Delayed clamping of the umbilical cord improves hematologic status of Guatemalan infants at 2 mo of age. *Am J Clin Nutr.* 1997;65(2): 425-431.

113. Alexeev EE, He X, Slupsky CM, et al. Effects of iron supplementation on growth, gut microbiota, metabolomics and cognitive development of rat pups. *PLOS One.* 2017;12(6): e0179713.

114. Brannon PM, Taylor CL. Iron supplementation during pregnancy and infancy: uncertainties and implications for research and policy. *Nutrients.* 2017;9(12):1327.

115. Wu Y, Song J, Wang Y, et al. The potential role of ferroptosis in neonatal brain injury. *Front Neurosci.* 2019;13:115.

116. Gies S, Roberts SA, Diallo S, et al. Risk of malaria in young children after periconceptional iron supplementation. *Matern Child Nutr.* 2020;17(2):e13106.

117. Sazawal S, Black RE, Ramsan M, et al. Effects of routine prophylactic supplementation with iron and folic acid on admission to hospital and mortality in preschool children in a high malaria transmission setting: community-based, randomised, placebo-controlled trial. *Lancet.* 2006;367(9505):133-143.

118. O'Brien KO, Zavaleta N, Caulfield LE, et al. Prenatal iron supplements impair zinc absorption in pregnant Peruvian women. *J Nutr.* 2000;130(9):2251-2255.

119. Majumdar I, Paul P, Talib VH, et al. The effect of iron therapy on the growth of iron-replete and iron-deplete children. *J Trop Pediatr.* 2003;49(2):84-88.

120. Dewey KG, Domellöf M, Cohen RJ, et al. Iron supplementation affects growth and morbidity of breast-fed infants: results of a randomized trial in Sweden and Honduras. *J Nutr.* 2002;132(11):3249-3255.

121. Cantor AG, Bougatsos C, Dana T, et al. Routine iron supplementation and screening for iron deficiency anemia in pregnancy: a systematic review for the US Preventive Services Task Force. *Ann Int Med.* 2015;162(8):566-576.

122. Kortman GAM, Boleij A, Swinkels DW, et al. Iron availability increases the pathogenic potential of Salmonella typhimurium and other enteric pathogens at the intestinal epithelial interface. *PLoS One.* 2012;7(1):e29968.

123. Jaeggi T, Kortman GAM, Moretti D, et al. Iron fortification adversely affects the gut microbiome, increases pathogen abundance and induces intestinal inflammation in Kenyan infants. *Gut.* 2015;64(5):731-742.

124. Keir AK, Yang J, Harrison A, et al. Temporal changes in blood product usage in preterm neonates born at less than 30 weeks' gestation in Canada. *Transfusion.* 2015;55(6):1340-1346.

125. Puia-Dumitrescu M, Tanaka DT, Spears TG, et al. Patterns of phlebotomy blood loss and transfusions in extremely low birth weight infants. *J Perinatol.* 2019;39(12):1670-1675.

126. Koury MJ, Bondurant MC. Erythropoietin retards DNA breakdown and prevents programmed death in erythroid progenitor cells. *Science.* 1990;248(4953):378-381.

127. Juul SE, Vu PT, Comstock BA, et al. Effect of high-dose erythropoietin on blood transfusions in extremely low gestational age neonates: post hoc analysis of a randomized clinical trial. *JAMA Pediatr.* 2020;174(10):933-943.

128. Juul SE, Comstock BA, Wadhawan R, et al. A randomized trial of erythropoietin for neuroprotection in preterm infants. *N Engl J Med.* 2020;382:233-243.

129. Juul SE. Nonerythropoietic roles of erythropoietin in the fetus and neonate. *Clin Perinatol.* 2000;27(3):527-541.

Chapter 7

Risk Factors for Iron Deficiency in Neonates

Pamela J. Kling, MD

Chapter Outline

Introduction

Iron, although critically necessary, is both a good and a bad actor because excess unbound iron may be toxic. The physiologic window between the extremes of iron deficiency (ID) and excess is narrow. Official guidelines for identifying and managing iron status in ill neonates are based on limited research data and thus are nonspecific and incomplete, especially with parenteral iron administration.

Eighty percent of placental-fetal iron transfer occurs during the last trimester. Preterm newborns without benefit of the third trimester are at great risk for ID, having accrued limited iron endowment to sustain the greater iron needs for rapid postnatal growth rates and critical neurodevelopment. In addition to prematurity, fetal conditions impacting iron status include multiple gestation and large or small for gestational age (LGA or SGA). Advances in clinical neonatal intensive care unit (NICU) practice patterns impact iron status in ill newborns. Even at term, maternal ID, alcohol intake, diabetes, obesity, hypertension, and/or placental dysfunction can substantially impair fetal iron endowment. Medically underserved populations are at risk for infantile ID and impaired fetal iron endowment. Although not currently a recognized diagnosis, perhaps neonatologists should recognize neonates with low fetal iron endowment (i.e., diagnose congenital ID).

Defining the Controversies

Iron is critically necessary for sustaining most body processes and in neonates to sustain both growth and neurodevelopment. Developing ID in early life can impair neurodevelopment, cognition, and behavior. Although critically necessary, iron is both a good and a bad actor because excess unbound iron is toxic. In ill neonates, free unbound iron is particularly problematic and may raise risk for infection and generate excessive oxidant stress that may worsen lung disease.

Recent advances in contemporary NICU practice may either negatively or positively impact iron status in ill newborns. Both delayed umbilical cord clamping (DCC) and red blood cell (RBC) transfusions increase total body iron. Conversely, iron demands are increased by greater postnatal phlebotomy losses relative to body weight, especially with extremely low gestation preterm neonates. Iron demands also rise with transfusion preventative strategies by erythropoietic stimulating agents (ESAs) and with recent nutritional strategies to improve postnatal growth rates.

Maternal diagnoses that impair fetal iron endowment are increasingly common contributors to preterm birth and/or ill NICU neonates. Even in apparently well-appearing term neonates, maternal or placental conditions such as severe maternal ID, alcohol intake, diabetes, obesity, hypertension, and/or placental dysfunction can substantially impair fetal iron endowment, promoting congenital ID. Fetal conditions place NICU neonates at risk for congenital ID, prematurity, multifetal gestation, LGA, or SGA. Medically underserved populations at risk for infantile ID anemia, such as low socioeconomic status (SES), maternal psychosocial stress, and/or ethnic minority status, are also at risk for congenital ID (Fig. 7.1). Multiple risk factors may be summative in term neonates. Although not current practice, it is important for clinicians to recognize and diagnose congenital ID.

Traditional tests of iron status in neonates may be challenging for clinicians to interpret because normal and threshold levels differ from those in older individuals. However, thresholds are known. In part due to limited data, official guideline recommendations for iron management in at-risk neonates are incomplete. Recommendations lack both clarity and specificity for managing early ID in at-risk neonates. Recommendations may be out of date based on contemporary NICU practice. Thus NICU and outpatient pediatric providers are left to approach iron status in at-risk infants without evidenced-based guidelines.

Perinatal Iron Physiology

If maternal iron status is normal and the placenta functional, fetal iron endowment rises in proportion to gestational age and birth weight, with 80% of iron endowed in the last trimester. At birth, healthy term newborns have accrued 75 mg of iron per kg of body weight.[1] Normally, fetal iron is endowed at 1.6 to 2.0 mg/kg daily.[2] Because 80% of fetal body iron resides within hemoglobin (Hb), iron is prioritized for erythropoiesis above other tissue needs. Most term neonates born after uncomplicated pregnancies have sufficient iron stores to support erythropoiesis and growth for only 4 to 6 months.[3,4]

Iron status is sensed in the liver by the master iron regulator, hepcidin, and controlled through cell-surface intestinal iron transporters making intestinal iron absorption efficient in infancy. When circulating hepcidin levels fall, iron enters the circulation, coming from both intestinal iron absorption and liver stores.[5] Maternal hepcidin levels normally fall to meet the sixfold higher pregnancy needs for iron absorption[6] facilitating placental iron transfer.[5] Higher maternal liver hepcidin (1) inhibits her iron absorption, (2) blocks iron trafficking from her reticular-endothelial system, and (3) blocks placental-fetal transfer. Obesity or rapid weight gain in pregnancy may cause sufficient inflammation to raise maternal hepcidin[7] and limit enteral absorption, placental transfer, and fetal iron delivery. Diabetes is a novel example in that the apical placenta transferrin receptor may be glycosylated in its active site, specifically inhibiting placental iron transfer.[8] Even with normal maternal iron, placental dysfunction, especially with hypertension sufficiently severe for fetal growth restriction, may also limit placental iron transfer.[9] Other inflammatory maternal, placental, and/or fetal mechanisms may force the iron balance

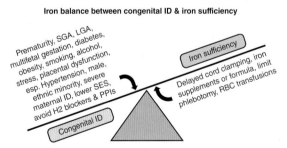

Iron balance between congenital ID & iron sufficiency

Prematurity, SGA, LGA, multifetal gestation, diabetes, obesity, smoking, alcohol, stress, placental dysfunction, esp. Hypertension, male, ethnic minority, severe maternal ID, lower SES, avoid H2 blockers & PPIs

Congenital ID

Iron sufficiency

Delayed cord clamping, iron supplements or formula, limit phlebotomy, RBC transfusions

Fig. 7.1 Balance of forces promoting or preventing congenital iron deficiency (ID). The forces that predispose to congenital ID *(down arrow)* include multiple perinatal-neonatal risk factors compared to forces *(up arrow)* that bolster neonatal iron status into iron sufficiency commonly are greater than those that outweigh the modifiable factors that improve iron status in at-risk infants.

into congenital ID that is unable to offset interventions that promote iron sufficiency (see Fig. 7.1).

Risk Factors for Congenital, Neonatal, and Infantile ID

Because congenital ID may lead to infantile ID, risks are similar and can be demarcated relating to (1) maternal supply, (2) dysfunctional placental logistics, and/or (3) fetal factors representing demands (see Fig. 7.1).

MATERNAL IRON SUPPLY

Although maternal ferritin is directly associated with fetal iron endowment,[10] treating mild ID during pregnancy may not improve either maternal or fetal iron status, although birth weights and gestational age may be higher.[11] The US Preventative Services Task Force (USPSTF) reports insufficient literature evidence for routine screening or iron supplementation in pregnancy,[12] whereas the American College of Obstetrics and Gynecology recommends routine screening and supplementation of iron during pregnancy. Pregnancy complicated by anemia of chronic disease or obesity can cause maternal hepcidin levels to rise, blocking either maternal iron absorption and/or placental iron transfer.[7] In extreme obesity at delivery, cord blood hepcidin levels fell in relationship to fetal iron status,[13] supporting that the fetal needs for iron transfer not met due to either placental dysfunction or poor maternal supply. In practice, congenital ID has become common due to the common diagnoses of diabetes, obesity ± maternal ID, smoking, alcohol ingestion, and untreated or severe maternal ID.

DYSFUNCTIONAL PLACENTAL IRON TRANSPORT

Risk for congenital ID occurs due to decreased fetal supply, even with normal maternal iron measures. Decreased fetal supply can be seen in diabetes, obesity or other inflammatory disorders, placental insufficiency, hypertensive disorders of pregnancy causing intrauterine growth restriction (IUGR), and severe psychosocial stressors.[14,15]

FETAL RISK FACTORS FOR ID

Fetal characteristics that limit fetal iron endowment include LGA or SGA, male sex, preterm birth, and/or multifetal gestation.[14,16-20] Preterm neonates are particularly at risk for congenital ID,[21] and without the third trimester transfer to iron they have relatively lower liver iron than term newborns and poorer tests of iron status than term newborns. Preterm birth is their major risk, with many risk factors less predictive because risks may become physiologically important in later gestation.[22] However, combining SGA with preterm birth also predicts poorer iron, with maternal hypertension/preeclampsia a dominant contributor.[22]

HEALTH DISPARITIES AND RISK FACTORS FOR ID

Many risk factors are also health disparity issues in the United States. Maternal anemia, maternal diabetes, maternal obesity, young maternal age, maternal minority status (especially of Mexican descent), lower SES, maternal psychosocial stressors, Medicaid status, being SGA, and prematurity can be more frequent in medically underserved populations.[17]

SUMMATIVE RISK FACTORS

In term or late preterm deliveries, having multiple risk factors increased the risk for low cord iron status in a summative fashion up to three risks,[23] but we also found that indices were poorest with the combined risks of maternal obesity, diabetes, and LGA,[17] likely from decreased supply and increased demand.[24] In a composite cohort of women in whom potential risk factors were collected, 31% had congenital ID, and nearly 24% of those breastfed for any length of time also tested as ID by ferritin at 6 to 12 months.[25] In preterm cord blood, SGA was a strong predictor, but maternal hypertension was a driver of congenital ID in SGA preterm neonates.

RISK FACTORS AND INFANTILE ID

In addition to factors influencing congenital ID, postnatal exposures can promote progression from congenital ID to neonatal ID and then to infantile ID in the at-risk NICU population (Fig. 7.2). Mathematically, a typical 1000-g preterm neonate has a 40-mL RBC mass (hematocrit × blood volume). Their iron loss approximates 13.8 mg due to cumulative phlebotomy loss (18% of the original iron endowment). If NICU RBC transfusions can be avoided, this child will need 1 mg per day iron accretion for the first year of life to offset losses and meet growth needs (Table 7.1).[26] Representative late preterm and term newborns are also included for comparison. Table 7.2 summarizes the medical and dietary risk factors and clinical presentation of ID in early and late infancy.

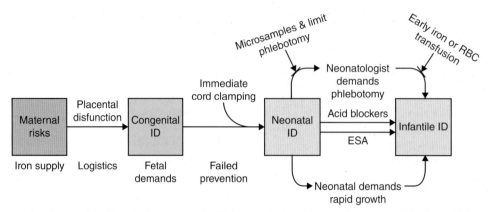

Fig. 7.2 Iron supply and demand. Problems in the supply chain of fetal-neonatal iron delivery that may lead to infantile iron deficiency *(ID)*. Congenital ID can be due to either maternal risks representing potential problems with iron supply, placental dysfunction representing potential logistical problems, and/or greater fetal demands. Immediate cord clamping represents a failed initial neonatal ID prevention strategy. In ill neonatal intensive care unit neonates, neonatal demand for rapid growth and neonatologist demand for phlebotomy, treatment with either stomach acid blockers and/or erythrocyte stimulating agents *(ESA)* can all lead to infantile ID. Tools to prevent infantile ID include microsampling and limiting phlebotomy losses or, alternatively, early iron and red blood cell *(RBC)* transfusions to compensate for phlebotomy losses.

TABLE 7.1	Iron Acquisition in the First Year		
	IRON ACQUISITION IN THE FIRST YEAR		
	Term	**Late Preterm**	**Preterm**
Weight at birth	3.5 kg	2.5 kg	1.0 kg
Body iron at birth	268 mg	183 mg	76.6 mg
Weight at 1 yr	10.5 kg	10.0 kg	9.5 kg
Body iron at 12 mo	377 mg	362 mg	344 mg
Body iron increment first year	109 mg	179 mg	276 mg
Iron losses first year (-)	91 mg	91 mg	104.8 mg
Total iron need first year	200 mg	270 mg	381 mg
Iron needs per day first year	0.55 mg/d	0.75 mg/d	1.04 mg/d

Adapted from Fomon SJ. Iron. In: Fomon S, ed. *Nutrition of Normal Infants.* Mosby; 1993:239-260.

Sequelae of ID

Although not the goal of this chapter, potential sequelae of congenital or acquired ID are important and include impaired neurocognition, metabolic disturbances, and/or other developmental organ structural and functional defects. In acute or chronic fetal hypoxia, including in diabetes and placental insufficiency, fetal erythropoietin prioritizes available iron for RBC production at the expense of brain and other organs. A growing body of literature also supports that ID fundamentally impacts the developing brain, altering sensitive neural processes, including dopamine synthesis, myelination, and hippocampal structure and function, involving both short- and some long-term neurocognitive sequelae.[27] However, research regarding preventative or treatment strategies is limited. Research is also underway to identify potential peripheral tests that are early and specific predictors of central nervous system ID.

Prevention and/or Treatment of ID

PREVENTION OF ID

At preterm delivery, an autologous transfusion by DCC prevents RBC transfusions,[28] augments RBC mass by 10% to 15%,[29] lessens anemia of prematurity, and improves short- and long-term iron status.[28,30,31] DCC in late preterm and term SGA infants improved iron status at 3 to 6 months (number needed to benefit [NNTB] of 16).[32] DCC in preterm neonates was associated with a lower incidence of intracranial hemorrhage[28] and higher overall survival.[33] In very preterm infants, DCC decreased death or adverse neurodevelopmental outcome at 2 years (NNTB of 8).[34] DCC post cesarean section

TABLE 7.2	Medical and Dietary Risk Factors and Clinical Presentation		
Age Group	**Medical Risk Factors**	**Dietary Risk Factors**	**Clinical Presentation**
Birth–4 mo	Prematurity, IUGR, SGA, LGA, twin, maternal diabetes, maternal obesity, immediate cord clamping, milk protein allergy, ethnic minority (especially Mexican), low socioeconomic status, PPI or H2 acid blockers	Exclusive breast milk for 4 mo	Asymptomatic, sleep disturbance, irritability, breath-holding spells, febrile seizures
4–12 mo	Rapid growth, lead exposure, cow's milk protein allergy, PPI or H2 acid blockers, lead exposure	Exclusive breast milk without iron supplements, early cow milk, restrictive diet	Asymptomatic, sleep disturbance, irritability, breath-holding spells, febrile seizures, restless legs, pica, decreased energy, pallor

IUGR, Intrauterine growth restrictions; *LGA*, large for gestational age; *PPI*, proton pump inhibitor; *SGA*, small for gestational age.
Adapted from Baker RD, Greer FR. Diagnosis and prevention of iron deficiency and iron-deficiency anemia in infants and young children (0-3 years of age). *Pediatrics*. 2010;126(5):1040-1050. doi:10.1542/peds.2010-2576.

deliveries were comparable to DCC after vaginal deliveries, with better iron status at 4 months of age.[33] Although unknown whether it is specifically due to increased iron, neurocognitive function improved in term infants after DCC (NNTB of 10).[36] After DCC in preterm newborns, myelination improved and intracranial hemorrhage or decreased.[37] Better iron status at 4 months in term infants after DCC was directly related to myelin content in regions associated with motor, visual, and sensory processing,[38] and the composite of severe neurologic injury.[39] The American Academy of Pediatrics (AAP) and American College of Obstetricians and Gynecologists[40] recommend DCC at nearly all vaginal births to improve RBC iron endowment.

TREATMENT OF ID

Current practice emphasizes feeding premature or ill infants with donor or maternal milk, with limited iron in any of the commercial human milk fortifiers. Human milk is a negligible iron source because content is relatively low (0.35 mg/L), insufficient for either premature infants or compensation for a poor endowment (i.e., congenital ID).[16] Nearly all ill NICU neonates able to be fed are fed human milk. It is important to note that published guidelines are no longer contemporary, being published before standardization of the clinical practice of DCC (better iron endowment), use of human milk (lower iron content than premature formulas), goals of promoting increased brain and somatic growth rates (higher iron demands for RBC expansion), initiatives to improve survival of

the most preterm infants, and understanding that lower transfusion thresholds are less concerning than earlier appreciated.

Two contemporary independent quality improvement studies reported guidelines for both starting iron supplementation at 2 weeks (or full feeds) and iron screening at 1 month in at-risk NICU infants. Our study held iron supplements immediately post RBC transfusion,[23] and the other study did not.[41] Despite high compliance with DCC, supplementation by 2 weeks, and screening at 1 month, both studies found at least 16% of infants were still diagnosed with ID.[23,41]

The effect of early enteral iron supplementation on neurocognitive outcome has been studied. Preterm and late-preterm infants given early vs. late iron experienced neither harm nor benefit in one study,[42] improved behavior in a second study,[43] and better neurologic exams in a third study[44] with a NNTB of 5.[45] Although SGA infants[19] and LGA infants of diabetic mothers[46,47] are also at risk for congenital ID, any benefit from early iron supplements is yet to be established. Breastfed term neonates with early iron supplements exhibited better visual acuity in one study[48] and better Bailey psychomotor indices in a meta-analysis (NNTB of 14).[49] In a long-term study, socioemotional advantages were found in iron-supplemented infants that persisted into 10 years of life.[50]

IRON SOURCES

Human milk is low in iron, with the 2010 AAP clinical report recommending breastfed newborns supplemented with iron by 4 months of age and iron in premature infants by 1 month.[16] Packed RBC transfusion infuses up to 1 mg of iron per mL transfused (3.47 mg iron per g of hemoglobin), a substantial amount, as plasma ferritin levels rise with transfusion or fall with transfusion avoidance or ESA administration.[51] Clinical practice guidelines support administering at least 2 to 6 mg/kg daily enteral iron supplements to preterm newborns at 2 to 4 weeks of life continuing until 1 year of life.[16] Long-term iron status is of concern in preterm NICU graduates due to limited available data on iron levels in infants receiving ESAs postdischarge. The 2010 AAP Committee on Nutrition clinical report recommended screening earlier than 12 months for ID for preterm and late-preterm infants, or also for term infants with accompanying risk factors.[16] Obtaining reticulocyte hemoglobin (RET-He) or plasma ferritin levels at 1 month of life or near hospital discharge can better estimate incorporated RBC iron or iron stores in preterm infants,[52] especially those avoiding RBC transfusions. Testing can guide postdischarge nutritional recommendations, but monitoring iron status of NICU graduates at both 6 and 12 months is also appropriate.

The AAP and European Society of Pediatric Gastroenterology, Hepatology, and Nutrition (ESPGHAN) recommended that preterm infants be provided at least 2 mg/kg/day elemental iron through 12 months of age in breasted infants.[16,53] Iron-fortified formulas for term and preterm supply 2 to 3 mg/kg/day.[16,53] Iron in US formulas is only 10% bioavailable; US infant formulas may contain sufficient iron for some preterm and at-risk term NICU graduates. If giving erythropoietin or darbepoetin (ESAs), 2 to 6 mg/kg daily elemental iron is recommended.

However, ID-erythropoiesis can still be seen, making it important to monitor iron status in ESA therapy. Parenteral iron is of concern, but can be given with early ESA treatment,[54,55] but due to theoretical iron toxicity risks, caution should be used when combining parenteral iron and RBC transfusions. Due to the iron load received from multiple RBC transfusions (spread out over the life of the transfused cells), some NICUs hold iron supplements for 1 to 2 weeks after transfusions.

PARENTERAL IRON SUPPLEMENTATION

Combining parenteral iron with ESAs is effective and improves iron status in other patient populations. Limited research data are available to inform the optimal timing and dosage of parenteral iron in preterm neonates. In preterm newborns, ESAs combined with parenteral vs. enteral iron resulted in comparable hematocrit percentages between the two routes of administration,[55-57] but higher reticulocytes and plasma ferritin when parenteral iron was administered.[55] No clinical iron toxicity was identified in these original studies. Pollak et al. examined and found a transient rise in malondialdehyde levels (a marker of oxidative stress).[55] Concerns for parenteral iron toxicity are important due to deficient antioxidant capabilities in preterm neonates, which may result in increased bronchopulmonary dysplasia, retinopathy of prematurity, and necrotizing enterocolitis.[58-60] In contrast to the study by Pollak et al., contemporary reports of parenteral iron have not shown toxicity.[41,61] Historical data showed that transferrin saturations can reach 100% in multiple transfused infants with bronchopulmonary dysplasia, so monitoring transferrin saturations in at-risk preterm infants may be helpful. Due to the potential of hemolysis with RBC transfusions,[62] we measured and found transiently elevated malondialdehyde levels following transfusion.[63] Holding parenteral or enteral iron administration for 1 to 2 days posttransfusion may avoid transient elevations in oxidative products.

Supplemental iron should be continued in breastfed preterm infants until weaning to either iron-fortified formula or complementary foods that supply 2 mg/kg/day of iron.[16] Both the USPSTF and AAP agree on special considerations for supplementing LGA babies remaining above the 95th percentile during infancy and low birth weight/late preterm infants, due to iron needs for growth.[16,64] Both societies agree that human milk is an inadequate iron source for low birth weight late preterm infants, a population unlikely to be transfused, reinforcing the need for early supplementation.[21] The AAP recommends 2 to 4 mg/kg/d by 1 month, continuing for 12 months, and both the ESPGHAN and Canadian Pediatric Society recommend supplemental iron for the first 6 months at 2 to 3 mg/kg/day if less than 2000 g and at 1 to 2 mg/kg/d if 2000 g or above,[65] especially if exclusively breastfeeding (summarized in Table 7.3). The AAP recommends supplements of 1 mg/kg/day elemental iron starting at 4 months in healthy exclusively breastfed infants,[16] whereas the USPSTF does not.

TABLE 7.3 Dietary Iron and Screening Recommendations for At-Risk Neonates			
Recommendation Source	**Age**	**Elemental Iron (mg/day)**	**Special Screening**
American Academy of Pediatrics	Preterm <37 wk, except those multiply transfused	2–4 mg/kg/day by 1 mo, continuing 12 mo	At any age, no regimen for test or follow-up, include universal anemia screening at 12 mo
Nutrition and Gastroenterology Committee, Canadian Pediatric Society	No recommendation	1–2 mg/kg/day if 2–2.5 kg; 2–3 mg/kg/day if <2 kg	Not addressed
European Society for Pediatric Gastroenterology, Hepatology, and Nutrition	Premature infants, <2 kg @ 1–6 mo	2–3 mg/kg up to 15 mg/day at 2–6 wk until 6–12 mo	Not addressed
European Society for Pediatric Gastroenterology, Hepatology, and Nutrition	Low birth weight infants, at 2–2.5 kg 1–6 mo	1–2 mg/kg/day at 2–6 wk to 6 mo	Not addressed

Adapted from Baker RD, Greer FR. Diagnosis and prevention of iron deficiency and iron-deficiency anemia in infants and young children (0-3 years of age). *Pediatrics*. 2010;126(5):1040-1050. doi:10.1542/peds.2010-2576; Domellof M, Braegger C, Campoy C, et al. ESPGHAN Committee on Nutrition: Iron requirements of infants and toddlers. *J Pediatr Gastroenterol Nutr*. 2014;58(1):119-129. doi:10.1097/MPG.0000000000000206; Lodha A, Shah PS, Soraisham AS, et al. for the Canadian Neonatal Network Investigators. Association of Deferred vs Immediate Cord Clamping with Severe Neurological Injury and Survival in Extremely Low-Gestational-Age Neonates. *JAMA Network Open*. Mar 1;2(3):e191286.

Indices of Iron Status

HEMOGLOBIN NADIR AND GROWTH RATE

After term birth, erythropoiesis is suppressed by improved oxygen delivery, resulting in a physiologic nadir in hemoglobin accompanying growth. A more exaggerated drop is seen in preterm newborns due to small circulating blood volume, relative greater growth rates and iatrogenic phlebotomy losses, and shortened RBC survival, termed anemia of prematurity.[66] The anemia of prematurity is traditionally described as nutritionally insensitive, although adequate iron contributes to the recovery of hemoglobin. Hemoglobin is a poor surrogate of iron status at any age but poorer yet in preterm or ill neonates. Because iron sufficiency during early life may improve neurocognitive outcomes,[27] precisely defining iron status in at-risk infants should be considered when pursuing a neuroprotective strategy. In healthy infants, although the USPSTF cited insufficient evidence for universal ID screening,[64] the AAP recommends universal hemoglobin screening at 9 to 12 months, utilizing hemoglobin less than 110 g/L (11 g/dL), as a surrogate for ID at 1 year of age.[16] However, it is unclear that hemoglobin is a good surrogate for iron status. Recent published work showed a nonlinear relationship between ferritin and hemoglobin in infancy with extremely low ferritin of 4.6 µg/L corresponding to a hemoglobin of 110 g/L.[67] We confirmed the same low ferritin, concluding that hemoglobin was a poor surrogate of iron status.[68]

MEASURING IRON STATUS

Research data on actionable iron status indices are limited. The 2010 AAP clinical guideline acknowledged that prematurity and other medical factors increase risk for developing infantile ID, but recommendations lacked specificity regarding frequency of initial and follow-up testing. At birth and early infancy, normative values for tests of iron status differ from those in later life.[14,22,24,69] Understanding threshold levels is necessary to guide interpretation. Ferritin levels differ as gestational age decreases and postnatal age increases. Threshold levels by postnatal and gestational ages have been published.[70-73] Ranges for cord ferritin levels differ with increasing gestational age: The 95% confidence interval (CI) for term infants is 40 to 309 µg/L, whereas the 95% CI for preterm infants is 35 to 267 µg/L.[69] Akkermans et al. examined ferritin levels that might predict the development of ID in exclusively breast-milk fed, late preterm infants without iron supplementation. They found that a concentration of less than 155 µg/L in the first week or less than 70 µg/L at 6 weeks of life predicted ID later on.[52] During ESA trials in preterm neonates, thresholds of 65 to 100 µg/L were used to increase iron therapy.[74] Ferritin is problematic due to artifactual elevation by infection, inflammation, or childhood immunization. Although so-called normal levels differ in preterm and term neonates, it is unknown whether the goal for preterm neonates should be to match term levels because they grow at a faster rate, needing more, not less, iron. Traditional RBC indices are less useful because they are complicated by normally high reticulocyte counts, with higher mean cell volume (MCV) and red cell distribution width (RDW) values.[75] Many automated hematology counters report RET-He content, a more sensitive measure of iron-deficient erythropoiesis.[76] RET-He is advantageous after 1 week of life because it is performed on the same microtube as the complete cell count and has threshold levels for ID of 29 pg that remain unchanged throughout childhood.[77] At birth, the 95% CI for cord blood RET-He is 33 to 38.1 pg, and at 1 month is 23.2 to 30.4 pg.[75] Two independent NICU quality improvement initiatives in preterm, SGA, and infants of diabetic mothers neonates found at least 16% of the NICU cohort had infantile ID at 1 month, despite iron supplementation at 2 weeks. One employed RET-He level of 29 pg as the threshold for defining ID.[41] Our study employed a ferritin threshold of 70 µg/L, finding 16% rate for ID, but our rate rose to 32% if the ferritin threshold of 100 µg/L was used.

Although not yet recommended by the AAP, very preterm infants may benefit from a personalized approach, screening at 1 month, hospital discharge, and 6 months, as well as universal screening around 1 year, especially with human milk feeding. Late preterm infants or ill term infants may benefit from screening at discharge and at both 6 and 12 months. It is also possible that newborn screening for iron status may become commonplace in at-risk infants.

Summary

Preterm infants and those with clinical and demographic risk factors for ID are at risk for congenital ID, and at risk for developing neonatal and infantile ID. Risk factors include maternal conditions that decrease iron supply, impact dysfunctional placental iron transport, or are a result of fetal and neonatal factors. Many of these risk factors are overrepresented in women with perinatal heath disparities. Potential sequelae include impaired neurocognitive development. Neonatal care may improve iron status such as with DCC, early iron supplementation, and RBC transfusions. Neonatal care may also accelerate iron losses through phlebotomy or result in greater demand due to greater growth rates or ESA treatment. Iron status can readily be monitored in neonates and early infancy. However, normal and threshold levels for iron sufficiency may differ from levels in older infants and children. Threshold levels for a new index, reticulocyte hemoglobin, changes little after 1 week of life and provides promise in monitoring at-risk neonates and infants.

REFERENCES

1. Oski FA. Iron deficiency in infancy and childhood. *New Engl J Med*. 1993;329:190-193.
2. Harthoorn-Lasthuizen EJ, Lindemans J, Langenhuijsen MM. Does iron-deficient erythropoiesis in pregnancy influence fetal iron supply? *Acta Obstet Gynecol Scand*. 2001;80:392-396.
3. Fomon SJ, Ziegler EE, Nelson SE, et al. Erythrocyte incorporation of iron by 56-day-old infants fed a 58Fe-labeled supplement. *Pediatr Res*. 1995;38:373-378.
4. Widness JA, Lombard KA, Ziegler EE, et al. Erythrocyte incorporation and absorption of 58Fe in premature infants treated with erythropoietin. *Pediatr Res*. 1997;41:416-423.
5. Rehu M, Punnonen K, Ostland V, et al. Maternal serum hepcidin is low at term and independent of cord blood iron status. *Eur J Haematol*. 2010;85(4):345-352. doi:10.1111/j.1600-0609.2010.01479.x.
6. O'Brien KO, Zavaleta N, Abrams SA, et al. Maternal iron status influences iron transfer to the fetus during the third trimester of pregnancy. *Am J Clin Nutr*. 2003;77:924-930.
7. Dao MC, Sen S, Iyer C, et al. Obesity during pregnancy and fetal iron status: is hepcidin the link? Research Support, N.I.H., Extramural Research Support, Non-U.S. Gov't Research Support, U.S. Gov't, Non-P.H.S. *J Perinatol*. 2013;33(3):177-181. doi:10.1038/jp.2012.81.
8. Petry CD, Wobkin JD, McKay H, et al. Placental transferrin receptor in diabetic pregnancies with increased fetal iron demand. *Am J Physiol*. 1994;267:E507-E517.
9. Briana DD, Boutsikou T, Baka S, et al. Perinatal role of hepcidin and iron homeostasis in full-term intrauterine growth-restricted infants. *Eur J Haematol*. 2013;90(1):37-44. doi:10.1111/ejh.12035.
10. Shao J, Lou J, Rao R, et al. Maternal serum ferritin concentration is positively associated with newborn iron stores in women with low ferritin status in late pregnancy. *J Nutr*. 2012;142(11):2004-2009. doi:10.3945/jn.112.162362.
11. Cogswell ME, Parvanta I, Ickes L, et al. Iron supplementation during pregnancy, anemia and birth weight: a randomized controlled trial. *Am J Clin Nutr*. 2003;78:773-781.

12. Siu AL, Force USPST. Screening for iron deficiency anemia and iron supplementation in pregnant women to improve maternal health and birth outcomes: U.S. Preventive Services Task Force Recommendation Statement. *Ann Intern Med.* 2015; 163(7):529-536. doi:10.7326/M15-1707.

13. Dosch NC, Guslits EF, Weber MB, et al. Maternal obesity affects inflammatory and iron indices in umbilical cord blood. *J Pediatr.* 2016;172:20-28. doi:10.1016/j.jpeds.2016.02.023.

14. Lott DG, Zimmerman MB, Labbe' RF, et al. Erythrocyte zinc protoporphyrin ratios are elevated with prematurity and with fetal hypoxia. *Pediatrics.* 2005;116:414-422.

15. Lesser KB, Schoel SB, Kling PJ. Elevated zinc protoporphyrin/heme ratios in umbilical cord blood after diabetic pregnancy. *J Perinatol.* 2006;26(11):671-676. doi:10.1038/sj.jp.7211600.

16. Baker RD, Greer FR. Diagnosis and prevention of iron deficiency and iron-deficiency anemia in infants and young children (0-3 years of age). *Pediatrics.* 2010;126(5):1040-1050. doi:10.1542/peds.2010-2576.

17. McLimore HM, Phillips AK, Blohowiak SE, et al. Impact of multiple prenatal risk factors on newborn iron status at delivery. *J Pediatr Hematol Oncol.* 2013;35:473-477. doi:10.1097/MPH.0b013e3182707f2e.

18. MacQueen BC, Christensen RD, Ward DM, et al. The iron status at birth of neonates with risk factors for developing iron deficiency: a pilot study. *J Perinatol.* 2017;37(4):436-440. doi:10.1038/jp.2016.234.

19. Mukhopadhyay K, Yadav RK, Kishore SS, et al. Iron status at birth and at 4 weeks in preterm-SGA infants in comparison with preterm and term-AGA infants. *J Matern Fetal Neonatal Med.* 2012;25(8):1474-1478. doi:10.3109/14767058.2011.643328.

20. Carter RC, Jacobson JL, Molteno CD, et al. Effects of heavy prenatal alcohol exposure and iron deficiency anemia on child growth and body composition through age 9 years. *Alcohol Clin Exp Res.* 2012;36(11):1973-1982. doi:10.1111/j.1530-0277.2012.01810.x.

21. Akkermans MD, Uijterschout L, Abbink M, et al. Predictive factors of iron depletion in late preterm infants at the postnatal age of 6 weeks. *Eur J Clin Nutr.* 2016;70(8):941-946. doi:10.1038/ejcn.2016.34.

22. McCarthy PJ, Zundel HR, Johnson KR, et al. Impact of growth restriction and other prenatal risk factors on cord blood iron status in prematurity. *J Pediatr Hematol Oncol.* 2016;38(3):210-215. doi:10.1097/MPH.0000000000000536.

23. Brichta CE, Godwin J, Norlin S, et al. Impact and interactions between risk factors on the iron status of at-risk neonates. *J Perinatol.* 2022;42(8):1103-1109.

24. Rao R, Georgieff MK. Iron in fetal and neonatal nutrition. *Semin Fetal Neonatal Med.* 2007;12(1):54-63. doi:10.1016/j.siny.2006.10.007. Epub 2006 Dec 6.

25. Rendina DN, Blohowiak SE, Coe CL, et al. Maternal perceived stress during pregnancy increases risk for low neonatal iron at delivery and depletion of storage Iron at one year. *J Pediatr.* 2018;200:166-173.e2. doi:10.1016/j.jpeds.2018.04.040.

26. Fomon SJ. Iron. In: Fomon S, ed. *Nutrition of Normal Infants.* St. Louis, MO: Mosby; 1993:239-260.

27. Georgieff MK. Long-term brain and behavioral consequences of early iron deficiency. *Nutr Rev.* 2011;69(1):S43-S48. doi:10.1111/j.1753-4887.2011.00432.x.

28. Rabe H, Diaz-Rossello JL, Duley L, et al. Effect of timing of umbilical cord clamping and other strategies to influence placental transfusion at preterm birth on maternal and infant outcomes. *Cochrane Database Syst Rev.* 2012;8:CD003248. doi:10.1002/14651858.CD003248.pub3.

29. Strauss RG, Mock DM, Johnson KJ, et al. A randomized clinical trial comparing immediate versus delayed clamping of the umbilical cord in preterm infants: short-term clinical and laboratory endpoints. *Transfusion.* 2008;48:658-665. doi:10.1111/j.1537-2995.2007.01589.x.

30. Aladangady N, McHugh S, Aitchison TC, et al. Infants' blood volume in a controlled trial of placental transfusion at preterm delivery. *Pediatrics.* 2006;117(1):93-98. doi:10.1542/peds.2004-1773.

31. Hutton EK, Hassan ES. Late vs early clamping of the umbilical cord in full-term neonates: systematic review and meta-analysis of controlled trials. *JAMA.* 2007;297(11):1241-1252. doi:10.1001/jama.297.11.1241.

32. McDonald SJ, Middleton P, Dowswell T, et al. Effect of timing of umbilical cord clamping of term infants on maternal and neonatal outcomes. *Cochrane Database Syst Rev.* 2013;(7):CD004074. doi:10.1002/14651858.CD004074.pub3.

33. Backes CH, Rivera BK, Haque U, et al. Placental transfusion strategies in very preterm neonates: a systematic review and meta-analysis. *Obstet Gynecol.* 2014;124(1):47-56. doi:10.1097/AOG.0000000000000324.

34. Armstrong-Buisseret L, Powers K, Dorling J, et al. Randomised trial of cord clamping at very preterm birth: outcomes at 2 years. *Arch Dis Child Fetal Neonatal Ed.* 2020;105(3):292-298. doi:10.1136/archdischild-2019-316912. Epub 2019 Aug 1.

35. Andersson O, Hellström-Westas L, Domellof M. Elective caesarean: does delay in cord clamping for 30 s ensure sufficient iron stores at 4 months of age? A historical cohort control study. *BMJ Open.* 2016;6(11):e012995. doi:10.1136/bmjopen-2016-012995.

36. Rana N, Kc A, Malqvist M, et al. Effect of delayed cord clamping of term babies on neurodevelopment at 12 months: a randomized controlled trial. *Neonatology.* 2019;115(1):36-42. doi:10.1159/000491994.

37. Chiruvolu A, Tolia VN, Qin H, et al. Effect of delayed cord clamping on very preterm infants. *Am J Obstet Gynecol.* 2015;213(5):676.e1-e7. doi:10.1016/j.ajog.2015.07.016.

38. Mercer JS, Erickson-Owens DA, Deoni SCL, et al. Effects of delayed cord clamping on 4-month ferritin levels, brain myelin content, and neurodevelopment: a randomized controlled trial. *J Pediatr.* 2018;203:266-272.e2. doi:10.1016/j.jpeds.2018.06.006.

39. Lodha A, Shah PS, Soraisham AS, et al. Association of deferred vs immediate cord clamping with severe neurological injury and survival in extremely low-gestational-age neonates. *JAMA Netw Open.* 2019;2(3):e191286. doi:10.1001/jamanetworkopen.2019.1286.

40. Committee on Obstetric Practice ACOG. Committee Opinion No. 684: Delayed umbilical cord clamping after birth. *Obstet Gynecol.* 2017;129(1):e5-e10. doi:10.1097/AOG.0000000000001860.

41. Bahr TM, Carr NR, Christensen TR, et al. Early iron supplementation and iron sufficiency at one month of age in NICU patients at-risk for iron deficiency. *Blood Cells Mol Dis.* 2021. Available at: https://doi.org/10.1016/j.bcmd.2021.102575.

42. Joy R, Krishnamurthy S, Bethou A, et al. Early versus late enteral prophylactic iron supplementation in preterm very low birth weight infants: a randomised controlled trial. *Arch Dis Child Fetal Neonatal Ed.* 2014;99(2):F105-F109. doi:10.1136/archdischild-2013-304650.

43. Berglund SK, Westrup B, Hagglof B, et al. Effects of iron supplementation of LBW infants on cognition and behavior at 3 years. *Pediatrics.* 2013;131(1):47-55. doi:10.1542/peds.2012-0989.

44. Steinmacher J, Pohlandt F, Bode H, et al. Randomized trial of early versus late enteral iron supplementation in infants with a birth weight of less than 1301 grams: neurocognitive development

at 5.3 years' corrected age. *Pediatrics*. 2007;120(3):538-546. doi:10.1542/peds.2007-0495.

45. Long H, Yi JM, Hu PL, et al. Benefits of iron supplementation for low birth weight infants: a systematic review. Review. *BMC Pediatr*. 2012;12:99. doi:10.1186/1471-2431-12-99.

46. Siddappa AM, Georgieff MK, Wewerka SW, et al. Iron deficiency alters auditory recognition memory in newborn infants of diabetic mothers. *Pediatr Res*. 2004;55:1034-1041.

47. Riggins T, Miller NC, Bauer PJ, et al. Consequences of low neonatal iron status due to maternal diabetes mellitus on explicit memory performance in childhood. Research Support, N.I.H., Extramural. *Dev Neuropsychol*. 2009;34(6):762-779. doi:10.1080/87565640903265145.

48. Friel JK, Aziz K, Andrews WL, et al. A double-masked, randomized control trial of iron supplementation in early infancy in healthy term breast-fed infants. *J Pediatr*. 2003;143:582-586.

49. Cai C, Granger M, Eck P, et al. Effect of daily iron supplementation in healthy exclusively breastfed infants: a systematic review with meta-analysis. *Breastfeed Med*. 2017;12(10):597-603. doi:10.1089/bfm.2017.0003.

50. Lozoff B, Castillo M, Clark KM, et al. Iron supplementation in infancy contributes to more adaptive behavior at 10 years of age. *J Nutr*. 2014;144(6):838-845. doi:10.3945/jn.113.182048.

51. Brown MS. Effect of transfusion and phlebotomy on serum ferritin levels in low birth weight infants. *J Perinatol*. 1996;16:39-42.

52. Akkermans MD, Uijterschout L, Abbink M, et al. Predictive factors of iron depletion in late preterm infants at the postnatal age of 6 weeks. *Eur J Clin Nutr*. 2016;70(8):941-946. doi:10.1038/ejcn.2016.34.

53. Domellof M, Braegger C, Campoy C, et al. ESPGHAN Committee on Nutrition: Iron requirements of infants and toddlers. *J Pediatr Gastroenterol Nutr*. 2014;58(1):119-129. doi:10.1097/MPG.0000000000000206.

54. Ohls RK, Ehrenkranz RA, Wright LL, et al. The effects of early erythropoietin therapy on the transfusion requirements of preterm infants below 1250 grams birthweight: a multicenter, randomized controlled trial. *Pediatrics*. 2001;108:934-942.

55. Pollak A, Hayde M, Hayn M, et al. Effect of intravenous iron supplementation on erythropoiesis in erythropoietin-treated premature infants. *Pediatrics*. 2001;107:78-85.

56. Meyer MP, Haworth C, Meyer JH, et al. A comparison of oral and intravenous iron supplementation in preterm infants receiving recombinant erythropoietin. *J Pediatr*. 1996;129:258-263.

57. Kivivuori SM, Virtanen M, Raivio KO, et al. Oral iron is sufficient for erythropoietin treatment of very low birth-weight infants. *Eur J Pediatr*. 1999;158:147-151.

58. Sullivan JL. Iron, plasma antioxidants and the 'oxygen radical disease of prematurity. *Am J Dis Child*. 1988;142:1341-1344.

59. Evans PJ, Evans R, Kovar IZ, et al. Bleomycin-detectable iron in the plasma of premature and full-term neonates. *FEBS Lett*. 1992;303:210-212.

60. Miller NJ, Rice-Evans C, Davies MJ, et al. A novel method for measuring antioxidant capacity and its application to monitoring the antioxidant status in premature neonates. *Clin Sci*. 1993;84:407-412.

61. Ohls RK, Ehrenkranz RA, Wright LL, et al. Effects of early erythropoietin therapy on the transfusion requirements of preterm infants below 1250 grams birth weight: a multicenter, randomized, controlled trial. *Pediatrics*. 2001;108(4):934-942.

62. Humphrey MJ, Harrell-Bean HA, Eskelson C, et al. Blood transfusion in the neonate: effects of dilution and age of blood on hemolysis. *J Pediatr*. 1982;101:605-607.

63. Kling PJ, Reichard RD, Roberts RA, et al. The effects of transfusions on oxidative stress and plasma erythropoietin levels in premature infants. *Ann Hematol*. 2000;79:B13.

64. Siu AL. Screening for iron deficiency anemia in young children: USPSTF recommendation statement. *Pediatrics*. 2015;136(4):746-752. doi:10.1542/peds.2015-2567.

65. Lapillonne A, Bronsky J, Campoy C, et al. Feeding the late and moderately preterm infant: a position paper of the European Society for Paediatric Gastroenterology, Hepatology and Nutrition Committee on Nutrition. *J Pediatr Gastroenterol Nutr*. 2019;69(2):259-270. doi:10.1097/MPG.0000000000002397.

66. Ohls RK. Evaluation and treatment of anemia in the neonate. In: Christensen RD, ed. *Hematologic Problems of the Neonate*. Philadelphia, PA: WB Saunders; 2000:137-169.

67. Abdullah K, Birken CS, Maguire JL, et al. Re-evaluation of serum ferritin cut-off values for the diagnosis of iron deficiency in children aged 12-36 months. *J Pediatr*. 2017;188:287-290. doi:10.1016/j.jpeds.2017.03.028.

68. Mukhtarova N, Ha B, Diamond CA, et al. Seru ferritin threshold for infantile iron deficiency screening in one-year-olds. *J Pediatr*. 2022;245:217-221. Available at: https://doi.org/10.1016/j.jpeds.2022.01.050.

69. Siddappa AM, Rao R, Long JD, et al. The assessment of newborn iron stores at birth: a review of the literature and standards for ferritin concentrations. *Neonatology*. 2007;92:73-82.

70. Maier RF, Obladen M, Scigalla P, et al. The effect of epoetin beta (recombinant human erythropoietin) on the need for transfusion in very-low-birth-weight infants. *N Engl J Med*. 1994;330:1173-1178.

71. Meyer MP, Meyer JH, Commerford A, et al. Recombinant human erythropoietin in the treatment of the anemia of prematurity: results of a double-blind, placebo-controlled study. *Pediatrics*. 1994;93:918-923.

72. Bader D, Blondheim O, Jonas R, et al. Decreased ferritin levels, despite iron supplementation, during erythropoietin therapy in anaemia of prematurity. *Acta Paediatr*. 1996;85:496-501.

73. Bechensteen AG, Halvorsen S, Haga P, et al. Erythropoietin, protein and iron supplementation and the prevention of anaemia of prematurity: effects on serum immunoreactive Epo, growth and protein and iron metabolism. *Acta Paediatr*. 1996;85:490-495.

74. Kling PJ, Roberts RA, Widness JA. Plasma transferrin receptor levels and indices of erythropoiesis and iron status in healthy term infants. *Am J Pediatr Hematol Oncol*. 1997;20:309-314.

75. Christensen RD, Henry E, Bennett ST, et al. Reference intervals for reticulocyte parameters of infants during their first 90 days after birth. *J Perinatol*. 2016;36(1):61-66. doi:10.1038/jp.2015.140.

76. Goodnough LT, Skikne B, Brugnara C. Erythropoietin, iron and erythropoiesis. *Blood*. 2000;96:823-833.

77. Kasper DC, Widness JA, Haiden N, et al. Characterization and differentiation of iron status in anemic very low birth weight infants using a diagnostic nomogram. *Neonatology*. 2009;95:164-171. doi:10.1159/000153101.

Chapter 8

Using Targeted Genetic Panels to Find the Causes of Neonatal Hemolytic Anemia

Archana M. Agarwal, MD and Anton Rets, MD, PhD

Chapter Outline

Definition, Etiologies, and Implications of Neonatal Hemolytic Anemia

Neonatal hemolytic anemias (NHA) are a group of pathologic conditions manifesting with low hemoglobin (Hb) levels and/or red blood cell (RBC) counts due to premature destruction of erythrocytes during the perinatal period. These RBCs may be destroyed in the intravascular or the extravascular compartments. Generally, hemolysis is evidenced by anemia and hyperbilirubinemia in this period. RBCs are known to be relatively more fragile even in healthy neonates than in older children or adults, possibly because of lower resistance of the RBC membrane to oxidizing factors, differences in Hb fractions, and a shorter RBC lifespan due to various other intrinsic reasons. The typical RBC lifespan for a term neonate is 60 to 80 days, as compared to 100 to 120 days for an adult.[1-3] In preterm neonates, it is even shorter (35–50 days).

Depending on the cause, NHAs are divided into two main categories: immune mediated and nonimmune mediated. The former results from a maternal immunoglobulin G (IgG) antibody-mediated isoimmunization to antigens expressed on the neonate's RBCs.[4] Hemolytic disease of the fetus and neonate/newborn (HDFN) is a term commonly used in this setting. The most severe type of HDFN is seen in Rhesus-mediated hemolysis (RhD), but other RBC antigen systems such as the ABO system can also be involved.[5] Immune-mediated NHAs can be diagnosed by serologic testing. The molecular studies are not a part of the standard laboratory workup of immune-mediated NHA, so detailed discussions of these topics are beyond the scope of this chapter.

Neonates can develop nonimmune NHAs due to acquired factors such as infections or exposure to toxins or secondary to inherited conditions. The latter group of disorders typically involves mutations in many genes such as those encoding structural proteins, enzymes, and transcription factors. Recent advances in molecular sequencing technologies have enabled rapid, reliable identification of these inherited nonimmune NHAs.

The three main categories of inherited NHAs include (1) RBC membrane disorders; (2) quantitative/qualitative defects of hemoglobin, including conditions that reduce hemoglobin stability[6,7]; and (3) RBC enzyme deficiencies.[8-10] We will also discuss congenital disorders of bilirubin metabolism that manifest with neonatal hyperbilirubinemia, as hyperbilirubinemia is frequently an important manifestation of hemolytic anemia (HA). Finally, congenital dyserythropoietic anemia (CDA),[6] an inherited condition characterized by an ineffective erythropoiesis presenting in some cases as NHA, will be reviewed.

RBC MEMBRANE DISORDERS

RBC membrane disorders are relatively common inherited conditions. These can be divided into genetic defects that (1) alter cytoskeleton scaffolding and, consequently, the shape of RBCs; and (2) alter the regulation of RBC volume. The best-known examples of the first group include hereditary spherocytosis (HS), hereditary elliptocytosis (HE), and hereditary pyropoikilocytosis (HPP). The second group is exemplified by hereditary stomatocytosis.

The major determinants of RBC shape and flexibility are the structure of the cytoskeleton and its interaction with the lipid bilayer of the membrane. Adequate amounts of structurally intact proteins, particularly α-spectrin (encoded by *SPTA1*), β-spectrin (*SPTB*), ankyrin-1 (*ANK1*), band 3, also known as anion exchanger 1 (*SLC4A1*), and protein 4.2 (*EPB42*), are essential for normal RBC functioning and lifespan. Mutations in these genes can cause RBC membrane defects.[11,12] Fig. 8.1 depicts the interaction between RBC membrane proteins and lipid bilayer.

HS has a high prevalence, especially in infants of Northern European ancestry; the frequency may be as high as 1:1000 to 1:3000. It is the most common cause of hereditary HA in the Western population. The pattern of inheritance may be autosomal dominant (AD; 75% of cases) or autosomal recessive (AR; 25% cases). HS is caused by altered "vertical" protein-lipid interactions involving ankyrin (40–65%), band 3 (20–35%), β spectrin (15 30%), α spectrin, and protein 4.2 (<5%).[11] HS presenting in AD inheritance pattern is usually caused by mutations in *ANK1*, *SLC4A1,* and *SPTB*. Most *ANK1* mutations are point mutations that can suppress the synthesis of ankyrin. Unfortunately,

up to 15% to 20% of these mutations occur de novo, and the lack of a family history can cause diagnostic difficulties.[13] As ankyrin is the principal binding site for spectrin on the membrane, its inadequate production results in functional deficiency of the spectrin scaffold. Large deletions within *ANK1* gene are rare and may be associated with a larger loss of chromosome 8p11.2 and a contiguous gene syndrome (*FGFR1*, *ANK1*, and possibly other genes) clinically manifesting as a combination of Kallmann syndrome and HS.[14]

Mutations in *SLC4A1* (band 3) are usually missense or frameshift in nature, affecting both the exons and splice sites. The mutations have a deleterious effect on band 3 expression and produce a mild to moderate HA with an AD pattern of inheritance. *SLC4A1* mutations can also cause distal renal tubular acidosis.[11,15] The AR forms causing severe transfusion-dependent anemia in neonates are usually caused by compound heterozygote mutations in α-spectrin. Since α-spectrin is usually produced in high amounts with considerable reserve, heterozygote mutations are typically not symptomatic. However, two low-expression alleles in α-spectrin need mention[16,17]; the α LELY (low-expression Lyon) can be seen in up to one third of the normal population and can reduce α-spectrin expression by up to 50%. Neonates with these genetic abnormalities can develop severe transfusion-dependent HPP (discussed later) in conjunction with an HE allele in trans that gradually improves with time. Another low-expression allele, the α LEPRA (low-expression PRAgue) is an intronic mutation and can cause a severe form of HS if inherited with a pathogenic *SPTA1* allele in trans. Protein 4.2 functions as a binding protein between ankyrin and band 3. Most mutations in the *EPB42* gene are missense or nonsense, and cause protein 4.2 deficiency. HS associated with *EPB42* mutations is more frequent in the Japanese population and shows AR inheritance and mild to moderate hemolytic anemia.[18]

HE and HPP are caused by altered "horizontal" protein-protein interactions in the RBC cytoskeleton negatively affecting RBC deformability and producing misshapen erythrocytes: ovalocytes or elliptocytes in HE and numerous nonspecific poikilocytes in HPP. From a clinical and pathogenetic perspective, HE and HPP are viewed as two entities on a continuous spectrum, ranging from asymptomatic with a mild phenotype in HE to severe anemia, hemolysis, and transfusion dependency in HPP.[11,12] The key abnormality is in

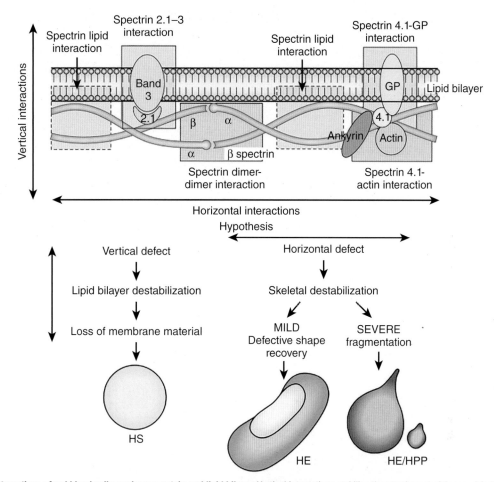

Fig. 8.1 Interactions of red blood cell membrane protein and lipid bilayer. Vertical interactions stabilize the attachment of the spectrin lattice to the lipid bilayer. Abnormalities in this attachment result in destabilization of the lipid bilayer, membrane loss during splenic conditioning, and hereditary spherocytosis. Horizontal interactions reversibly hold spectrin dimers and tetramers together, allowing stretching and distortion of the red blood cell membrane during circulation. Weakening of these interactions results in loss of elasticity. *GP*, Glycoproteins; *HE*, hereditary elliptocytosis; *HPP*, hereditary pyropoikilocytosis; *HS*, hereditary spherocytosis. (Reproduced with permission and minor modifications from Letterio et al. Hematologic and oncologic problems in the fetus and neonate. In: *Fanaroff and Martin's Neonatal-Perinatal Medicine*, 79, 1416-1475. Originally adapted from Palek J. Red cell membrane disorders. In: Hoffman R, et al., eds., *Hematology: Basic Principles and Practice*. New York: Churchill Livingstone; 1991:472.)

formation of α-β spectrin heterodimers or their self-association into tetramers. The principal genes involved in HE/HPP are *SPTA1*, *SPTB*, or *EPB41*. *SPTA1* and *SPTB* mutations account for 60% to 75% of these patients.[8,19]

SPTA1 gene mutations are classically missense, affecting the dimer-tetramer self-association site. Because α-spectrin chains are produced in excess, an isolated heterozygous pathogenic mutation in *SPTA1* is unlikely to produce a clinical condition. However, a compound heterozygosity with another pathogenetic

mutation or, what happens more frequently, with a common *SPTA1* low expression allele with decreased α-spectrin production, can result in an overt HPP.[16] *SPTB* mutations are seen in approximately 30% of HE patients. The effect of these mutations also alters the association of spectrin heterodimers to tetramers. Alterations of protein 4.1 due to *EPB41* mutations result in its quantitative or qualitative deficiencies. The types of mutations vary, ranging from point mutations to large deletions. The heterozygous state is asymptomatic, but homozygotes can experience a severe disease. Characteristically, the elliptocytes in patients with mutated *EPB41* are numerous (almost 100% of RBCs) and slender.[11,12,19]

RBC volume disorders are caused by an inability to regulate water and ion transport through the membrane, which introduces overhydration or dehydration of the cell. Thus the conditions in this group are broadly divided into overhydrated and dehydrated stomatocytosis. Dehydrated stomatocytosis (hereditary xerocytosis [HX]) is more prevalent and presents as a HA of variable degree and unexplained iron overload.[20] The most commonly mutated gene in HX is *PIEZO1*, which encodes for a mechanically activated cation channel. The pathogenic *PIEZO1* mutations are usually gain-of-function.[20] Fig. 8.2 depicts the peripheral smear and osmotic gradient ektacytometry result from a patient with HS. A few patients with HX have mutations in *KCNN4* that encodes the Gardos channel.[21] Overhydrated stomatocytosis is a very rare disorder with only approximately 100 patients described worldwide. Heterozygous mutations in the Rh-associated glycoprotein (*RHAG*) are commonly associated with overhydrated stomatocytosis.[20]

INHERITED HEMOGLOBIN DEFECTS

Abnormalities of globin chains are broadly divided into quantitative (thalassemias) and qualitative (hemoglobinopathies or variant hemoglobins). Most hemoglobin variants are clinically benign and asymptomatic, but some hemoglobinopathies and thalassemias can present as NHA. In a normal neonate, RBCs contain predominantly Hb F ($\alpha_2\gamma_2$) at approximately 70% to 80%, followed by Hb A ($\alpha_2\beta_2$) at 20%, and Hb A2 ($\alpha_2\delta_2$) at 0.5% to 1%. Due to a relatively low amount of β-globin chains, both β-thalassemia and β-chain variants do not manifest in neonates. However, development of anemia with or without hemolysis at about 6 months of age should raise a suspicion of a β-globin chain disorder. Individuals with α-thalassemia demonstrate a wide spectrum of genotypes and clinical presentations, ranging from asymptomatic individuals with or without changes in the blood counts (usually associated with a silent carrier state, -α/αα), to varying degrees of anemia and hemolysis (like those with Hb H disease, --/-α).[22] Neonates with Hb H disease show increased Hb Bart (γ_4), which is switched to Hb H (β_4) at a later age.[23] Some variant hemoglobins, including the α- and γ-chain variants, may result in NHA due to low stability.

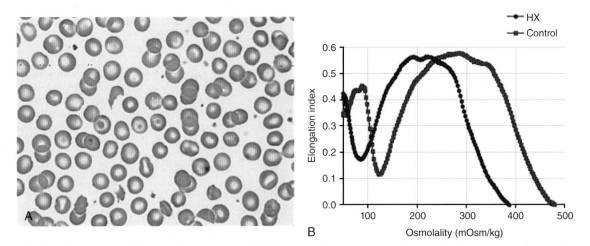

Fig. 8.2 **Hereditary xerocytosis (HX) caused by heterozygous *PIEZO1* mutation.** Chronic hemolysis compensated with reticulocytosis (hemoglobin 14 g/dL, reticulocytes 16%). The patient had a PIEZO1 mutation (c.7367G>A; p.R2456H) causing HX. **(A)** Blood smear with macrocytosis (MCV 96 fL) showing occasional stomatocytes, target cells, and dense fragmented cells. **(B)** Osmotic gradient ektacytometry showing the typical HX curve with left shift attributable to decreased O_{min} and O_{hyp} (O_{min} = osmolality at which 50% red blood cells (RBCs) hemolyze in the osmotic fragility test; value affected by the surface area to volume ratio). EI_{max} is maximum elongation that the RBCs can achieve under shear stress and relates cytoskeletal properties. The declining portion shows the O_{hyp}, the osmolality value at which the cell's maximum diameter is half of EI_{max} and correlates with the initial intracellular viscosity. A left shift reflects increased intracellular viscosity of RBCs caused by increased intracellular hemoglobin concentration and/or a dehydration state. (Reproduced with permission and minor modifications from Risinger et al. Rare hereditary hemolytic anemias. Hematol Oncol Clin N Am. 2019;33[3]:373-392.)

One example is the Hb Hasharon, an α-chain variant (HBA2:c.142G>C)[24]; the point mutation introduces an amino acid substitution in the α-chain that weakens its interaction with a normal γ-globin chain. The unstable hemoglobin hybrid comprises 14% to 19% of the total hemoglobin. Such γ-globin variants can present with NHA and hyperbilirubinemia, but these clinical manifestations resolve by 4 to 6 months of age when γ-globin is replaced by β-globin.[25,26]

RBC ENZYME DEFICIENCIES

The inability of the RBCs to maintain protein synthesis throughout the lifespan results in progressive decline of enzymatic activity. Qualitative and quantitative enzymatic defects result in hemolysis and, consequently, anemia. RBCs contain only a limited number of active metabolic pathways, namely glycolysis (to generate adenosine triphosphate [ATP]), hexose monophosphate shunt (to protect against oxidative stress by generating nicotinamide adenine dinucleotide phosphate [NADPH] and reducing glutathione), Rapoport-Luebering shunt (to generate 2,3-biphosphoglycerate that modulates oxygen affinity), and nucleotide metabolism. Fig. 8.3 illustrates the glycolytic, pentose phosphate pathway and 2,3-biphosphoglycerate pathway and its deficiencies. There are over a dozen known

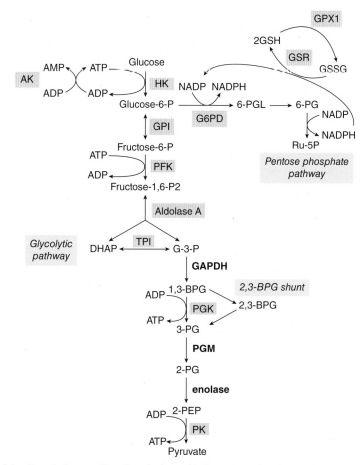

Fig. 8.3 The glycolytic (Embden-Meyerhof enzymatic pathway), along with the pentose phosphate pathway and the 2,3-BPG (2,3-bisphospho-glycerate) shunt. Deficiency of the enzymes shown in orange boxes causes hemolytic anemia. *AK*, Adenylate kinase; *G6PD*, glucose-6-phosphate dehydrogenase; *GPI*, glucose-6-phosphate isomerase; *GPX1*, glutathione peroxidase; *GSR*, glutathione reductase; *HK*, hexokinase; *PFK*, phosphofructokinase; *PGK*, phosphoglycerate kinase; *PK*, pyruvate kinase; *TPI*, triosephosphate isomerase. (Reproduced with permission and minor modifications from Risinger et al. Rare hereditary hemolytic anemias. Hematol Oncol Clin N Am. 2019;33[3]:373-392.)

inherited defects in these pathways, but only a few account for most cases of enzymopathic NHA: glucose-6-phosphate dehydrogenase (G6PD), pyruvate kinase (PK), and pyrimidine-5'-nucleotidase-1 (P5'N1).

G6PD is a key enzyme in the hexose monophosphate shunt pathway and is responsible for generation of NADPH, which maintains activity of three other enzymes: glutathione reductase, catalase, and a more recently recognized peroxiredoxin 2.[27] G6PD deficiency is a common condition affecting hundreds of millions of people worldwide. The prevalence varies from less than 1:1000 in Northern Europeans to 1:3 in the Arabian Peninsula or sub-Saharan Africa. The *G6PD* gene, located on chromosome Xq28, accounts for the X-linked recessive inheritance pattern of this condition. Most *G6PD* variants are due to single amino acid substitution. Other abnormalities such as nonsense, frameshift mutations, or large deletions are not known.[28] The mutations introduce qualitative defects by the means of decreased enzymatic activity or decreased stability. Mutations affecting the NADP-binding domain cause a more severe reduction in activity. The clinical presentation and the disease course vary from asymptomatic carriers to patients who become symptomatic only when challenged by the exposure to oxidizing agents, certain foods, or infection, up to severe lifelong hemolytic anemia. In neonates, G6PD deficiency may manifest either as an exaggerated hyperbilirubinemia without significant anemia or, in severe cases, marked anemia with a significant hemolytic component. In contrast to the early occurrence of hemolysis and hyperbilirubinemia in many hereditary HAs, the onset of hyperbilirubinemia in G6PD-deficient neonates may be delayed, becoming clinically apparent on days 2 to 3 of life, in which case it can be inaccurately considered a physiologic jaundice, resulting in a delayed diagnosis. Hemolytic events in breast-fed neonates can be associated with the maternal ingestion of fava beans or medications such as sulfa drugs.

PK deficiency is the most common enzymopathy of the glycolytic pathway and is very likely the most common enzyme deficiency causing hemolysis. The overall prevalence is estimated at 1:20,000. The enzyme provides the RBC with half of its ATP pool. The pathogenetic mechanism(s) of hemolysis is not clearly understood, but infants with PK deficiency can develop severe jaundice shortly after birth.

The *PKRL* gene consists of 12 exons and provides tissue-specific expression via facilitation of one of the two promoters: PK-R in erythrocytes and PK-L in the liver. Over 220 different *PKRL* mutations have been associated with HA. The most prevalent are single nucleotide missense mutations.[29,30] Other aberrancies include splice site mutations, small and large deletions, frameshifts, and insertions. The disorder is transmitted in AR fashion as either a homozygous or a compound heterozygous genotype. These neonates are prone to significant anemia and hyperbilirubinemia that may improve over time to a milder phenotype in later life.[31] Recently, an allosteric activator of both wild type and mutant PK enzymes, mitapivat, has been approved by Food and Drug Administration (FDA) as a therapeutic agent. The compound enhances the PK activity in erythrocytes treated ex vivo.[32]

P5'N1 deficiency is the third most common enzymopathy causing hemolysis, although the disease is quite rare. Clinical symptoms occur only in homozygous and compound heterozygous states (AR pattern). Most patients demonstrate a lifelong mild to moderate anemia with chronic hemolysis. Occasional exacerbations following infection can also occur. The *NT5C3* gene is located on chromosome 7p15 and contains 11 exons. It produces three transcripts by means of alternative splicing of exons 2 or R. The isoform lacking both exons is specifically expressed in RBCs. The enzyme facilitates metabolism of toxic pyrimidine nucleoside phosphates into cytidine and uridine, which can passively diffuse across the RBC membrane. The mutations of *NT5C3* gene include missense, nonsense, deletions and insertions, or splice site alterations.[29]

DISORDERS OF BILIRUBIN METABOLISM

Inherited defects of bilirubin metabolism can present with HA with jaundice or with NHA. There may be a higher possibility of bilirubin toxicity in the central nervous system in neonates. Neonates are particularly prone to developing hyperbilirubinemia as they have higher hemoglobin concentrations, shorter RBC lifespans, and less efficient bilirubin metabolism with lower bilirubin uptake, conjugation, and excretion; the activity of bilirubin conjugation enzymes may be only 1% of that seen in adults.[9,10,33] The alterations of the genes involved in bilirubin metabolism may affect many steps of normal bilirubin processing: uptake and intrahepatic storage of unconjugated bilirubin (glutathione S-transferase-μ-1 [*GSTM1*]), bilirubin conjugation (UDP glucuronosyltransferase [*UGT1A1*]), bile excretion (ATP-binding cassette transporters: *ABCC2* and *MRP2*), and hepatic reuptake (organic anion transport proteins: *SLCO1B1* and *SLCO1B3*). Fig. 8.4 depicts the schematic summary of the pathway of bilirubin transport and metabolism. By far, bilirubin conjugation disorder is the most common type of hereditary hyperbilirubinemia. It is caused by mutations of genes encoding UDP-glucuronosyltransferase (UGT) superfamily enzymes: UGT1, UGT2, UGT3, and UGT8.[34] Of those, UGT1A1 is responsible for bilirubin glucuronidation. Mutations of *UGT1A1* are associated with abnormal bilirubin conjugation, including Gilbert and Crigler-Najjar syndromes.[35,36] Gilbert syndrome is widely prevalent, occurring in 3% to 13% of the general population. There are geographical variations of the genetic alteration in Gilbert syndrome: In people of European descent there are one or more additional TA repeat(s) in the promoter region, whereas in the Asian population the mutations involve exon 1 of the gene. Classically, Gilbert syndrome is characterized by chronic or recurrent unconjugated hyperbilirubinemia of varying severity with otherwise normal liver function tests. Crigler-Najjar syndrome (types I and II) demonstrates a complete or near complete (<10%) loss of enzyme activity, respectively. It is a rare condition generally inherited in an AR manner. The patients have a significant block in bilirubin glucuronidation, producing severe neonatal jaundice with a risk of kernicterus. Their jaundice is recurrent and persistent despite therapeutic measures (phototherapy or exchange transfusion).

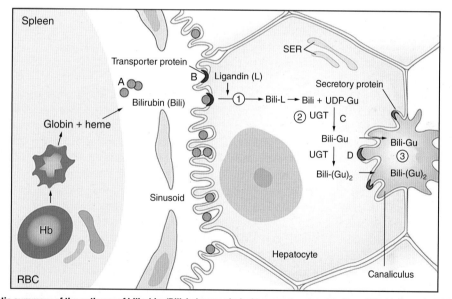

Fig. 8.4 Schematic summary of the pathway of bilirubin *(Bili, in brown circles)* **transport and metabolism.** Bilirubin is produced from metabolism of heme, primarily in the spleen, and is transported to the liver bound to albumin. It enters the hepatocyte by binding to a transporter protein *(red crescents)* and crosses the cell membrane *(circled 1)*, thus entering the cell. It binds to Y and Z proteins *(not shown)* and then to ligandin for transport to the smooth endoplasmic reticulum (SER). In the SER, bilirubin is conjugated to glucuronic acid by *(circled 2)* UDP-glucuronyl transferase 1 (UGT). Conjugated bilirubin is then secreted into the canaliculi *(circled 3)* by the ATP-binding cassette transporter protein MRP2/cMOAT/ABCC2 *(shown as blue crescents)*. In overproduction disease *(A)*, such as hemolytic anemia, unconjugated bilirubin is produced at rates that exceed the ability of the liver to clear it, leading to a usually transient increase in unconjugated bilirubin in serum. In both Gilbert and Crigler-Najjar syndromes, mutations in the gene encoding UDP glucuronyl transferase *(UDPGT1A1)*, shown at *C* in the figure, result in buildup of unconjugated bilirubin in hepatocytes and ultimately in serum. In Gilbert syndrome, there may also be a defect in the bilirubin transporter protein, shown at *B* in the figure. Mutations in the *MRP2/cMOAT/ABCC2* gene result in defective secretory proteins, causing buildup of conjugated bilirubin in hepatocytes and, ultimately, in serum, resulting in the Dubin-Johnson syndrome *(D)*, an autosomal-recessive disease. Conjugated hyperbilirubinemia is also found in Rotor syndrome, possibly virus induced. *Hb,* Hemoglobin; *RBC,* red blood cell. (Reproduced with permission and minor modifications from Daniels et al. Evaluation of liver function. In: *Henry's Clinical Diagnosis and Management by Laboratory Methods;* chapter 22:314-330.e4.)

Rotor syndrome is caused by a defect in hepatic uptake and storage. It is associated with mutations in *SLCO1B1* and *SLCO1B3*, which encode organic anion transport proteins expressed on hepatocytes and facilitate the reuptake of bilirubin glucuronides from the plasma. Homozygous or compound heterozygous mutations in these genes can lead to elevation in both conjugated and unconjugated bilirubin in otherwise asymptomatic individuals.[37]

CONGENITAL DYSERYTHROPOIETIC ANEMIA

CDAs are rare disorders characterized by ineffective erythropoiesis causing anemia with variable degree of hemolysis, erythroid hyperplasia in the bone marrow, and abnormal morphologic features of the cells in the erythroid lineage, also commonly associated with iron overload.[38] The initial classification is established based on the morphologic/ultrastructural features and include three types: CDA type I, type II, and type III. Type II is the most frequent of these conditions. More recently, cases that were not conforming to the criteria of these main types have been designated as CDA variants. Most CDA patients have mild to moderate anemia, but some may require blood transfusion, especially during the first months of life.[39] Mutations in several genes have been associated with CDA. Patients with CDA type I frequently have mutated *CDAN1* (80%) or *C15ORF41* gene. *SEC23B* is implicated in CDA type II, mostly due to missense followed by nonsense, intronic, and small indel mutations.[38-40] Mitotic protein MKLP1 encoded by *KIF23* is impaired in CDA type III. The CDA variant group seems to represent a "waste basket", including several potential subgroups (types IV, V, VI, and VII) with many responsible genes (*GATA-1*, *KLF1*, etc.).

General Diagnostic Approach and Considerations

Encountering HA or hyperbilirubinemia in a neonate generates an extensive list of possibilities and in many cases a significant diagnostic challenge. A thorough family history may be very helpful to steer the diagnostic process in a certain direction, but unfortunately it is often noncontributory. The patient's age also creates other important considerations. For example, the degree of anemia and hyperbilirubinemia or the trending of the laboratory results may impose a particular urgency on the timeliness of the definitive diagnosis as hyperbilirubinemia; if not addressed, it can result in

devastating consequences of kernicterus. Administered blood transfusions should also be kept in mind, as they can alter the results of many tests. The diagnostic approach may vary from case to case, but a stepwise algorithmic tactic has proven to be the most useful in most cases (see Fig. 8.5).[9,41,42]

The distinction between immune-mediated and nonimmune-mediated NHA can be made by a direct antiglobulin test (Coombs test). The positive result would suggest immune HA, triggering additional serologic workup to better characterize the nature of the antibodies.[41] To rule out acquired causes of nonimmune HA, one can consider the review of the family history with a close attention to the parent's exposure to toxins, medications, etc., as well as an infectious workup, if indicated. In parallel, hereditary causes must also be assessed. Peripheral blood smear evaluation by an experienced hematologist/pathologist is a fast and inexpensive test. Although a specific diagnosis is rarely made on the sole basis of morphology, some findings can provide guidance as to what type of testing to perform next. For example, numerous spherocytes in a setting of a negative Coombs test would favor HS, bite cells are present in unstable Hb and G6PD deficiency, echinocytes could suggest PK deficiency, and in some parts of the world certain infectious such as malaria can also be addressed at this point.[43] High suspicion for a hereditary HA should warrant appropriate screening tests. For RBC membrane disorders, osmotic fragility, band 3 by EMA flow cytometry, and ektacytometry are commonly performed.[11] Enzyme deficiency often requires measurement of the enzyme activity. Hb fractionation by high performance liquid chromatography (HPLC), capillary electrophoresis, gel electrophoresis, isoelectric focusing, or mass spectrometry are recommended when a Hb disorder is suspected. To identify an unstable Hb, Hb stability test and evaluation for Heinz bodies are also utilized. Although this approach can identify many causes of NHA, the definitive diagnosis of some of the rarer forms of HA can be elusive due to a lack of family history (AR in nature) and traditional diagnostic tests being unreliable due to frequent transfusions. Molecular testing can be particularly helpful in these scenarios.

TARGETED GENE PANEL APPROACH FOR DIAGNOSIS

Increasing availability and affordability of molecular testing has introduced major changes in the diagnostic

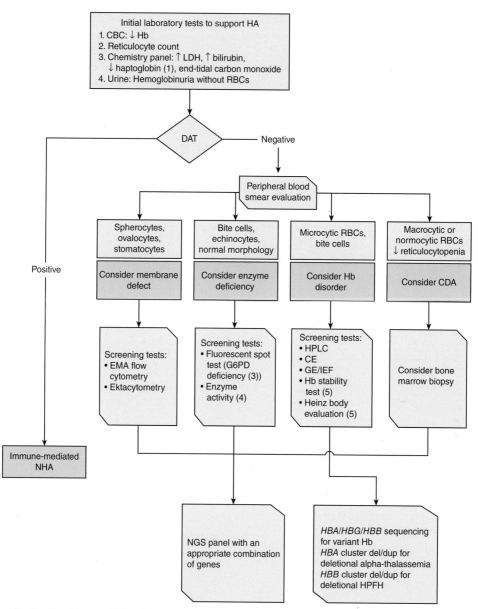

Fig. 8.5 Diagnostic algorithm for neonatal hemolytic anemia.

(1) The interpretation of haptoglobin in the neonatal population should be done with caution as normal neonates may have decreased to nearly absent haptoglobin.

(2) Osmotic fragility and membrane protein electrophoresis are unreliable in a recently transfused patient. Waiting for 4 weeks after transfusion is advised.

(3) Fluorescent spot test for G6PD deficiency has a good diagnostic performance in severe G6PD deficiency. In moderate or mild deficiency, false negative results are common.

(4) Enzyme activity evaluation can yield false negative results in cases with reticulocytosis (reticulocytes have a significantly higher enzyme activity) and after transfusion. PK activity measurements can be falsely high due to inadequate removal of the leukocytes from the specimen.

(5) Heinz body and Hb stability tests are not recommended for children younger than 6 months of age due to high Hb F, which causes falsely positive results.

CBC, Complete blood count; CDA, congenital dyserythropoietic anemia; CE, capillary electrophoresis; DAT, direct antiglobulin test; EMA, eosin-5′-malemide; G6PD, glucose-6-phosphate dehydrogenase; GE, gel electrophoresis; Hb, hemoglobin; HPFH, hereditary persistence of fetal hemoglobin; HPLC, high performance liquid chromatography; IEF, isoelectric focusing; LDH, lactate dehydrogenase; NGS, next generation sequencing; NHA, neonatal hemolytic anemia; RBC, red blood cell.

workup of several conditions in the neonates, including NHA. Historically, karyotype analysis, microarray comparative hybridization, and single gene-based sequencing adopting Sanger technology and capillary sequencing have been the three pillars of molecular testing. The former two are suitable for a minority of genetic conditions associated with HNA, as they can only be useful for relatively large chromosomal alterations. The genetic basis of hereditary NHAs makes the gene sequencing approach most suitable. Traditional Sanger panels are limited by longer turnaround times that frequently run into weeks and small size that can cover only a few genes. These shortcomings can be overcome by next generation sequencing (NGS) technologies.[8,44,45] Whole genome sequencing (WGS) and whole exome sequencing (WES) hold promise in acutely ill infants and have a diagnostic yield of 25% to 60% depending on the patient selection and depth of coverage.[46,47] However, both techniques are technically demanding and need a sophisticated bioinformatics pipeline. Overall turnaround time is also longer, and there are limitations in our ability to identify variant(s) of unknown significance (VUS).

Targeted panel-based approach is a useful tool for analyzing disease- or phenotype-specific mutations, leading to a much higher diagnostic yield. It provides a cost-effective way of studying disease-specific genes. Targeted NGS panels with genes ranging from 28 to 217 have been evaluated since 2012.[44,48,49] Considering the significant overlap in HA phenotypes, the reliance on clinical evaluation and basic diagnostic tests such as complete blood count and peripheral smear evaluation are not likely to be enough. Russo et al.[48] have shown that an enzyme deficiency was mistakenly diagnosed as CDA in 10 patients with congenital HA. In our evaluation of 268 patients with unexplained HA, pathogenic and likely pathogenic variants were identified in 64/268 patients (24%), where half were novel mutations. Even though the overall diagnostic yield appears to be lower than expected, this can be explained by our setup as a tertiary reference laboratory where we have limited access to clinical information and biochemical testing.[50] In our cohort, 11% (29/264) patients were homozygous for a promoter polymorphism in the *UGT1A1* gene A(TA)7TAA (*UGT1A1*28*), suggesting that Gilbert syndrome was a likely cause of the hyperbilirubinemia. Moreover, 4

of 29 cases with *UGT1A1* polymorphisms were associated with hyperbilirubinemia along with pathogenic mutations in spectrin genes.[50] The diagnostic yield of targeted NGS can be improved with comprehensive information on the clinical and biochemical phenotype. The accurate classification of the variants in the genes and avoidance of frequent reporting of VUS depend on the availability of the complete clinical phenotype along with family history, peripheral smear evaluation, and other biochemical testing.

Molecular approach has a significant advantage as it is not affected by some preanalytical variables, such as blood transfusions. In this context, multiplex test panels can be useful for understanding the complex pathophysiology. As an example, Gilbert syndrome usually manifests with mild to minimal hyperbilirubinemia, but can cause disproportionately significant hyperbilirubinemia in patients with RBC membrane defect or enzyme deficiencies.

One of the challenges of the NGS panel is that it still takes up to 3 weeks to obtain the results. However, increasing efficiency of the NGS technology and information processing is encouraging. It will likely become the preferred test in conjunction with the traditional biochemical tests. Targeted NGS sequencing for HA is available for the diagnosis and management of these conditions from major commercial laboratories (e.g., Mayo Medical Laboratories, Cincinnati Children's Molecular Genetics Laboratory, Yale University Blood Disease Reference Laboratory, and ARUP Laboratories).

Conclusion

The molecular basis of NHA is complex, causing a wide spectrum of disorders with clinical presentation ranging from completely asymptomatic to life threatening (hydrops fetalis or bilirubin encephalopathy). Hyperbilirubinemia may lead to an increased hospital stay and produce significant anxiety for the newborn's parents. Many NHAs have a nonspecific phenotype, which together with negative family history make it difficult to arrive at the correct and definitive diagnosis. Furthermore, the diagnosis is challenging in neonates as some of the biochemical tests are affected by naturally high Hb F and frequent blood transfusions. NGS-based targeted panels can circumvent these confounding factors and are beneficial in these scenarios due to a relatively short turnaround time and the ease of incorporating multiple genes of interest, including those involved in bilirubin metabolism. In addition to therapeutic implications for the patient, an accurate diagnosis can provide a basis for genetic counseling and disease prevention. Furthermore, with decreasing cost and increasing throughput, a targeted NGS approach would likely become standard of care in conjunction with a standard biochemical test.

REFERENCES

1. Franco RS. The measurement and importance of red cell survival. *Am J Hematol.* 2009;84:109-114.
2. Pearson HA. Life-span of the fetal red blood cell. *J Pediatr.* 1967;70:166-171.
3. Mock DM, Matthews NI, Zhu S, et al. Red blood cell (RBC) survival determined in humans using RBCs labeled at multiple biotin densities. *Transfusion.* 2011;51:1047-1057.
4. de Haas M, Thurik FF, Koelewijn JM, et al. Haemolytic disease of the fetus and newborn. *Vox Sang.* 2015;109:99-113.
5. Moise KJ. Fetal anemia due to non-Rhesus-D red-cell alloimmunization. *Semin Fetal Neonatal Med.* 2008;13:207-214.
6. Risinger M, Emberesh M, Kalfa TA. Rare hereditary hemolytic anemias: diagnostic approach and considerations in management. *Hematol Oncol Clin North Am.* 2019;33:373-392.
7. Gallagher PG. Diagnosis and management of rare congenital nonimmune hemolytic disease. *Hematology Am Soc Hematol Educ Program.* 2015;2015:392-399.
8. Rets A, Clayton AL, Christensen RD, et al. Molecular diagnostic update in hereditary hemolytic anemia and neonatal hyperbilirubinemia. *Int J Lab Hematol.* 2019;41(1):S95-S101.
9. Christensen RD, Nussenzveig RH, Yaish HM, et al. Causes of hemolysis in neonates with extreme hyperbilirubinemia. *J Perinatol.* 2014;34:616-619.
10. Christensen RD, Yaish HM. Hemolytic disorders causing severe neonatal hyperbilirubinemia. *Clin Perinatol.* 2015;42:515-527.
11. Da Costa L, Galimand J, Fenneteau O, et al. Hereditary spherocytosis, elliptocytosis, and other red cell membrane disorders. *Blood Rev.* 2013;27:167-178.
12. Narla J, Mohandas N. Red cell membrane disorders. *Int J Lab Hematol.* 2017;39(1):S47-S52.
13. Gallagher PG. Hematologically important mutations: ankyrin variants in hereditary spherocytosis. *Blood Cells Mol Dis.* 2005;35:345-347.
14. Vermeulen S, Messiaen L, Scheir P, et al. Kallmann syndrome in a patient with congenital spherocytosis and an interstitial 8p11.2 deletion. *Am J Med Genet.* 2002;108:315-318.
15. Chu C, Woods N, Sawasdee N, et al. Band 3 Edmonton I, a novel mutant of the anion exchanger 1 causing spherocytosis and distal renal tubular acidosis. *Biochem J.* 2010;426:379-388.
16. Delaunay J, Nouyrigat V, Proust A, et al. Different impacts of alleles alphaLEPRA and alphaLELY as assessed versus a novel, virtually null allele of the SPTA1 gene in trans. *Br J Haematol.* 2004;127:118-122.
17. Randon J, Boulanger L, Marechal J, et al. A variant of spectrin low-expression allele alpha LELY carrying a hereditary elliptocytosis mutation in codon 28. *Br J Haematol.* 1994;88:534-540.
18. Eber S, Lux SE. Hereditary spherocytosis—defects in proteins that connect the membrane skeleton to the lipid bilayer. *Semin Hematol.* 2004;41:118-141.
19. Niss O, Chonat S, Dagaonkar N, et al. Genotype-phenotype correlations in hereditary elliptocytosis and hereditary pyropoikilocytosis. *Blood Cells Mol Dis.* 2016;61:4-9.
20. Gallagher PG. Disorders of erythrocyte hydration. *Blood.* 2017;130:2699-2708.
21. Glogowska E, Lezon-Geyda K, Maksimova Y, et al. Mutations in the Gardos channel (KCNN4) are associated with hereditary xerocytosis. *Blood.* 2015;126:1281-1284.
22. Tamary H, Dgany O. Alpha-thalassemia. In: Adam MP, Ardinger HH, Pagon RA, et al., eds. *GeneReviews((R)).* Seattle, WA; 1993.
23. Bender MA, Yusuf C, Davis T, et al. Newborn screening practices and alpha-thalassemia detection - United States, 2016. *MMWR Morb Mortal Wkly Rep.* 2020;69:1269-1272.
24. Ostertag W, Smith EW. Hb Sinai, a new alpha chain mutant alpha his 47. *Humangenetik.* 1968;6:377-379.
25. Lee-Potter JP, Deacon-Smith RA, Simpkiss MJ, et al. A new cause of haemolytic anaemia in the newborn. A description of an unstable fetal haemoglobin: F Poole, alpha2-G-gamma2 130 trptophan yeilds glycine. *J Clin Pathol.* 1975;28:317-320.
26. Pirastru M, Mereu P, Trova S, et al. Hb F-Avellino [(G)gamma41(C7)Phe --> Leu; HBG2: c.124 T > C]: a new hemoglobin variant observed in a healthy newborn. *Hemoglobin.* 2016;40:61-63.
27. Low FM, Hampton MB, Winterbourn CC. Peroxiredoxin 2 and peroxide metabolism in the erythrocyte. *Antioxid Redox Signal.* 2008;10:1621-1630.
28. Minucci A, Moradkhani K, Hwang MJ, et al. Glucose-6-phosphate dehydrogenase (G6PD) mutations database: review of the "old" and update of the new mutations. *Blood Cells Mol Dis.* 2012;48:154-165.
29. Koralkova P, van Solinge WW, van Wijk R. Rare hereditary red blood cell enzymopathies associated with hemolytic anemia - pathophysiology, clinical aspects, and laboratory diagnosis. *Int J Lab Hematol.* 2014;36:388-397.
30. Grace RF, Zanella A, Neufeld EJ, et al. Erythrocyte pyruvate kinase deficiency: 2015 status report. *Am J Hematol.* 2015;90:825-830.
31. Delivoria-Papadopoulos M, Oski FA, Gottlieb AJ. Oxygen-hemoglobulin dissociation curves: effect of inherited enzyme defects of the red cell. *Science.* 1969;165:601-602.
32. Kung C, Hixon J, Kosinski PA, et al. AG-348 enhances pyruvate kinase activity in red blood cells from patients with pyruvate kinase deficiency. *Blood.* 2017;130:1347-1356.
33. Wong RJ, Stevenson DK. Neonatal hemolysis and risk of bilirubin-induced neurologic dysfunction. *Semin Fetal Neonatal Med.* 2015;20:26-30.
34. Kaplan M, Hammerman C, Beutler E. Hyperbilirubinaemia, glucose-6-phosphate dehydrogenase deficiency and Gilbert syndrome. *Eur J Pediatr.* 2001;160:195.
35. Clarke DJ, Moghrabi N, Monaghan G, et al. Genetic defects of the UDP-glucuronosyltransferase-1 (UGT1) gene that cause familial non-haemolytic unconjugated hyperbilirubinaemias. *Clin Chim Acta.* 1997;266:63-74.
36. Bosma PJ, Chowdhury JR, Bakker C, et al. The genetic basis of the reduced expression of bilirubin UDP-glucuronosyltransferase 1 in Gilbert's syndrome. *N Engl J Med.* 1995;333:1171-1175.
37. van de Steeg E, Stranecky V, Hartmannova H, et al. Complete OATP1B1 and OATP1B3 deficiency causes human Rotor

syndrome by interrupting conjugated bilirubin reuptake into the liver. *J Clin Invest.* 2012;122:519-528.

38. Heimpel H, Kellermann K, Neuschwander N, et al. The morphological diagnosis of congenital dyserythropoietic anemia: results of a quantitative analysis of peripheral blood and bone marrow cells. *Haematologica.* 2010;95:1034-1036.

39. Wickramasinghe SN, Wood WG. Advances in the understanding of the congenital dyserythropoietic anaemias. *Br J Haematol.* 2005;131:431-446.

40. Iolascon A, Heimpel H, Wahlin A, et al. Congenital dyserythropoietic anemias: molecular insights and diagnostic approach. *Blood.* 2013;122:2162-2166.

41. Yaish HM, Christensen RD, Lemons RS. Neonatal nonimmune hemolytic anemia. *Curr Opin Pediatr.* 2017;29:12-19.

42. Christensen RD, Yaish HM. Hemolysis in preterm neonates. *Clin Perinatol.* 2016;43:233-240.

43. Christensen RD, Yaish HM, Gallagher PG. A pediatrician's practical guide to diagnosing and treating hereditary spherocytosis in neonates. *Pediatrics.* 2015;135:1107-1114.

44. Agarwal AM, Nussenzveig RH, Reading NS, et al. Clinical utility of next-generation sequencing in the diagnosis of hereditary haemolytic anaemias. *Br J Haematol.* 2016;174:806-814.

45. Bianchi P, Vercellati C, Fermo E. How will next generation sequencing (NGS) improve the diagnosis of congenital hemolytic anemia? *Ann Transl Med.* 2020;8:268.

46. Meng L, Pammi M, Saronwala A, et al. Use of exome sequencing for infants in intensive care units: ascertainment of severe single-gene disorders and effect on medical management. *JAMA Pediatr.* 2017;171:e173438.

47. Woerner AC, Gallagher RC, Vockley J, et al. The use of whole genome and exome sequencing for newborn screening: challenges and opportunities for population health. *Front Pediatr.* 2021;9:663752.

48. Russo R, Andolfo I, Manna F, et al. Multi-gene panel testing improves diagnosis and management of patients with hereditary anemias. *Am J Hematol.* 2018;93:672-682.

49. Vives-Corrons JL, Krishnevskaya E, Rodriguez IH, et al. Characterization of hereditary red blood cell membranopathies using combined targeted next-generation sequencing and osmotic gradient ektacytometry. *Int J Hematol.* 2021;113:163-174.

50. Agarwal A, Patel JL, Clayton A, et al. Use of next generation sequencing panel for routine diagnosis of hereditary hemolytic anemias. *Blood.* 2018;132:2325.

Transfusion Medicine

Chapter 9

Erythropoietin and Darbepoetin Use in the NICU

Robin K. Ohls, MD

Chapter Outline

Introduction

Premature infants receive a greater number of transfusions and are exposed to a greater number of donors compared to any other hospitalized population. Transfusion guidelines are now used in many neonatal units; however, the search for the most appropriate transfusion guidelines continues. Recently, two of the largest randomized controlled trials (RCTs) to date enrolled over 2800 extremely low birth weight (ELBW) infants and showed similar 2-year outcomes between those infants transfused using liberal (higher) hematocrit strategies compared to restrictive (lower) hematocrit strategies[1,2] (see Chapter 10). Despite these efforts, the fact remains that in the smallest preterm infants there is a positive correlation between the amount of blood removed for laboratory evaluation and the volume of blood replaced via red cell transfusion (Fig. 9.1). When restrictive transfusion guidelines are applied, greater phlebotomy losses (and lower hematocrits) are tolerated before transfusions are ordered. The use of red cell growth factors provides increased red cell mass, thereby delaying the need for transfusions even further, resulting in lower total transfusion volumes.

Erythropoiesis Stimulating Agents

Erythropoiesis stimulating agents (ESAs) to improve red cell mass have been studied for over 40 years. ESAs such as erythropoietin (Epo) and darbepoetin (Darbe) have proven successful in decreasing transfusion number, transfusion volume, and donor exposures in adults, children, and the smallest, most critically ill infants. Epo, a 34-kD glycoprotein whose gene is located on the long arm of chromosome 7, was first purified in the 1970s by Goldwasser and Miyake, who isolated 8 mg of Epo from 2500 L of urine from patients with aplastic anemia.[3] Epo is made up of a 165–amino acid backbone chain with four carbohydrate groups attached (three N-linked carbohydrates and one O-linked carbohydrate). The *Epo* gene was cloned

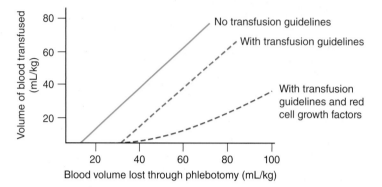

Relationship between phlebotomy and transfusion volumes

Fig. 9.1 Red cell transfusion volumes are directly related to phlebotomy losses. In neonates, and especially in extremely low birth weight infants, a direct (positive) relationship exists between the amount of blood drawn for phlebotomy *(shown on the X axis)* and the volume of blood returned in the form of a packed red cell transfusion *(shown on the Y axis)*. The *black solid line* represents the general relationship: Without the institution of transfusion guidelines nearly all blood lost is replaced through transfusions. The *blue dashed line* represents an estimated relationship when instituting restrictive transfusion guidelines, resulting in a lag in transfusing despite ongoing losses, and decreased blood transfused. The *red hatched line* represents the relationship between phlebotomy and transfusions when red cell growth factors are used. There is a decrease in the slope due to the increased red cell mass as a result of administering red cell growth factors; therefore less volume of blood is required per volume lost through phlebotomy.

in 1985[4] and soon thereafter approved by the US Food and Drug Administration in 1989 for adults with anemia due to end stage renal disease (ESRD). Studies performed in the pediatric population expanded the use of Epo to stimulate red cell production and decrease transfusions in children with ESRD.

Amgen, the company that originally marketed and produced Epo, recognized a direct relationship between Epo's sialic acid–containing carbohydrate content and the serum half-life. They altered 5 of the 165 amino acids to produce two additional N-linked carbohydrate sites, resulting in a 37-kD biologically modified ESA, darbepoetin alfa (Darbe), trade named Aranesp. Studies confirmed the longer serum half-life and greater biologic activity of Darbe.[5] Clinical trials in adults with ESRD reported adequate hematopoietic responses when Darbe was administered every 1 to 4 weeks.[6]

Preterm ESA Studies

Interest in administering Epo to preterm infants began in the late 1980s. Initial studies in the early 1990s evaluated Epo doses that were effective in adults, but were lower than doses required for preterm infants, given the differences in clearance and

volume of distribution that were not identified until later in the 1990s (see Pharmacokinetics).

Maier et al. were one of the first European neonatal investigative groups to publish a large multicenter RCT on Epo in very low birth weight (VLBW) infants.[7] Investigators reported improved hematocrits and decreased transfusions in infants weighing less than 1500 g who received subcutaneous (SC) Epo, 250 units/kg three times weekly, starting by day 3 of life. Numerous randomized trials (reviewed previously) in Europe, Australia, New Zealand, the United States, and South America followed, evaluating different dosing regimens and lengths of treatment.[8] To varying degrees, depending on dosing and the population studied, Epo administration stimulated erythropoiesis and decreased transfusion number and volume.

By the mid-1990s researchers identified nonhematopoietic effects of ESAs. Over the next 10 years they determined that ESAs in animal models were protective in the developing brain, suggesting the possibility that they might be of benefit to very premature infants at risk for intraventricular hemorrhage (IVH), hypoxic-ischemic injury, and developmental delay. Neuroprotective mechanisms of ESAs included decreased neuronal apoptosis, decreased inflammation, promotion of oligodendrocyte differentiation and maturation, and improved white matter survival.[9-14] Based on preliminary in vitro evaluations of Darbe dose effects on marrow progenitors[15] and our previous work comparing Epo concentrations to cognitive outcome,[16] we designed a multicenter, randomized, placebo-controlled study of Darbe and Epo administration to preterm infants to evaluate both hematopoietic and neuroprotective effects of ESAs. Infants with birth weights 500 to 1250 g and 48 hours or less of age were randomized to Darbe (10 μg/kg, 1x/week SC), Epo (400 units/kg, 3x/week SC), or placebo (sham dosing) through 35 weeks corrected gestation. All infants were transfused according to a restrictive protocol and received supplemental iron, folate, and vitamin E. Transfusions, complete blood counts, absolute reticulocyte counts (ARC), phlebotomy losses, common neonatal morbidities, and adverse effects were recorded. We powered the study for two primary outcomes. The primary outcome for the hospital phase of the study was number of transfusions, while the primary outcome for the follow-up phase of the study was cognitive composite score on the Bayley Scales of Infant Development, Third Edition (Bayley III). We hypothesized that infants receiving Epo or Darbe would have decreased transfusions during hospitalization and improved cognitive outcomes at 18 to 22 months corrected age compared to the placebo group.

Hospital Outcomes

Infants in the Epo and Darbe groups received significantly fewer transfusions (p=0.015) and were exposed to fewer donors (p=0.044) than the placebo group (Darbe: 1.2±2.4 transfusions and 0.7±1.2 donors/infant; Epo: 1.2±1.6 transfusions and 0.8±1.0 donors/infant; placebo: 2.4±2.9 transfusions and 1.2±1.3 donors/infant).[17] Transfusions and donor exposures were reduced by 50% in ESA-treated infants compared to placebo-treated infants. Hematocrit and ARC were higher in the Darbe and Epo groups compared to placebo (p=0.001, Darbe and Epo vs. placebo for both hematocrit and ARC). Morbidities were similar among groups, including the incidence of retinopathy of prematurity (ROP). We concluded that

infants receiving ESAs received fewer transfusions and fewer donor exposures, with fewer injections given to Darbe recipients. Importantly, 56% of VLBW infants in the ESA group remained transfusion free during their neonatal intensive care unit (NICU) stay.

Neurodevelopmental Outcomes

Neurodevelopmental follow-up was performed on 80 (29 Epo, 27 Darbe, 24 placebo) of 92 surviving infants enrolled in the above-mentioned study.[18] After adjusting for sex and maternal education, infants who had received Darbe or Epo had significantly higher cognitive composite scores on the Bayley III (96.2±7.3 and 97.9±14, respectively; mean ± standard deviation) in comparison to placebo recipients (88.7±13.5; p=0.01 vs. ESA recipients) (Table 9.1). The ESA group also scored significantly higher on object permanence, an early test of executive function (p=0.05). None of the ESA recipients were diagnosed with cerebral palsy, while five cases of cerebral palsy were identified in the placebo group (p<0.001). The incidence of neurodevelopmental impairment in the ESA group was significantly lower compared to placebo (odds ratio 0.18; 95% confidence interval 0.05–0.63).[24] There were no differences in visual or hearing impairment among groups.

Funding from the National Institutes of Health (NIH) was obtained to continue evaluating neurodevelopment in the former preterm population, with the addition of control children who had been born healthy at term.[19,20] Children were followed at preschool age and compared to healthy children previously born at term. Again, ESA recipients scored higher than placebo recipients on tests of cognition, and of executive function (EF; working memory, cognitive flexibility, and impulse control), and had less neurodevelopmental impairment at 4 years of age.[19] Cognitive and EF test scores remained similar between 4 and 6 years within each group (ESA, placebo, term).[20] There were significant differences between the three groups on tests of full-scale IQ (FSIQ: p=0.004), performance IQ (PIQ: p=<.001), word memory (p=0.001), and gift delay (measuring impulsivity: p=0.001) (see Table 9.1). At 6 years of age the ESA group scored significantly higher than the placebo

TABLE 9.1 Neurodevelopment at 18 to 22 Months, and at 4 and 6 Years With Term Comparison

	ESA[a]		Placebo		P VALUE[e] ESA vs. Placebo	
Subjects at 18-22 Months (N)	Darbe[b] (27)	Epo[c] (29)	24			
Composite cognitive	96.2 (7.3)	97.9 (14.3)	88.7 (13.5)		0.01	
Composite language	92.4 (15.2)	89.9 (18.4)	83.6 (13.1)		0.06	
Object permanence	2.8 (0.4)	2.4 (0.9)	2.2 (1.0)		0.05	
NDI[d] (%)	3 (11)	2 (6.9)	9 (37.5)		0.008	
Cerebral palsy	0 (0)	0 (0)	5 (20.8)		<0.001	
Subjects at 4 years (N)	**ESA (39)**		**Placebo (14)**	**Term (24)**	**ESA vs. Placebo**	**ESA vs. Term**
Full-scale IQ	91.5 (18.1)		79.1 (18.5)	102.6 (12.8)	0.034	0.011
Verbal IQ	93.0 (17.0)		79.1 (19.6)	103.9 (10.6)	0.015	0.006
Performance IQ	91.7 (18.3)		82.9 (16.9)	100.8 (15.2)	0.12	0.071
General language comprehension	89.8 (17.0)		84.8 (17.1)	101.8 (15.1)	0.35	0.006
Executive function	99.9 (11.7)		91.5 (13.3)	105.2 (7.8)	0.035	0.083
Working memory	100.6 (14.6)		91.6 (17.2)	103.9 (12.4)	0.047	0.35
Inhibition	99.1 (15.2)		91.5 (17.6)	106.4 (10.0)	0.11	0.066
Subjects at 6 years (N)	**ESA (34)**		**Placebo (17)**	**Term (20)**	**ESA vs. Placebo**	**ESA vs. Term**
Full-scale IQ	94.3 (19.4)		77.3 (13.4)	97.9 (15.9)	0.019	0.49
Verbal IQ	92.9 (20.7)		82.4 (15.3)	98.0 (15.5)	0.155	0.34
Performance IQ	98.0 (16.8)		76.6 (10.7)	99.1 (16.4)	0.0008	0.81
Executive function Inhibition	96.9 (33.9)		71.6 (46.7)	112.3 (24.6)	0.07	0.09

Values represent mean±standard deviation.
[a]Erythropoiesis stimulating agents
[b]Darbepoetin
[c]Erythropoietin
[d]Neurodevelopmental impairment, defined as having either cerebral palsy, visual deficit, hearing deficit, or a cognitive score <70
[e]P values based on odds ratios, adjusted for maternal education and sex
Data compiled from Ohls RK, Kamath-Rayne BD, Christensen RD, et al. Cognitive outcomes of preterm infants randomized to darbepoetin, erythropoietin, or placebo. *Pediatrics.* 2014;133:1023-1030; Ohls RK, Cannon DC, Phillips J, et al. Preschool assessment of preterm infants treated with darbepoetin and erythropoietin. *Pediatrics.* 2016;137:1-9; Ohls RK, Lowe J, Yeo RA, et al. Longitudinal assessment of preterm infants treated with erythropoiesis stimulating agents. *Curr Pediatr Rev.* 2023;19:417-424.

group on FSIQ (mean: placebo: 82.9; ESA: 94.9, p=0.038), PIQ (placebo: 83.3; ESA: 98.1, p=0.008), and EF tests of working memory, attention, and verbal fluency (placebo: 71.3; ESA: 95.2, p=0.008). Term controls scored better than placebo on all cognitive and EF measures, while ESA and term controls scored similarly on all intellectual tests and on tests of EF.

The preschool and school-age follow-up portions of the study were limited by low reenrollment, as a number of families were unable to be contacted. Nonetheless, the improvements in cognition over time in the ESA group (catching up to term control scores by 6 years of age) provided enough evidence of the potential for neuroprotection to obtain NIH funding for a multicenter Darbe trial to improve red cell mass and neurodevelopment. This trial randomized 650 infants 23 to 28 6/7 weeks gestation to Darbe or placebo through 35 weeks corrected gestation. Two-year follow-up was recently completed by the NICHD Neonatal Research Network, with determination of the primary outcome (performed in 90% of the participants) available in 2023.

Pharmacokinetics

Studies evaluating neonatal Epo pharmacokinetics were performed in the 1990s after initial pilot studies evaluating adult Epo doses in preterm infants were unsuccessful. Studies in newborn monkeys and sheep demonstrated that neonates had a larger volume of distribution and a more rapid elimination of Epo, necessitating the use of higher doses than required for adults.[21,22] Similarly, in preterm infants, the volume of distribution of Epo was three- to four-fold greater than that seen in adults, and the clearance was also three to four times greater.[21-23] Epo pharmacokinetics were confirmed in VLBW infants.[23]

In adults, Darbe pharmacokinetics demonstrated a half-life ($t_{1/2}$) of 49 hours after a single SC dose and 25 hours after intravenous (IV) dosage.[24] We anticipated that a similar relationship in pharmacokinetics between adults and infants would exist with Darbe, such that the volume of distribution and the clearance would be greater. Our group evaluated pharmacokinetics in 12 neonates (birth weights 1129 ± 245 g, and 29.2 ± 1.2 weeks) who received a single SC dose of Darbe at 1 or 4 μg/kg.[25] Darbe concentrations peaked 6 to 12 hours after administration. A single SC dose resulted in serum concentrations 54 to 308 mU/mL with a 1-μg/kg dose and 268 to 980 mU/mL with a 4-μg/kg dose. The $t_{1/2}$ was 26 hours (range 10–50 hours, mean 29.6 for the 1-μg/kg group and 21.5 for the 4-μg/kg group). Clearance was 17.1 mL/hr/kg for the 1-μg/kg group and 20.7 mL/hr/kg for the 4-μg/kg group. Clinically, both immature reticulocyte counts (IRC) and ARC significantly increased.

Pharmacokinetics after administration of a single, 4-μg/kg IV dose of Darbe were also evaluated. Ten neonates were enrolled, with gestational ages between 26 and 40 weeks (7 neonates <32 weeks, 3 neonates >32 weeks). Doses administered between 3 and 28 days showed a $t_{1/2}$ of 10.1 hours, a volume of distribution of 0.77 L/kg (range 0.180–3.05 L/kg), and a clearance of 52.8 mL/hr/kg (range 22.4–158.0 mL/kg/hr). Both volume of distribution and clearance were increased in comparison to older children and adults. In comparison to SC dosing, there was a less consistent rise in both IRC and ARC,[26] which may have reflected the variability in IV dosing. Both studies suggested that Darbe doses needed to be greater and administered more frequently in neonates than that used in children and adults. Population pharmacokinetics confirmed a two-compartment model with first-order elimination.[27]

To evaluate in vitro marrow responsiveness to Darbe, reticulocyte responses were measured in preterm infants administered SC Darbe in a randomized, blinded Darbe dose-response study.[15] Preterm infants weighing 1500 g or less and 10 or more days of age were randomized to placebo or a 2.5-, 5-, or 10-μg/kg/dose Darbe, given once a week SC for 4 weeks. Complete blood counts, reticulocyte counts, transfusions, and adverse events (AE) were recorded. Eighteen preterm infants (896 ± 59 g, 28.7 ± 0.7 weeks of gestation, 13 ± 1 days of age at study entry) were enrolled. Infants randomized to 10 μg/kg/dose achieved the highest reticulocyte counts by day 14 of the study. Infants receiving 5 or 10 μg/kg/dose required fewer transfusions during the study period (p=0.006). No AEs were reported. We concluded that preterm infants respond to Darbe by increasing erythropoiesis in a dose-dependent fashion, with the greatest reticulocyte response occurring in infants receiving 10 μg/kg/dose.

Circulating Erythrocyte Volume

Pharmacokinetic analyses are useful in determining differences between adult, pediatric, and neonatal dosing. For red cell growth factors, erythrokinetics—the response of red cell progenitors to various doses and dosing schedules—can be useful as well. We evaluated three-times-a-week dosing with once-a-week dosing of Epo in preterm infants to determine if the increase in red cell mass, termed circulating erythrocyte volume (CEV), was similar between the two dosing schedules with the same total weekly dose of Epo.[28] Infants were enrolled between 1 and 4 weeks of age and randomized to receive "standard" Epo dosing (400 units/kg/dose administered SC three times weekly) or a single weekly dose of Epo, 1200 units/kg administered SC once weekly. The CEV was calculated by multiplying the daily weight by the hematocrit and the estimated blood volume (85 mL/kg) and was plotted as percent over baseline (set at 100%). Infants in both groups had similar increases in CEV (Fig. 9.2, right panel), showing that the erythrokinetics were similar whether the infants received the total weekly dose of 1200 units/kg as a once-a-week dosing or more frequently as three-times-per-week dosing.

Similar CEV calculations were performed on infants receiving 10-ug/kg/dose Darbe (see Fig. 9.2, left panel), showing significant increases in CEV over 4 week dosing period compared to placebo, and showing similar erythrokinetics of weekly Darbe to weekly Epo (1200 units/kg/week) and three times weekly Epo (400 units/kg). Despite differences in pharmacokinetics, the erythroid progenitor responsiveness to different dosing schedules of Epo or Darbe were similar, in that the red cell mass increased significantly, nearly doubling over the 4-week period.

Side Effects

Although monitored for closely in clinical studies, side effects of ESAs in neonates are rare. ESA side effects seen in adults (hypertension and thromboses) appear at similar rates in ESA recipients and placebo recipients. One side effect specifically monitored in preterm neonatal ESA studies is ROP. Our study and other recent studies have not observed any differences in the incidence of any stage of ROP during hospitalization, and no differences have been reported in visual impairment at 18 to 22 months corrected age.[18,29-31] Hesitancy in the use of ESAs over concerns for increased ROP developed following publication of a 2006 Cochrane meta-analysis, which suggested an association between early (first week of life) Epo administration and ROP greater than stage 2[32] compared with late Epo administration.[33] However, this meta-analysis reflected a misclassification of a single center Epo study by Romagnoli et al. into the early Epo administration group.[34] When this study was correctly

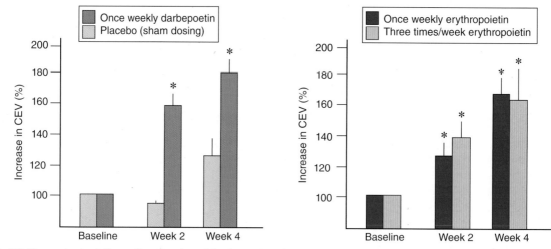

Fig. 9.2 Changes in circulating erythrocyte volume following erythropoietin and darbepoetin administration. The *left panel* shows the percent increase in circulating erythrocyte volume *(CEV)* compared to baseline in preterm infants administered darbepoetin *(blue bars)* compared to placebo *(grey bars)*. CEV nearly doubles over 4 weeks. The *right panel* shows the percent increase in CEV compared to baseline in preterm infants administered once weekly erythropoietin *(red bars)* compared to standard three times weekly dosing *(coral bars)*. There was no difference between treatment strategies during the 4-week period. Both treatment strategies increased CEV significantly over baseline. (From Patel S, Ohls RK. Darbepoetin administration in term and preterm neonates. *Clin Perinatol.* 2015;42:557-566; Ohls RK, Roohi M, Peceny HM, et al. A randomized, masked study of weekly erythropoietin dosing in preterm infants. *J Pediatr.* 2012:160:790-795.)

BOX 9.1 UPDATED ANALYSIS OF 2722 PRETERM INFANTS ENROLLED IN ESA STUDIES

Studies	ESA[a] ROP[b]	ESA Total	Placebo/ Control ROP	Placebo/ Control Total
Cochrane	38	410	26	391
Fauchère et al.	2	212	5	191
Song et al.	79	366	97	377
PENUT	60	426	70	421
Total	**179**	**1414**	**198**	**1308**

ANALYSIS (FISHER EXACT TEST)

	ROP	No ROP		
ESA	179	1235	1414	Incidence of ROP in ESA recipients: 12%
Placebo	198	1110	1308	Incidence of ROP in placebo recipients: 15%
Total	**377**	**2345**	**2722**	**p=0.067**

[a]Erythropoiesis stimulating agents
[b]Retinopathy of prematurity
Data from Juul SE, Comstock BA, Wadhawan R, et al. A randomized trial of erythropoietin for neuroprotection in preterm infants. *N Engl J Med.* 2020;382:233-243; Song J, Sun H, Xu F, et al. Recombinant human erythropoietin improves neurological outcomes in very preterm infants. *Ann Neurol.* 2016;80:24-34; Fauchère JC, Koller BM, Tschopp A, et al., with Swiss Erythropoietin Neuroprotection Trial Group. Safety of early high-dose recombinant erythropoietin for neuroprotection in very preterm infants. *J Pediatr.* 2015;167:52-57; Ohlsson A, Aher SM. Early erythropoietin for preventing red blood cell transfusion in preterm and/or low birth weight infants. *Cochrane Database Syst Rev.* 2006:CD004863.

grouped with other studies of late Epo use, the revised meta-analysis showed no significant difference in ROP with the use of early or late Epo.[35] When data from recent RCTs are included in analyses, the evidence for ESAs providing protection from ROP nears statistical significance (p=0.067) (Box 9.1). This lack of ESA effect on ROP was confirmed in a recent meta-analysis.[36] Despite this, care providers unaware of recent studies continue to site "concerns for ROP" as a reason not to use ESAs in preterm infants.

Cost Effectiveness

Transfusion numbers have decreased in preterm infants over the last several years compared to previous decades, in part due to an increased awareness of morbidities, including intraventricular hemorrhage, transfusion-related lung injury, donor exposure, and transfusion-related intestinal injury.[37] The development

and adherence to transfusion guidelines, the implementation of cord milking or delayed cord clamping, and reduction in phlebotomy losses have all contributed to an overall decrease in transfusions. Recent well-powered RCTs demonstrated that the more liberal use of blood transfusions did not improve outcomes.[1,2] (See Chapter 10 for review.)

A comparative effectiveness study sought to determine if the addition of red cell growth factors (Darbe in this case) could decrease transfusions to an even greater extent when coupled with blood-sparing strategies.[38] Henry et al. performed the study across four Utah NICUs and demonstrated that transfusion rates were decreased to a greater extent over baseline with the use of anemia prevention guidelines, including instituting delayed cord clamping/cord milking, introducing policies for limiting phlebotomy losses, and initiating iron and Darbe treatment (Fig. 9.3). The study found that the NICUs that adhered to both anemia-preventing guidelines and used Darbe also had lower rates of neonatal morbidities, such as necrotizing enterocolitis (≥ Bell stage 2), ROP (≥ stage 3), or severe IVH (≥ grade 3).

Preterm High-Dose Epo Studies

Recent clinical trials have been published that evaluated significantly higher Epo doses, in the hopes of providing a similar neuroprotective effect as that reported in animal models. The first high-dose Epo study was performed from 2005 to 2012 by Fauchère et al. in Switzerland.[31] Investigators randomized 448 VLBW preterm infants (26–32 weeks of gestation) during the first 3 hours after birth to receive IV Epo (3000 U/kg body weight) or placebo for a total of three doses, administered at 3, 12 to 18, and 36 to 42 hours after birth. Infants underwent early head ultrasound imaging, and those with preexisting grade 3 or 4 IVH were excluded. The primary outcome of the study was the Bayley Scales of Infant Development, Second Edition, mental developmental index (BSID II MDI) at 24 months corrected age.

There were no differences in common preterm morbidities, including IVH or ROP during hospitalization. Among 448 preterm infants randomized (mean gestational age, 29.0 weeks; mean birth weight, 1210 g; 59% female), 228 were randomized to Epo

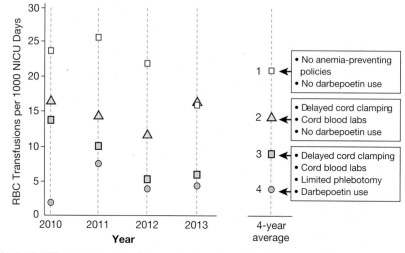

Fig. 9.3 Annual red blood cell *(RBC)* transfusion rates. Rates reported in number of transfusions per 1000 neonatal intensive care unit *(NICU)* days, shown from 2010 to 2013 for four NICUs in Utah. The 4-year average for each NICU is shown on the right of the graph. NICUs are labeled 1 through 4. NICU 1 employed no anemia-preventing policies and did not use darbepoetin. NICU 2 practiced delayed cord clamping and obtained initial labs from cord blood but did not use darbepoetin. NICUs 3 and 4 employed delayed cord clamping, obtained initial labs from cord blood, limited phlebotomy, and used darbepoetin to increase red cell mass. (Data from Henry E, Christensen RD, Sheffield MJ, et al. Why do four NICUs using identical RBC transfusion guidelines have different gestational age-adjusted transfusion rates? *J Perinatol.* 2015;35:132-136.)

and 220 to placebo, with outcome data available for 365 infants (81%) at a mean age of 23.6 months.[39] There were no significant differences in the neurodevelopmental outcome between the two groups: The mean MDI was 93.5 in the Epo group (95% CI, 91.2–95.8) and 94.5 in the placebo group (95% CI, 90.8–98.5) (difference, -1.0 [95% CI, -4.5–2.5]; $p=0.56$). There were also no differences in secondary outcomes. Interestingly, early subgroup analyses of magnetic resonance images (MRIs) obtained at term equivalent age revealed improved outcomes among Epo-treated subjects,[40,41] which led to optimism among investigators that developmental differences would be identified at 2 years of age.

A similar patient population in China was evaluated by Song et al.[30] These investigators administered Epo at lower "hematopoietic" doses (500 units/kg IV every other day for 2 weeks) in a preterm population (26–32 weeks of gestation; infants with grade 3 or 4 IVH prior to randomization were excluded). A total of 800 infants were randomly assigned to receive Epo (n=366) or placebo (n=377) within 72 hours after birth. Neurodevelopmental outcome data were available for 668 infants

(83.5%). The primary outcome of death or moderate/severe neurologic disability was significantly different between groups at 18 months corrected age, with only 43 of 330 infants (13%) in the Epo group compared to 91 of 338 infants (26.9%) in the placebo group having the primary outcome (relative risk [RR] = 0.40, 95% CI 0.27–0.59, $p<0.001$). The rate of moderate/severe neurologic disability was lower in the infants receiving Epo (22 of 309 infants, 7.1%) compared to the infants receiving placebo (57 of 304 infants, 18.8%, RR=0.32, 95% CI 0.19–0.55, $p<0.001$). There were no excess adverse events observed, and the infants in the Epo group had significantly fewer total number of blood transfusions compared to the placebo group ($p<0.001$). Despite excluding infants with preexisting grade 3 or 4 IVH, the incidence of IVH was significantly higher than comparable populations of preterm infants in NICUs in the United States, and higher than the population studied by Fauchère et al. This may explain (in part) the differences in outcomes that were found between the two studies.

Juul et al. designed the multicenter PENUT (Preterm Epo for Neuroprotection) trial to evaluate high-dose

Epo administered to ELGANs infants.[29] Doses were chosen based on preclinical studies that showed neuroprotective effects in animal models at Epo doses of 1000 to 2500 units/kg/dose.[42] A total of 941 infants 24 to 27 6/7 weeks of gestation from 19 sites in the United States were randomized to receive Epo or placebo. Infants randomized to Epo received 1000 units/kg IV every other day for six doses, followed by 400 units/kg three times weekly through 32 weeks corrected gestational age. Transfusion guidelines and iron supplementation were advised but not mandated. The primary outcome was death or severe neurodevelopmental impairment at 22 to 26 months of postmenstrual age. Severe neurodevelopmental impairment was defined as severe cerebral palsy or a composite motor or composite cognitive score of less than 70 (which corresponds to 2 SD below the mean, with higher scores indicating better performance) on the Bayley III.

There was no significant difference between the Epo group (26%) and the placebo group (26%) in the incidence of death or severe neurodevelopmental impairment at 2 years of age, and no differences in ROP, IVH, or other common neonatal morbidities. The Epo recipients received half the number of transfusions and were exposed to fewer donors, so erythropoietic effects were present. Post hoc analyses of the entire cohort revealed that increased numbers of transfusions were associated with worse developmental scores,[43] while increased iron supplementation was associated with improved developmental outcomes.[44] Speculation on why high-dose Epo did not show efficacy included the challenges of accurate developmental testing at 2 years and the possibility that the higher Epo doses considered neuroprotective in animals were outside the neuroprotective range for human neonates.

Term ESA Studies

Many multicenter clinical trials evaluating Epo in term infants with hypoxic ischemic encephalopathy (HIE) have been performed in the last 20 years, either alone or in conjunction with therapeutic hypothermia. Recent reviews and meta-analyses have been published.[45-47] Data from these meta-analyses were optimistic that ESAs might provide additional neuroprotection above and beyond therapeutic hypothermia. All but

one study evaluated Epo. The DANCE study (Darbepoetin administered to neonates undergoing cooling for encephalopathy)[48] evaluated Darbe as a potential neuroprotective agent in term infants undergoing hypothermia as treatment for HIE. No side effects attributable to Darbe were reported, and the dose appeared safe in this population; however, systematic neurodevelopmental evaluations after discharge were not performed.

Wu et al. performed a series of preliminary studies evaluating Epo in term infants undergoing cooling for moderate to severe HIE.[49,50] The results of those studies provided evidence and optimism that high-dose Epo would improve neurodevelopmental outcomes in term infants with moderate to severe HIE. The investigators designed the HEAL trial (High Dose Erythropoietin for Asphyxia and Encephalopathy; NCT02811263) to confirm their initial findings. A total of 500 infants 36 weeks or older gestation undergoing therapeutic hypothermia were randomized to high-dose Epo (1000 units/kg/dose) or placebo for a total of five doses over 7 days.[51] Of those 500 infants enrolled, 257 received Epo and 243 received placebo.

The primary outcome of death or NDI was similar in the two groups (52.5% of the Epo recipients and 49.5% of the placebo recipients [RR, 1.03; 95% CI 0.86–1.24; P=0.74). The incidence of serious adverse events (AE) was higher in the Epo group (0.86 Epo vs. 0.67 placebo; RR, 1.26; 95% CI 1.01–1.57). These results contrasted results of previous trials. Known AE of long-term use of erythropoietin in adults (hypertension, thrombosis, and polycythemia) were not more common in the Epo recipients, and the investigators could not attrite their findings to any one mechanism. Additionally, no differences were identified on MRI findings of the brain or functional outcomes. The investigators concluded that high-dose Epo administered to newborns undergoing therapeutic hypothermia for hypoxic–ischemic encephalopathy did not result in a lower risk of death or neurodevelopmental impairment than placebo and was associated with a higher rate of serious AE.

Despite the lack of efficacy in HEAL, studies evaluating ESA administration to neonatal populations continue. One such population that might benefit from ESA therapy are term infants with mild encephalopathy who do not qualify for cooling, thus no current evidence-based therapy exists. A pilot study was performed by DuPont et al. in neonates 34 weeks and older gestation diagnosed with mild encephalopathy by metabolic analysis and Sarnat staging.[52] Neonates were randomized in the first 24 hours of age to receive one dose of Darbe (10 µg/kg IV) or placebo. Clinical and laboratory data on neonates and their mothers were collected. The Bayley III and a standardized neurologic examination at 8 to 12 months corrected age were performed.

The authors found no differences in baseline characteristics of the 21 infants randomized (9 Darbe, 12 placebo). No adverse events were reported. Bayley III scores were average in both Darbe and placebo groups (see Table 9.2) and were not statistically different, although there was a trend in improved cognitive scores in the Darbe recipients. As anticipated, Darbe recipients had a shorter length of stay (p<0.05) and achieved full feedings more rapidly (p<0.01). Further study is needed to determine what treatment (Darbe, cooling, or expectant management) provides the best outcomes for neonates with mild HIE.

Rationale for ESA Dosing

Similar to findings in the PENUT trial, high-dose Epo in term infants with HIE did not improve neurodevelopmental outcomes, and high-dose ESAs are not currently recommended for this population of term infants with moderate to severe encephalopathy. Based on preclinical studies in animals showing improved neurodevelopmental outcomes,[42] the 1000 units/kg/dose tested in PENUT and HEAL might have been above the range needed in preterm and term infants to provide optimal neuroprotection. However, studies

TABLE 9.2 Characteristics and Outcomes of Neonates Enrolled in Darbepoetin for Mild Encephalopathy Study		
Patient Characteristics	**Placebo (n=12)**	**Darbe (n=9)**
Male: number (%)	6 (50.0)	6 (66.7)
Gestational age (weeks):	39.3 (1.9)	39.5 (1.5)
Cord blood pH	7.1 (0.1)	7.0 (0.0)
Cord blood base deficit	11.8 (4.3)	15.7 (3.3)
1 min Apgar	2.5 (1, 3)	2.0 (2.0, 4.5)
5 min Apgar	4 (3, 6)	6 (4.5, 7)
Time from birth to dose given (hour)	16.8 (14.8, 20.6)	13.8 (12.2, 24.9)
Hospital Outcomes		
Day of life enteral feedings started	2.0 (1.8, 2.0)	1.0 (1.0, 2.0)
Days to full feeding	6 (4, 13)[†]	3 (1.5, 4.5)**
Length of stay*	8.5 (7.0, 16.0)	5.0 (4.0, 5.0)
Follow-up Outcomes	**Placebo (n=11)**	**Darbe (n=9)**
Age at testing (months)	10.4 (1.7)	10.9 (1.7)
Bayley III Cognitive Composite	95.0 (95.0, 102.5)	100.0 (95.0, 115.0)
Bayley III Language Composite	89.0 (87.5,95.5)	94.0 (89.0, 97.0)

*p<0.05
**p<0.01
[†]n=11 (excluded the one infant who was discharged on home gavage feeding); values are mean (standard deviation) or median (interquartile range).
Data compiled from DuPont TL, Baserga M, Lowe J, et al. Darbepoetin as a neuroprotective agent in mild neonatal encephalopathy: a randomized, placebo-controlled, feasibility trial. *J Perinatol.* 2021;41:1339-1346.

Effects of ESAs that improve neurodevelopment

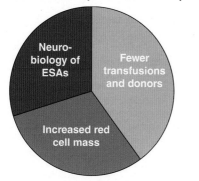

Fig. 9.4 Mechanisms of erythropoiesis stimulating agents *(ESAs)* **that may result in improved neurodevelopmental outcomes.** Preclinical and clinical studies evaluating ESA administration report improvements in cognition, executive function, and a decrease in the diagnosis of cerebral palsy. These improvements are likely a result of multiple mechanisms: the neurobiology of ESAs that decrease neuronal apoptosis and stimulate neurogenesis and oligodendrogenesis, the increase in red cell mass that may provide improved oxygen availability to brain and other organs, and the decrease in red cell transfusions and donor exposures.

using hematopoietic doses of Epo or Darbe have shown promise in improving neurodevelopmental outcomes in preterm infants.[53] The use of hematopoietic doses over a longer period (weeks instead of days) provides benefits that may lead to improved neurodevelopment (Fig. 9.4). In addition to the potential biologic activity on developing neurons and oligodendrocytes, there is a significant body of evidence

reporting increased hematocrits and decreased transfusions in ESA recipients, without adverse effects. Higher hematocrits increase oxygen availability, although it is unknown if greater oxygen utilization occurs, especially in the preterm brain. Decreased transfusions are associated with improved developmental outcomes[44,54] and decreased BPD rates.[55,56]

ESAs administered to increase red cell mass are safe and effective, and guidelines for ESA dosing as well as supplemental iron dosing have been established for preterm infants in our NICUs (Box 9.2). ESAs can also benefit infants with other neonatal anemias that put them at risk for transfusions (Box 9.2), including anemia due to ABO or Rh incompatibility,[57] infants awaiting surgery,[58] or the anemia associated with BPD.[59,60] Box 9.2 provides guidelines for ESA treatment in neonatal populations at risk for transfusion.

Summary

Clinical studies in preterm and term infants have shown ESAs to be safe and effective. There is evidence of neuroprotection in preterm infants when ESAs are administered in hematopoietic doses[53]: Preterm infants administered Darbe during their NICU stay received fewer transfusions and in smaller clinical studies had higher cognitive scores and a lower incidence of neurodevelopmental impairment into school age. Darbe is consequently being used as an ESA in several NICUs in the United States. Primary outcomes

BOX 9.2 INDICATIONS FOR ERYTHROPOIESIS STIMULATING AGENT (ESA) USE IN NEONATES

Populations	*Monitoring and Considerations*	*Treatment Length*
Very low birth weight infants	Monitor reticulocyte hemoglobin (RetHe) for Fe sufficiency (goal 29–35 pg). Check RetHe at 14 days of age. Repeat every 2–4 wk as needed to follow iron dosing. Increase oral iron by 2–4 mg/kg/day for RetHe <29 pg. Consider a single dose of iron sucrose if on 12 mg/kg/day enteral iron and RETHe is not increasing. Monitor hematocrit every 2–4 wk	Continue treatment through 34–36 corrected weeks gestation, and until infant is no longer at risk for transfusion. Continue iron supplementation after ESA is discontinued
Congenital surgical conditions	Monitor reticulocyte hemoglobin (RetHe) for Fe sufficiency (goal 29–35 pg). Check RetHe at 14 days of age. Repeat every 2–4 wk as needed to follow iron dosing. For infants who are nil per os (NPO), treat with parenteral iron (2–3 mg/kg 1–2 times weekly), monitor RetHe every 2 wk	Begin in first week of life, continue treatment until adequate hematocrit has been achieved following surgery and until infant is no longer at risk for transfusion

Continued

BOX 9.2 INDICATIONS FOR ERYTHROPOIESIS STIMULATING AGENT (ESA) USE IN NEONATES—cont'd

Populations	Monitoring and Considerations	Treatment Length
Late anemia of ABO/Rh disease	Monitor hematocrit and bilirubin every 1–2 wk	Begin ESAs when phototherapy is completed, continue treatment until adequate hematocrit has been achieved
Infants awaiting surgery	Monitor RetHe every 2 wk, consider checking ferritin if infant is NPO on prolonged total parenteral nutrition and has received >2 doses of parenteral iron; monitor hematocrit every 2 wk and preoperatively	Begin 2–4 wk prior to surgery, may continue treatment following surgery for significant blood loss until adequate hematocrit has been achieved
Infants with anemia of bronchopulmonary dysplasia	Monitor RetHe every 2 wk, consider checking ferritin if infant is requiring significant iron supplementation and has received >2 doses of parenteral iron	Continue treatment until adequate hematocrit has been achieved and until infant is no longer at risk for transfusion

of the 650 infants enrolled in the NRN Darbe trial will be available this year. Pilot studies of Darbe administration in term infants with mild HIE who do not qualify for cooling show promise. Due to the lack of efficacy of high-dose Epo in the PENUT and HEAL trials, further large RCTs are on hold until results of the NRN Darbe study are reported.

While ESAs hold promise in providing neuroprotection and improving neurodevelopmental outcomes of preterm neonates, the hematopoietic effects are clearly proven. ESAs administered to term and preterm infants increase red cell mass and decrease transfusions and donor exposures. Both mechanisms benefit infants who experience prolonged NICU stays and may ultimately improve long-term developmental outcomes.

REFERENCES

1. Franz AR, Engel C, Bassler D, et al. Effects of liberal vs restrictive transfusion thresholds on survival and neurocognitive outcomes in extremely low-birth-weight infants: the ETTNO randomized clinical trial. *JAMA*. 2020;324:560-570.
2. Kirpalani H, Bell EF, Hintz SR, et al. Higher or lower hemoglobin transfusion thresholds for preterm infants. *N Engl J Med*. 2020; 383:2639-2651.
3. Miyake T, Kung CK, Goldwasser E. Purification of human erythropoietin. *J Biol Chem*. 1977;252:5558-5564.
4. Erslev AJ, Caro J. Physiologic and molecular biology of erythropoietin. *Med Oncol Tumor Pharmacother*. 1986;3:159-164.
5. Egrie JC, Browne JK. Development and characterization of novel erythropoiesis stimulating protein (NESP). *Nephrol Dial Transplant*. 2001;16(3):S3-S13.
6. Overbay DK, Manley HJ. Darbepoetin-alpha: a review of the literature. *Pharmacotherapy*. 2002;22:889-897.
7. Maier RF, Obladen M, Scigalla P, et al. The effect of epoetin beta (Recombinant Human Erythropoietin) on the need for transfusion in very-low-birth-weight infants. *N Engl J Med*. 1994;330:1173-1178.
8. Bishara N, Ohls RK. Current controversies in the management of the anemia of prematurity. *Semin Perinatol*. 2009;33:29-34.
9. Zhang L, Chopp M, Zhang RL, et al. Erythropoietin amplifies stroke-induced oligodendrogenesis in the rat. *PLoS One*. 2010;5:e11016.
10. Iwai M, Stetler RA, Xing J, et al. Enhanced oligodendrogenesis and recovery of neurological function by erythropoietin after neonatal hypoxic/ischemic brain injury. *Stroke*. 2010;41:1032-1037.
11. Vairano M, Dello Russo C, Pozzoli G, et al. Erythropoietin exerts anti-apoptotic effects on rat microglial cells in vitro. *Eur J Neurosci*. 2002;16:584-592.
12. Sugawa M, Sakurai Y, Ishikawa-Ieda Y, et al. Effects of erythropoietin on glial cell development; oligodendrocyte maturation and astrocyte proliferation. *Neurosci Res*. 2002;44:391-403.
13. Jantzie LL, Miller RH, Robinson S. Erythropoietin signaling promotes oligodendrocyte development following prenatal systemic hypoxic-ischemic brain injury. *Pediatr Res*. 2013;74:658-667.
14. Jantzie LL, Corbett CJ, Firl DJ, et al. Postnatal erythropoietin mitigates impaired cerebral cortical development following subplate loss from prenatal hypoxia-ischemia. *Cereb Cortex*. 2015;9:2683-2695.
15. Patel S, Ohls RK. Darbepoetin administration in term and preterm neonates. *Clin Perinatol*. 2015;42:557-566.
16. Bierer R, Peceny MC, Harenberger CH, et al. Erythropoietin concentrations and neurodevelopmental outcome in preterm infants. *Pediatrics*. 2006;118:e635-640.
17. Ohls RK, Christensen RD, Kamath-Rayne BD, et al. A randomized, masked, placebo-controlled study of darbepoetin alfa in preterm infants. *Pediatrics*. 2013;132:e119-e127.
18. Ohls RK, Kamath-Rayne BD, Christensen RD, et al. Cognitive outcomes of preterm infants randomized to darbepoetin, erythropoietin, or placebo. *Pediatrics*. 2014;133:1023-1030.
19. Ohls RK, Cannon DC, Phillips J, et al. Preschool assessment of preterm infants treated with darbepoetin and erythropoietin. *Pediatrics*. 2016;137:1-9.
20. Ohls RK, Lowe J, Yeo RA, et al. Longitudinal assessment of preterm infants treated with erythropoiesis stimulating agents. *Curr Pediatr Rev*. 2023;19:417-424.
21. Widness JA, Veng-Pedersen P, Peters C, et al. Erythropoietin pharmacokinetics in premature infants: developmental, nonlinearity, and treatment effects. *J Appl Physiol*. 1996;80: 140-148.
22. George JW, Bracco CA, Shannon KM, et al. Age related differences in erythropoietic response to recombinant human erythropoietin: comparison in adult and infant rhesus monkeys. *Pediatr Res*. 1990;28:567-571.
23. Ohls RK, Veerman MW, Christensen RD. Pharmacokinetics and effectiveness of recombinant erythropoietin administered to

preterm infants by continuous infusion in parenteral nutrition solution. *J Pediatr.* 1996;128:518-523.

24. Zamboni WC, Stewart CE. An overview of the pharmacokinetic disposition of darbepoetin alfa. *Pharmacotherapy.* 2002; 22:133S-140S.

25. Warwood TL, Ohls RK, Wiedmeier SE, et al. Single-dose darbepoetin administration to anemic preterm neonates. *J Perinatol.* 2005;25:725-730.

26. Warwood TL, Ohls RK, Lambert DK, et al. Intravenous administration of darbepoetin to NICU patients. *J Perinatol.* 2006; 26:296-300.

27. An G, Ohls RK, Christsensen RD, et al. Population pharmacokinetics of darbepoetin in infants following single intravenous and subcutaneous dosing. *J Pharm Sci.* 2017;106:1644-1649.

28. Ohls RK, Roohi M, Peceny HM, et al. A randomized, masked study of weekly erythropoietin dosing in preterm infants. *J Pediatr.* 2012:160:790-795.

29. Juul SE, Comstock BA, Wadhawan R, et al. A randomized trial of erythropoietin for neuroprotection in preterm infants. *N Engl J Med.* 2020;382:233-243.

30. Song J, Sun H, Xu F, et al. Recombinant human erythropoietin improves neurological outcomes in very preterm infants. *Ann Neurol.* 2016;80:24-34.

31. Fauchère JC, Koller BM, Tschopp A, et al. with Swiss Erythropoietin Neuroprotection Trial Group. Safety of early high-dose recombinant erythropoietin for neuroprotection in very preterm infants. *J Pediatr.* 2015;167:52-57.

32. Ohlsson A, Aher SM. Early erythropoietin for preventing red blood cell transfusion in preterm and/or low birth weight infants. *Cochrane Database Syst Rev.* 2006;(3):CD004863.

33. Aher S, Ohlsson A. Late erythropoietin for preventing red blood cell transfusion in preterm and/or low birth weight infants. *Cochrane Database Syst Rev.* 2006;(3):CD004868.

34. Romagnoli C, Zecca E, Gallini F, et al. Do recombinant human erythropoietin and iron supplementation increase the risk of retinopathy of prematurity? *Eur J Pediatr.* 2000;159:627-628.

35. Ohlsson A, Aher SM. Early erythropoiesis-stimulating agents in preterm or low birth weight infants. *Cochrane Database Syst Rev.* 2020;2(2):CD004863.

36. Chou HH, Chung MY, Zhou XG, et al. Early erythropoietin administration does not increase the risk of retinopathy in preterm infants. *Pediatr Neonatol.* 2017;58:48-56.

37. Ohls RK. *Red Cell Transfusions in the Neonate.* UpToDate; August 18, 2022. https://www.uptodate.com/contents/red-blood-cell-rbc-transfusions-in-the-neonate?search=anemia%20of%20prematurity&source=search_result&selectedTitle=3~26&usage_type=default&display_rank=3

38. Henry E, Christensen RD, Sheffield MJ, et al. Why do four NICUs using identical RBC transfusion guidelines have different gestational age-adjusted RBC transfusion rates? *J Perinatol.* 2015;35:132-136.

39. Natalucci G, Latal B, Koller B, et al. with Swiss EPO Neuroprotection Trial Group. Effect of early prophylactic high-dose recombinant human erythropoietin in very preterm infants on neurodevelopmental outcome at 2 years: a randomized clinical trial. *JAMA.* 2016;315:2079-2085.

40. O'Gorman RL, Bucher HU, Held U, et al. with Swiss EPO Neuroprotection Trial Group. Tract-based spatial statistics to assess the neuroprotective effect of early erythropoietin on white matter development in preterm infants. *Brain.* 2015;138: 388-397.

41. Leuchter RH, Gui L, Poncet A, et al. Association between early administration of high-dose erythropoietin in preterm infants and brain MRI abnormality at term-equivalent age. *JAMA.* 2014;312:817-824.

42. Juul SE, Beyer RP, Bammler TK, et al. Microarray analysis of high-dose recombinant erythropoietin treatment of unilateral brain injury in neonatal mouse hippocampus. *Pediatr Res.* 2009;65:485-492.

43. Vu P, Ohls RK, Mayock DE, et al. Transfusions and neurodevelopmental outcomes in extremely low gestation neonates enrolled in the PENUT trial: a randomized clinical trial. *Pediatr Res.* 2021;90:109-116.

44. German KR, Vu PT, Comstock BA, et al. Enteral iron supplementation in infants born extremely preterm and its positive correlation with neurodevelopment; post hoc analysis of the preterm erythropoietin neuroprotection trial randomized controlled trial. *J Pediatr.* 2021;238:102-109.

45. Maxwell JR, Ohls RK. Update on erythropoiesis-stimulating agents administered to neonates for neuroprotection. *Neoreviews.* 2019;20:e622-e635.

46. McNally MA, Soul JS. Pharmacologic prevention and treatment of neonatal brain injury. *Clin Perinatol.* 2019;46:311-325.

47. Perrone S, Lembo C, Gironi F, et al. Erythropoietin as a neuroprotective drug for newborn infants: ten years after the first use. *Antioxidants.* 2022;11:652-681.

48. Baserga MC, Beachy JC, Roberts JK, et al. Darbepoetin administration to neonates undergoing cooling for encephalopathy: a safety and pharmacokinetic trial. *Pediatr Res.* 2015;78:315-322.

49. Wu YW, Bauer LA, Ballard RA, et al. Erythropoietin for neuroprotection in neonatal encephalopathy: safety and pharmacokinetics. *Pediatrics.* 2012;130:683-691.

50. Wu YW, Mathur AM, Chang T, et al. High-dose erythropoietin and hypothermia for hypoxic-ischemic encephalopathy: a phase II trial. *Pediatrics.* 2016;137:e20160191.

51. Wu YW, Comstock BA, Gonzalez FF, et al. Trial of erythropoietin for hypoxic-ischemic encephalopathy in newborns. *N Engl J Med.* 2022;387:148-159.

52. DuPont TL, Baserga M, Lowe J, et al. Darbepoetin as a neuroprotective agent in mild neonatal encephalopathy: a randomized, placebo-controlled, feasibility trial. *J Perinatol.* 2021;41:1339-1346.

53. Fischer HS, Reibel NJ, Bührer C, et al. Prophylactic erythropoietin for neuroprotection in very preterm infants: a meta-analysis update. *Front Pediatr.* 2021;9:657228.

54. Shah P, Cannon DC, Lowe JR, et al. Effect of blood transfusions on cognitive development in very low birth weight infants. *J Perinatol.* 2021;41:1412-1418.

55. Patel RM, Knezevic A, Tang J, et al. Enteral iron supplementation, red blood cell transfusion and risk of bronchopulmonary dysplasia in very low birth weight infants. *Transfusion.* 2019;59: 1675-1682.

56. Garcia MR, Comstock BA, Patel RM, et al. Iron supplementation and the risk of bronchopulmonary dysplasia in extremely low gestational age newborns. *Pediatr Res.* 2023;93(3):701-707.

57. Ohls RK, Wirkus PE, Christensen RD. Recombinant erythropoietin as treatment for the late hyporegenerative anemia of Rh hemolytic disease. *Pediatrics.* 1992;90:678-680.

58. Bierer R, Roohi M, Peceny C, et al. Erythropoietin increases reticulocyte counts and maintains hematocrit in neonates requiring surgery. *J Pediatr Surg.* 2009;44:1540-1545.

59. Christensen RD, Hunter DD, Goodell H, et al. Evaluation of the mechanism causing anemia in infants with bronchopulmonary dysplasia. *J Pediatr.* 1992;20:593-598.

60. Ohls RK, Hunter DD, Christensen RD. A randomized, double-blind, placebo-controlled trial of recombinant erythropoietin in treatment of the anemia of bronchopulmonary dysplasia. *J Pediatr.* 1993;123:996-1000.

Chapter 10

NICU Transfusion Guidelines and Strategies to Minimize Transfusions

Patrick D. Carroll MD, MPH and Robin K. Ohls MD

Chapter Outline

Introduction

Pathologic anemia is defined by a red blood cell (RBC) mass inadequate to meet the oxygen needs of tissues. Neonates often require red cell transfusions due to a decreased red cell mass brought about by acute blood loss. Preterm infants frequently experience a decline in red cell mass due to phlebotomy, a shortened red cell lifespan, and lack of erythropoietic response to a dropping hematocrit due to lack of erythropoietin (Epo) production, termed the anemia of prematurity. Target hemoglobin and hematocrit have been used as an indicator for a red cell transfusion in preterm neonates. Recently published data from two large multicentered trials in Europe and the United States showed that a restrictive approach (using a lower hematocrit to trigger a transfusion) resulted in fewer transfusions without an increase in death or serious neurodevelopmental impairment. The identification of individualized markers for transfusion need, beyond hematocrit triggers, that optimally balance the risk and benefits of transfusion, coupled with strategies to increase red cell mass to minimize transfusions, will serve to improve "transfusion stewardship," the appropriate and judicious use of transfusions in the neonatal intensive care unit (NICU).

The Development of Neonatal Transfusion Guidelines

Approaches to RBC transfusions in neonates have changed significantly over the last 40 years. In the 1970s and 1980s, phlebotomy losses in NICU patients were carefully recorded, and losses replaced when they reached 10 mL/kg. Transfusions were generally administered when the hematocrit dropped below 40%, and top-off transfusions (5–10 mL/kg volumes) were common in the later weeks of NICU hospitalization. Signs ascribed to anemia in preterm infants—apnea, poor feeding, tachycardia, and poor weight gain—would result in frequent transfusions over a wide range of hematocrits, without clear evidence of benefit.[1] A focused approach to developing transfusion guidelines was initiated in Canada in the 1990s after thousands of Canadians were exposed to hepatitis C and human immunodeficiency virus from contaminated blood.[2] Major Canadian multicentered trials evaluating restrictive vs. liberal transfusion triggers in adult (TRICC) and pediatric critical care patients (TRIPICU) both showed that a hemoglobin threshold of 7 g/dL for red cell transfusions decreased the number of transfusions received without increasing adverse outcomes.[3,4]

Since the early 2000s a number of studies have been performed evaluating hematocrit thresholds for transfusion in preterm infants. Bell et al. randomized 100 preterm infants 500 to 1300 g birth weight to a liberal (higher hematocrit) or restrictive (lower hematocrit) transfusion threshold strategy and compared clinical outcomes.[5] Infants in the liberal-transfusion group received more RBC transfusions (5.2±4.5) compared to the restrictive-transfusion group (3.3±2.9). There were no differences in pretransfusion cardiac output, hospital days, or survival to discharge. Investigators found an increase in grade 3 or 4 intraventricular hemorrhage (IVH) or periventricular leukomalacia (PVL) in the restrictive group (6/28 vs. 0/24 in the liberal group). They concluded that the more frequent major adverse neurologic imaging findings in the restrictive group suggested restrictive transfusions might be harmful. Long-term follow-up of infants enrolled in the Iowa trial was performed on a subset of children available for evaluation at 12 years. Both cognitive function (based on developmental assessment) and magnetic resonance imaging (MRI) outcome were actually better in the restrictive group, lessening the initial concerns that a restrictive strategy would impair long-term neurodevelopment.[6,7]

Canadian investigators for the Premature Infants in Need of Transfusion (PINT) Study[8] randomized 451 extremely low birth weight (ELBW) infants to a high or low threshold transfusion strategy within 48 hours of birth to determine effects of transfusion thresholds on hospital outcomes. Infants in the low threshold group received fewer transfusions and were transfused at a later age. There were no differences in morbidities or mortality between the low and high hemoglobin threshold groups, resulting in no difference in the composite outcome of death and serious morbidity at the time of discharge (bronchopulmonary dysplasia [BPD], severe retinopathy of prematurity [ROP], or, importantly, brain injury identified on ultrasound). At 18 to 21 months corrected age there were no differences between the two groups in the composite outcome of death or neurodevelopment impairment, defined as cerebral palsy (CP), significant visual or hearing impairment, or a Bayley Scales of Infant Development II (BSID II) Mental Development Index (MDI) score below 70.[9] In post hoc analyses using an MDI score <85 instead of <70, the primary outcome of death or neurodevelopmental impairment (NDI) was more likely in the low hematocrit group (45%) compared to the high hematocrit group (34%), leading investigators to hypothesize that maintaining a higher hematocrit would decrease the incidence of neurodevelopmental impairment in preterm infants.

A 2012 meta-analysis included both the Iowa and PINT studies and reported no difference in morbidities or mortality rates between high and low threshold transfusion groups.[10] Similar to adult and pediatric critical care populations, a restrictive (low) hematocrit threshold compared with a liberal (high) threshold (hematocrit 35–40%) resulted in fewer transfusions with no increase in mortality or serious morbidity.[10,11]

Recently, two similarly designed, large multicenter randomized trials were performed to confirm previous findings and determine effects of transfusion strategies on long-term outcomes. The Transfusion of Prematures (TOP) trial was designed by the principal investigators of the PINT and Iowa studies to test the hypothesis that maintaining a higher hematocrit would result in decreased NDI, by comparing neurodevelopmental outcomes of ELBW infants randomized to a high or low hematocrit threshold for transfusion.[12] This hypothesis was based on concerns over the increased IVH identified in the Iowa study, and the post hoc finding of increased percentage of infants in the low hematocrit group scoring below 85 in the PINT trial. Similarly, European investigators performing the Effects of Liberal vs. Restrictive Transfusion Thresholds on Survival and Neurocognitive Outcomes (ETTNO) study evaluated higher and lower hematocrit strategies for red cell transfusions, testing the hypothesis that the lower hematocrit strategy would lead to an increase in the primary outcome of death or neurodevelopmental disability.[13]

For the TOP trial, neonatologists were surveyed to determine an acceptable range of hematocrits that could be used to trigger transfusions,[14] and triggers were chosen to achieve a statistical difference in hemoglobin of 2 to 2.5 g/dL between groups (hematocrit 5–6%). In the ETTNO study, transfusion triggers were guided by current clinical practice in Germany.[15] The high and low thresholds chosen also aimed to produce a clinically relevant difference in mean hemoglobin concentrations between treatment groups of about 2 g/dL, to improve recognition of any effect of hemoglobin thresholds on neurocognitive outcome compared with the PINT trial, where differences between high and low thresholds were narrower.

Enrollment criteria and study methods for the two studies are shown in Table 10.1. In the ETTNO trial, transfusions prior to enrollment did not preclude participation in the study, and approximately 25% of infants received least one transfusion prior to randomization (24% vs. 25%, low vs. high). In TOP, transfusions could be given emergently prior to 6 hours of age (this occurred in 5% of the high group and 4% of the low group), but infants were ineligible if they received a transfusion after 6 hours of age. Transfusion triggers for each study are shown in Table 10.2.

The primary outcome for both trials was the combined outcome of NDI or death. NDI was defined in similar fashion in both trials: cognitive score less than 85 (on the composite cognitive score of the BSID III for TOP; BSID II MDI for ETTNO), moderate or severe CP (gross motor function classification system [GMFCS] ≥2 in TOP; Surveillance of Cerebral Palsy in Europe network definition for ETTNO), severe vision impairment, or severe hearing impairment.

Outcomes for both trials are shown in Table 10.3. Both trials found no differences between high and low groups in the primary outcome. In fact, outcomes were basically identical between groups for both studies. There were also no differences between groups in the individual components (death or NDI) of the

TABLE 10.1	Enrollment Criteria and Study Methodology for ETTNO and TOP	
	ETTNO	**TOP**
Gestational age	--	23 0/7–28 6/7 wk
Birth weight	400–999 g	--
Enrollment period	Within 72 hr of birth	Within 48 hr of birth
Length of study protocol	Transfused per protocol until discharge	Transfused per protocol through 36 completed wk
Stratification	400–749 g; 750–999 g	23–25 wk; 26–28 wk
Delayed cord clamping/milking	Recommended for sites; occurred in 627/1011 (62%)	Per site guidelines; occurred in 439/1684 (25%)
Transfusion volume	20 mL/kg	15 mL/kg
Transfusions mandated	Yes, within 72 hr of transfusion trigger	Yes, within 12 hr of identifying transfusion trigger
Epo administration allowed	No	No
Follow-up blinded	Yes	Yes
Primary outcome	Death or neurodevelopmental impairment	Death or neurodevelopmental impairment

g, grams; hr, hours; mL/kg, milliliters per kilogram; wk, weeks.
Data from Franz AR, Engel C, Bassler D, et al. Effects of liberal vs restrictive transfusion thresholds on survival and neurocognitive outcomes in extremely low-birth-weight infants: the ETTNO randomized clinical trial. *JAMA.* 2020;324:560–570; Kirpalani H, Bell EF, Hintz SR, et al. Higher or lower hemoglobin transfusion thresholds for preterm infants. *N Engl J Med.* 2020;383:2639–2651.

TABLE 10.2	Transfusion Triggers for ETTNO and TOP							
	ETTNO high critical	ETTNO high non-critical	ETTNO low critical	ETTNO low non-critical	TOP high respiratory support	TOP high no respiratory support	TOP low respiratory support	TOP low no respiratory support
0-7 days	<41	<35	<34	<28	38	35	32	29
8-14 days (TOP) 8-21 days (ETTNO)	<37	<31	<30	<24	37	32	29	25
≥15 days (TOP) >21 days (ETTNO)	<34	<28	<27	<21	32	29	25	21

ETTNO, Effects of Transfusion Thresholds on Neurocognitive Outcomes; *TOP*, Transfusions of Prematures.

For ETTNO: "critical" was defined as an infant having at least one of the following criteria: invasive mechanical ventilation, continuous positive airway pressure with fraction of inspired oxygen >0.25 for >12 out of 24 hours, treatment for patent ductus arteriosus, acute sepsis or necrotizing enterocolitis with circulatory failure requiring inotropic/vasopressor support, >6 nurse-documented apneas requiring intervention per 24 hours, or >4 intermittent hypoxemic episodes with pulse oximetry oxygen saturation <60%.

For TOP: respiratory support was defined as mechanical ventilation, continuous positive airway pressure, FiO2 >0.35, or nasal cannula ≥1 L/min (room air nasal cannula ≥1 L/min was considered respiratory support).

Transfusion triggers stayed in placed through 36 completed weeks gestation (TOP) or until discharge (ETTNO).

Data compiled from Franz AR, Engel C, Bassler D, et al. Effects of liberal vs restrictive transfusion thresholds on survival and neurocognitive outcomes in extremely low-birth-weight infants: the ETTNO randomized clinical trial. *JAMA.* 2020;324:560–70, and Kirpalani H, Bell EF, Hintz SR, et al. Higher or lower hemoglobin transfusion thresholds for preterm infants. *N Engl J Med.* 2020;383:2639–51. Hemoglobin values were converted to hematocrit by multiplying by 2.941.

primary outcome. Importantly, the percentage of infants with BSID III composite cognitive scores less than 85 was similar between groups: 269/695 (38.7%) in the high groups compared with 270/712 (37.9%) in the low group, with an adjusted relative risk (RR) of 1.04 (95% confidence interval [CI] 0.91–1.18). Concerns identified in the post hoc analyses performed in the PINT trial[9] were alleviated by this result. Cognitive delay was the primary factor determining NDI and was identified in 97% of the infants in the high groups and 91% of the infants in the low group who were designated as neurodevelopmentally impaired. No differences between groups were identified in common neonatal hospital morbidities (BPD, ROP, grade 3–4 IVH or PVL, or necrotizing enterocolitis [NEC]) (see Table 10.3). Metrics associated with severity of illness such as length of stay, time to full feeds, length of time on a ventilator, and duration of caffeine treatment were similar between low and high groups.

Similar to TOP, there were no differences between groups in the individual components (death or NDI) of the primary outcome for the ETTNO study. Importantly, the percentage of infants with BSID II MDI scores below 85 was similar between groups (37.8% high vs. 35.9% low), with an adjusted RR of 1.09

(95% CI 0.81–1.46). Cognitive delay (BSID II <85) was the primary factor determining NDI and was identified in 88% of the infants in the high group and 86% of the infants in the low group who were designated as neurodevelopmentally impaired.

The number of transfusions administered were significantly lower for both studies in the restrictive group compared to the liberal group: 4.4±4.0 vs. 6.2±4.3 transfusions in TOP; 1.7 vs. 2.6 transfusions in ETTNO. Moreover, a greater number of infants in the low threshold groups remained untransfused (see Table 10.3).

The results of these two well-designed, well-performed multicenter trials prove conclusively that transfusing critically ill ELBW infants at lower hematocrits did not result in adverse outcomes, while infants transfused at higher hematocrits did not do worse. Was there evidence that infants in either arm actually required a transfusion and improved following the transfusion? Aside from change in hematocrit, efficacy data were not collected. Because both studies relied on consensus in determining hematocrit thresholds, both studies likely ended up measuring what infants received, rather than what they needed. In promoting transfusion stewardship, documenting evidence of benefit should be a part of future studies.

TABLE 10-3 Two-Year and Hospital Outcomes for ETTNO and TOP

	ETTNO high	ETTNO low	TOP high	TOP low
2-yr outcomes:				
Number randomized	492	521	911	913
Number evaluated for primary outcome	450	478	845	847
Death/NDI	44.4% (200/450)	42.9% (205/478)	50.1% (423/845)	49.8% (422/847)
Death by 24 months	8.3% (38/460)	9.0% (44/491)	16.2% (146/903)	15.0% (135/901)
NDI	36% (162/450)	33.7% (161/478)	39.6% (277/699)	40.3% (287/712)
Cognitive score[a] mean	92.6±16.5	92.4±17.5	85.5±15	85.3±14.8
Cognitive score[a] <85	37.6% (154/410)	34.4% (148/430)	38.7% (269/695)	37.9% (270/712)
Cognitive score[a] <70			12.7% (88/695)	13.5% (96/712)
Cerebral palsy[b]	4.3% (18//419)	5.6% (25/443)	6.8% (48/711)	7.6% (55/720)
Hospital outcomes:				
Untransfused (%)	21	41*	3	12*
Transfusions (mean±SD)	2.6	1.7	6.2±4.3	4.4±4.0*
NEC	5.3%	6.2%	10.0%	10.5%
ROP > grade 2	15.9%	13.0%	19.7%	17.2%
Intraventricular hemorrhage grade 3–4[c]	8.1% (40/492)	6.7% (35/521)	17.1% (146/855)	17.9% (154/859)
Periventricular leukomalacia	23/492	30/521		
Bronchopulmonary dysplasia	28.4	26.0	59.0	56.3
Hospital days[d]	93±41	92±38	96 (72-129)	97 (75-127)

No differences between high and low groups in each study were identified in any of the measures listed above except number of transfusions (TOP) and percent untransfused (ETTNO and TOP).

No analyses have been performed between ETTNO and TOP studies.

[a]Bayley Scales of Infant Development III composite cognitive score for TOP; Bayley Scales of Infant Development II Mental Developmental Index for ETTNO.

[b]Gross motor function classification system ≥2 for TOP; Surveillance of Cerebral Palsy in Europe network definition for ETTNO.

[c]Numbers are combined for intraventricular hemorrhage and periventricular leukomalacia for TOP.

[d]Values are mean and interquartile range for TOP; mean and standard deviation for ETTNO.

ETTNO, Effects of Transfusion Thresholds on Neurocognitive Outcomes; *NDI,* Neurodevelopmental impairment; *NEC,* necrotizing enterocolitis; *ROP,* retinopathy of prematurity; *TOP,* Transfusions of Prematures.

Data from Kirpalani H, Bell EF, Hintz SR, et al. Higher or lower hemoglobin transfusion thresholds for preterm infants. *N Engl J Med.* 2020;383:2639–2651; Franz AR, Engel C, Bassler D, et al. Effects of liberal vs restrictive transfusion thresholds on survival and neurocognitive outcomes in extremely low-birth-weight infants: the ETTNO randomized clinical trial. *JAMA.* 2020;324:560–570.

Strategies to Minimize Transfusions

PREVALENCE OF ANEMIA

Although a physiologic decrease in hematocrit occurs universally following birth, identifying a true incidence of clinically significant anemia at various gestational ages is difficult. A variety of cutoff thresholds for anemia, inclusion or exclusion of infants receiving transfusion, and varying thresholds for transfusion makes identifying this incidence difficult. However, in a landmark study, Dallman published trends in anemia of prematurity.[16] In this study, he demonstrated that in term infants weighing more than 3000 g, the physiologic nadir of hemoglobin levels occurred at about 2 months of life, reaching 11.0 g/dL. The physiologic hemoglobin nadir was more pronounced and occurred slightly earlier in premature infants, with hemoglobin levels decreasing to 9.5 g/dL for infants 1500 to 2000 g and 9.0 g/dL for infants less than 1500 g.

The physiologic decrease in hemoglobin and hematocrit is largely due to a rapid decrease in endogenous erythropoietin levels just after birth. Following birth, the P_aO_2 (generally ~27 mm Hg before delivery) increases dramatically once the newborn infant has taken first breaths. With increased oxygenation there is a resultant rapid decrease in endogenous erythropoietin production, which is followed in 5 to 7 days by a decrease in reticulocyte count. These factors contribute to the physiologic anemia that universally occurs following birth.

Christensen et al. reported the trend in hematocrit and hemoglobin over the first 28 days of life among infants born at 35 to 42 weeks and 29 to 34 weeks of gestation.[17] This study included nearly 42,000 patients born at 35 to 42 weeks of gestation and nearly

40,000 patients born at 29 to 34 weeks of gestation (Fig. 10.1). Infants were excluded when their diagnosis included abruption, placenta previa, fetal anemia, or when a blood transfusion was given. In the 35- to 42-week cohort, the hemoglobin decreased from 18 g/dL to 13 g/dL, a decrease of 5 g/dL. Among the 29- to 34-week cohort, the initial hemoglobin decreased from approximately 17 g/dL to 11 g/dL.

Infants born more premature, smaller, and more critically ill undergo greater phlebotomy losses (both in number of times blood is sampled and in total volume/kg) to provide care. These phlebotomy losses exacerbate the likelihood of anemia. Estimates of NICU laboratory blood draws primarily in the first 2 weeks of life among premature VLBW infants are higher than the remainder of a neonate's hospitalization.[18] During the first 6 weeks of life laboratory blood losses have been reported to range from 11 to 22 mL/kg/week,

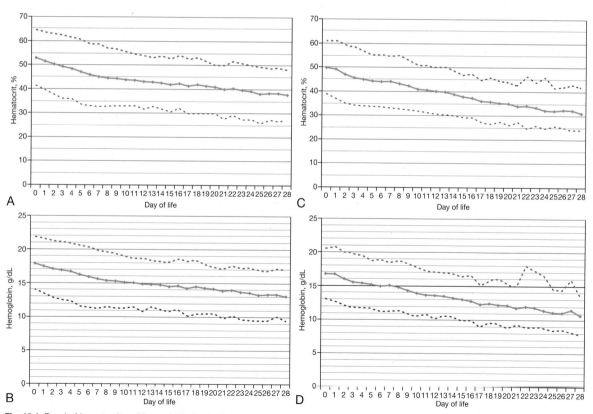

Fig. 10.1 Trend of hematocrit and hemoglobin for the first 28 days of life among infants born between 35 and 42 weeks **(A and B)** and between 29 and 34 weeks **(C and D)** of gestational age, respectively.

which is equivalent to 15% to 30% of the circulating blood volume.[19] There is a direct relationship between the volume of blood removed for laboratory testing and the volume of blood transfused from VLBW infants (Fig. 10.2).[20] In several studies, highly significant direct associations have been observed between volume of blood removed with that transfused (i.e., correlation coefficients of 0.75–0.90).[20-23] As described, phlebotomy loss is a significant contributor to anemia in ELBW and VLBW infants. Despite widespread acceptance of this practice, marked variation in blood lost due to laboratory testing has been noted. For example, in comparing laboratory blood loss over the first 2 weeks of life in infants weighing less than 1500 g, Ringer et al. reported that one NICU drew 17.5 mL/kg while another drew nearly twice as much (34.1 mL/kg).[24] After statistical adjustment for birth weight, gestational age, and severity of illness, laboratory blood loss remained 10.7 mL/kg per patient different between the two NICUs. Obladen et al. in the late 1980s reported blood loss of 24, 60, and 67 mL/kg for increasingly sick infants in their cohort.[21] In addition to reporting significant variation in phlebotomy loss (7–51 mL/kg) Nexo et al. reported that among 20 VLBW infants that 25% of the phlebotomy losses were in excess of the need for analytical procedures.[25] While variation in phlebotomy loss may in part be explained by differences in gestational age, birth weight, severity of illness, and other factors, the wide variation observed indicates considerable opportunity to limit phlebotomy loss.

Rates of phlebotomy vary greatly between hospitals. Rosebraugh et al. conducted a prospective study measuring the actual phlebotomy and "hidden" phlebotomy loss among ELBW infants in the first 28 days of life[26] and reported phlebotomy losses among VLBW infants in the first month of life of greater than 60 mL/kg, with blood loss of 10 mL/kg on the first day of life. A more recent study among 20 infants with an average birth weight of 836 g reported approximately 30 mL/kg cumulative iatrogenic blood loss in the first 28 days of life,[27] with 2.7 mL/kg blood loss on the first day of life. This institution routinely uses inline point of care for analysis of blood gas, glucose, and bilirubin.

TRANSFUSION RATES

Factors that include physiologic anemia, prematurity, and phlebotomy losses contribute to increased rates of transfusion. Early randomized trials (see earlier) evaluated restrictive vs. liberal transfusion guidelines for neonates.[5,8] The overwhelming majority of neonates received at least one transfusion whether in the liberal or restrictive transfusion arm. Retrospective analyses from nearly 1 million births between 2001 and 2011 in New South Wales, Australia, reported a rate of 331 transfusions per 1000 births less than 32 weeks gestational age and 4.8 per 1000 among term infants.[28] In a Canadian cohort, 44% of infants born at 23 to 29 weeks of gestation remained untransfused during their NICU stay.[29] This rate appears to be increasing among infants born at 26 to 29 weeks of gestation but remains unchanged or decreased for neonates born at

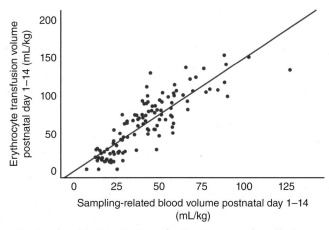

Fig. 10.2 Calculated blood volume of a 30-cm segment of umbilical cord.

23 to 25 weeks of gestation in 2010-2012 compared to prior years.

TRANSFUSION RISKS

Adopting strategies to prevent anemia is important to decrease risks associated with either anemia or transfusion. For many of these associations a cause-and-effect relationship remains to be determined.

Intraventricular Hemorrhage

In 2013 Christensen et al. reported an association between IVH and RBC transfusions given in the first days of life.[30] This finding was followed by a study from the same multicentered medical group in which a 75% decline in RBC transfusions occurred after adoption of a transfusion management program. In the same cohort of infants evaluated there was a decrease in IVH from 17% to 8%.[31] This association has not been replicated in other studies or at other hospitals.

Necrotizing Enterocolitis

Numerous studies have evaluated the association between red cell transfusions and NEC. This association, sometimes referred to as either transfusion-related acute gut injury (TRAGI) or transfusion-associated NEC (TANEC), was summarized in a 2012 report.[32] There were six factors discussed in support of a causative relationship between transfusions and NEC. A later study evaluated the relationship between RBC transfusion, anemia, and NEC. In this prospective study of 600 VLBW infants, no association was identified between RBC transfusion and NEC, although there was an association with severe anemia ($\leq$8 g/dL) and NEC (p=0.001).[33]

Bronchopulmonary Dysplasia

Several studies have reported a relationship between RBC transfusions and BPD. In a 2014 study of 231 preterm infants 32 weeks or less gestation, the rate of BPD was 9.8 times higher among 137 infants who had received a transfusion before the diagnosis of BPD, compared to the 94 who did not.[34] This difference remained after correction for other potential confounders, including gestational age, birth weight, no surfactant, mechanical ventilation 1 week or more, sepsis, aminophylline use, and NEC. Similar retrospective studies have also reported an increased incidence of BPD with transfusions,[20] and others have reported a decreased incidence of BPD in preterm infants receiving erythropoietin.[35]

Mortality

Investigators in Brazil evaluated outcomes in 1077 infants 1500 g or less. After adjusting for confounders, the RR of death during NICU hospitalization was 1.49 among infants who received at least one RBC transfusion in the first 28 days of life.[36]

Delayed Development

Given the evidence that transfusions themselves may lead to increased morbidities in adult and pediatric patients, several investigators evaluated the association between the number and volume of transfusions and developmental outcomes in preterm infants.[37,38] The impact of transfusions on developmental outcomes of preterm infants enrolled in a previous study was analyzed.[39,40] In that study, preterm infants were randomized to subcutaneous erythropoietin (400 units/kg three times weekly), darbepoetin (10 μg/kg once weekly), or placebo (sham injections) during their initial hospitalization, and the number and volume of red cell transfusions recorded. Children were evaluated using standard developmental tests of cognition at 18 to 22 months (56 infants in erythropoietin plus darbepoetin combined group, 24 infants in the placebo group). In a post hoc analysis,[37] cognitive scores on the BSID-III at 18 to 22 months were inversely correlated with transfusion volume (p=0.02). Infants receiving one or more transfusions in the placebo group had significantly lower cognitive scores than those that remained untransfused. Cognitive scores were similar between nontransfused and transfused subjects in the erythropoietin plus darbepoetin group, suggesting these red cell growth factors might provide neuroprotection from the effects of transfusions.

Results were analyzed in similar fashion in the Preterm Epo for Neuroprotection (PENUT) trial.[38] In that study, erythropoietin 1000 units/kg or placebo was given every 48 hours for a total of six doses, followed by 400 units/kg or sham injections three times a week through 32 weeks postmenstrual age. Six hundred and twenty-eight (315 placebo, 313 Epo) survived and were assessed at 2 years of age. Associations between BSID-III scores and the number and volume of pRBC transfusions were evaluated in a post hoc analysis. Each transfusion was associated with a decrease in composite cognitive score of 0.96 (95% CI: −1.34, −0.57), a decrease in composite motor score of 1.51 (−1.91, −1.12), and a decrease in composite language score of 1.10 (−1.54, −0.66). Significant negative associations between BSID-III score and transfusion volume and donor exposure were observed in the placebo group but not in the erythropoietin group. Similar to the previous study,[37] transfusions in ELBW infants were associated with worse neurodevelopmental outcomes.

Strategies to Minimize Transfusions

In general, there are three strategies to minimize transfusions in neonates: start with a greater volume of blood, decrease phlebotomy, and stimulate red cell production. Interventions that decrease anemia in the delivery room may decrease the likelihood of transfusion; these include delayed cord clamping or milking the umbilical cord and the use of umbilical cord blood for admission laboratory studies.

START WITH A GREATER BLOOD VOLUME

The term placental transfusion incorporates previously used terms, including delayed cord clamping (DCC) and milking the umbilical cord or cord blood milking (MUC), and less commonly cut umbilical cord milking.[41] Placental transfusion increases the initial complement of RBCs by effectively transfusing fetal blood from the placenta to the neonate.

The number of studies on placental transfusion have increased dramatically over the past 30 years. A recent Cochrane review for DCC and MUC in preterm infants published in 2019 included randomized trials in which DCC was defined as 30 to 180 seconds between the time of fetal delivery and clamping the umbilical cord.[42] Transfusions were significantly reduced in preterm infants undergoing DCC/MUC. Among infants less than 34 weeks of gestation, 45% in the DCC group received at least one transfusion compared to 56% undergoing early cord clamping (ECC), resulting in a RR for transfusion of 0.64 (0.47–0.87) favoring DCC. In the 2012 Cochrane review[43] infants undergoing DCC/MUC had higher hematocrit values at three different times relative to birth. Due to the significantly

lower incidence of transfusion, clinicians are generally not a focused on hematologic parameters among term infants. However, a 2013 Cochrane review evaluating delayed cord clamping in term infants demonstrated increased hemoglobin concentrations at 24 to 48 hours in this population as well.[44] Term infants undergoing DCC also experienced a persistent increase in iron stores.[44] Infants in the early cord clamping group were over twice as likely to be iron deficient at 3 to 6 months compared with infants undergoing DCC (RR 2.65, 1.04–6.73). A separate meta-analysis limited to umbilical cord milking reported initial hemoglobin that was 2 g/dL higher in the MUC group.[45] Among infants born at 33 weeks gestational age or greater, hemoglobin concentration remained higher by 1.2 g/dL and 1.1 g/dL at 48 hours and 6 weeks, respectively.

Studies nearly 50 years ago demonstrated incrementally increasing fetal blood volume and decreasing placental blood volume as a result of DCC for up to 180 seconds.[46] In term infants, Yao et al. demonstrated a correlation between infant blood volume and the duration between birth and clamping of the umbilical cord. DCC by 30, 60, or 180 seconds increased the infant blood volume by 6, 13.6, or 22.5 mL/kg, respectively. Adjusting the position of the infant relative to the mother in both vaginal and caesarean delivery was also reported in early studies to increase the volume of placental transfusion during DCC.[47,48] More recently, a multicenter randomized controlled trial (RCT) of term infants born by vaginal delivery demonstrated a similar volume of fetal blood transferred from the placenta to the infant independent of infant position suggesting gravity did not have an effect on transfused volume.[49]

MUC is another method of placental transfusion. This method offers the advantage of being completed more quickly than DCC. Some obstetricians more enthusiastically accept this approach due to the relative speed vs. DCC and the feeling of doing something rather than doing nothing as is perceived with DCC. However, this method has also been questioned due to the nonphysiologic manner of transfusing boluses of blood rather than gradual transfusion with DCC. In 2019 a multicenter randomized trial directly compared the outcomes following DCC and MUC among infants born between 23 and 34 weeks of gestation.[50] The Data Safety Monitoring Board stopped this trial early due to an increased risk of severe IVH among infants less than 28 weeks of gestation in the MUC group. This led to widespread recommendations to avoid MUC in infants less than 28 weeks of gestation. Additionally, the National Institute of Child Health and Human Development (NICHD) has approved a new trial of MUC vs. DCC in 30- to 32-week infants with cognitive status at 2 years as the primary outcome.

Several studies have sonographically investigated umbilical vessel sizes at various gestational ages. Using in situ umbilical vein and umbilical artery diameters,[51] cord blood volume was mathematically determined (Fig. 10.3). This model suggests that milking a 30-cm segment of umbilical cord may provide an additional 10 to 25 mL of blood to a neonate born at 23 to 34 weeks of gestation, respectively.

For DCC to effectively transfuse placental blood to the newly delivered neonate, fetal blood in the placenta must continue to transfer into the neonate for a period of time (i.e., potentially until the umbilical cord is clamped or cord pulsations cease). If the opposite results, the neonate would hemorrhage back into the placenta. To study this, the direction of blood flow during delayed cord clamping was evaluated using Doppler ultrasonography in term infants after vaginal delivery.[52] The duration of flow in the umbilical vein and both umbilical arteries varied among the 30 infants in this study. Ninety percent had venous flow toward the neonate noted immediately after birth, while the remaining 10% demonstrated no blood flow. Additional studies are needed to further clarify these blood flow patterns in premature infants following both vaginal and caesarean delivery.

Katheria et al. demonstrated improved superior vena cava blood flow and right ventricular output, both markers of systemic blood flow, in preterm infants following MUC compared to immediate cord clamping (ICC).[53] Additionally, the diastolic and mean blood pressure within the first 6 hours of life was increased in the MUC group. This finding is consistent with previous studies on MUC.[54,55] Although no studies on SVC flow have been done following DCC, blood pressure has been shown to be improved after DCC compared to ICC.[43]

Optimal Timing of Delayed Cord Clamping

The optimal timing for clamping the umbilical cord after birth has been a subject of controversy and debate.

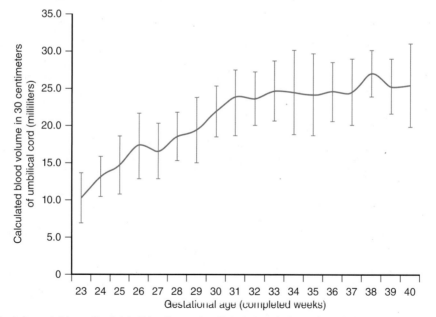

Fig. 10.3 Correlation between total sampling-related blood loss and erythrocyte transfusions volume during postnatal days 1 to 14 in a cohort of 149 extremely preterm infants. The volume of erythrocytes transfused during postnatal days 1 to 14 was highly correlated with the amount of sampling-related blood loss (mL/kg). rS = 0.870, *P*<.001

Although many RCTs in term and preterm infants have evaluated the benefits of DCC vs. ICC, the ideal timing for cord clamping has yet to be established. While a variety of durations of DCC has been used, these are typically compared to a control group undergoing ICC rather than a comparison of various durations of DCC. The majority of studies among preterm infants define DCC as between 30 and 120 seconds. Sixty seconds appears to be the most widely accepted duration of DCC, though this time versus other definitions of DCC is without strong scientific evidence.

Risks of Placental Transfusion

Physicians have raised concerns about potential risks of DCC. In particular, obstetricians reported concern that DCC may delay resuscitation, result in lower Apgar scores, and increase rates of hypothermia or cause IVH.[56,57] Neonatologists and pediatricians have reported concerns for hyperbilirubinemia and polycythemia as potential risks. When these outcomes were investigated,[58] it was found that there was no difference in the Apgar scores at 1, 5, or 10 minutes. There was also no difference in rates of hypothermia on admission. In fact, the average admission temperature was 0.14°C (95% CI -0.03–0.31) higher in the DCC/MUC group. The peak bilirubin level in the DCC/MUC group was higher by 0.88 mg/dL (15.01 µmol/L) than the ICC group. However, there was no difference in the frequency of phototherapy though there was a trend toward more phototherapy (RR 1.21; 95% CI 0.94–1.55). Finally, the cord pH between groups was not different. However, among infants requiring resuscitation, controversy remains whether placental transfusion practices provide more benefit than risk.[41,59] Perhaps the greatest demonstrated risk is severe IVH among infants less than 28 weeks undergoing MUC as described earlier.[50]

In a meta-analysis (prior to the 2019 DCC/MUC study) limited to infants less than 32 completed weeks of gestation who underwent either DCC or MUC, Backes et al. demonstrated that mortality was decreased by 58% (eight studies).[60] The finding of decreased mortality was also independently reported in a manuscript describing a quality improvement initiative following the implementation of MUC in all infants less than 30 weeks of gestation.[61] Compared to historical controls the rate of survival in the MUC group increased from 84% to 94% and 76% to 91% among infants less than 30 and less than 27 weeks of gestation, respectively. However, those findings were not replicated in a RCT performed by Tarnow-Mordi et al., in which over 1600 infants less than 30 weeks were randomized to ICC or DCC.[59] In this study there was no difference in the composite outcome of death or major morbidity between the two groups. There was a lower mortality rate in the DCC group (p=0.03), although this finding was found to be not statistically significant after correcting for multiple comparison of 13 secondary outcomes (p=0.39). Notably, among 784 infants randomized to the DCC cohort only 580 (74%) received at least 60 seconds of DCC. Seventy percent had their cord clamped prior to 60 seconds (including 97/209 prior to 10 seconds) due to clinical concern about the infant. It is possible that the infants for whom there was clinical concern would benefit most from DCC though this suggestion is speculative.

Long-Term Outcomes

Currently three studies have reported postdischarge outcomes for placental transfusion strategies. Mercer et al. reported 18-month outcomes among infants randomized to DCC compared to ICC.[62] In this study, the average length of DCC was 32 seconds. Infants in the DCC group were less likely to have motor scores below 85 on the BSID (odds ratio [OR] 0.32, 0.10–0.90). Rabe et al. examined neurodevelopmental outcomes at 2 and 3.5 years following either DCC or MUC.[63] No differences were seen in any of the three Bayley III composite scores when comparing DCC and MUC. Katheria et al. also compared neurodevelopmental outcomes at 22 to 26 months of infants randomized to DCC or MUC, and found that those in the MUC group had higher language and cognitive scores compared to the DCC group.[64] There was no difference in rates of mild or moderate to severe neurodevelopmental impairment. While studies continue to evaluate the short- and long-term outcomes of placental transfusion, there is wide agreement between various organizational recommendations, including the American Academy of Pediatrics, that DCC be performed in term infants and preterm infants who do not require resuscitation.[65]

DECREASE PHLEBOTOMY

With decreasing gestational age comes decreasing birth weight and therefore lower circulating blood volumes. Efforts have been made following delivery to preserve this limited blood volume. One such strategy to limit neonatal blood loss is cord blood sampling (CBS) using residual fetal blood in the umbilical cord and placenta for admission laboratory studies immediately after birth.

ELBW infants routinely have several laboratory tests sent immediately upon admission to the NICU. These generally include a blood culture, complete blood count (CBC), arterial and/or venous blood gas, and blood type and antibody screen. Less frequently, testing may include newborn metabolic screen, genetic testing, coagulation studies, and bilirubin. For the smallest neonates these admission laboratory studies may account for a significant percentage of their initial circulating blood volume.

Validation of Cord Blood Samples

Using residual fetal blood in the umbilical cord/placenta for these laboratory tests on admission is safe and valid (Table 10.4). Several studies have compared CBC parameters between CBS and a newborn blood

TABLE 10.4 Studies Evaluating the Validity of Cord Blood for Admission Laboratory Tests in Neonates

Laboratory Test	Author, Year	Comments
CBC	Hansen, 2005[66]	113 term infant paired samples. High correlation of WBC, hematocrit, platelets. I:T ratio reported.
	Carroll, 2011[67]	174 preterm infant paired samples. High correlation of WBC, hemoglobin, platelets. False positive thrombocytopenia on four cord samples.
	Christensen, 2011[68]	10 VLBW infant pilot study. No difference in CBC compared to historical controls.
	Beeram, 2012[69]	200 term and preterm infant paired samples. Similar results between sources. Higher rate of leukopenia in cord samples noted.
	Baer, 2013[70]	91 VLBW infants. No paired samples. Outcome study.
	Rotshenker-Olshinka, 2014[71]	305 term and preterm infant paired samples. Significant correlation between cord and infant CBC.
	Greer, 2019[72]	110 paired preterm and term cord blood and neonatal samples. Significant correlation between cord and infant WBC, hemoglobin, platelet count.
	Medeiros, 2021[73]	67 infants admitted to the NICU. Paired samples comparing umbilical venous and umbilical arterial blood with direct neonatal phlebotomy. High correlation of WBC, hemoglobin, I:T ratio, platelets.
Coagulation Studies, Platelet Count and Function	Raffaeli, 2021[75]	60 term and preterm neonates with paired cord or placental blood and neonatal blood. Placental blood had a procoagulant imbalance compared to neonatal draw on TEG and TGA. PT and APTT did not differ between samples.
	Grevsen, 2021[74]	20 paired term cord and peripheral samples. Platelet count and MPV did not differ. Fibrinogen, platelet aggregation differed.
Blood Culture	Polin, 1981[78]	200 cord blood cultures with 29 paired infant cultures. Cord sterilized with 2% tincture of iodine. One septic patient had positive cord and infant culture. Similar contamination rate between cord samples (2.5%) and infant samples (3.4%).

TABLE 10.4   Studies Evaluating the Validity of Cord Blood for Admission Laboratory Tests in Neonates—cont'd

Laboratory Test	Author, Year	Comments
	Herson, 1998[79]	81 term infants, 35 high-risk paired samples. Placental vein sterilized with povidone-iodine. 5 mL blood samples from cord obtained. 20% true positive from cord vs. 3% true positive from infant cultures of paired samples.
	Hansen, 2005[66]	113 term infants. Cord sterilized with alcohol. Zero contaminants or true positive cultures.
	Christensen, 2011[68]	10 VLBW infant pilot study. No positive cultures from cases or matched controls.
	Beeram, 2012[69]	200 term and preterm paired samples. Cord sterilized with povidone-iodine and then swabbed with alcohol. Two contaminants from cord blood. One contaminant and one pathogen from infant blood.
	Baer, 2013[70]	91 VLBW infants. No paired samples. Outcome study.
	Rotshenker-Olshinka, 2014[71]	223 term and preterm infant paired samples. Cord sterilized with chlorhexidine prior to placental delivery. No cases of sepsis. High contamination rate from both cord sample (12.5%) and infant sample (2.5%).
	Greer, 2019[72]	108 paired preterm and term cord blood and neonatal blood cultures. 3.7% true positive rate from cord blood 0.9% corresponding positive peripheral neonatal culture (3 false negatives). 4.6% contaminant cord blood culture rate vs. 0% contaminants from peripheral neonatal blood culture.
	Medeiros, 2021[73]	67 preterm infants. Cord/placenta sterilized with 70% isopropyl alcohol and 0.5% chlorhexidine. No true positives, 1 (1.5%) contaminant. Average cord blood culture volume 1.6 mL.
Blood Type	AAP, 2004[80]	Recommends "direct antibody test, blood type, and Rh (D) type on the infant's (cord) blood."
	Judd, 2001[83]	Practice guideline for immunohematology. Endorses obtaining blood type from cord blood or infant blood.
	Christensen, 2011[68]	10 VLBW infant pilot study.
	Baer, 2013[70]	91 VLBW infants. No paired samples. Outcome study.
	Alissa, 2021[82]	78 paired term samples compared ABO and Rh, DAT and antibody screen. Concordance demonstrated between cord and heel stick samples.
Antibody Screen	Josephson, 2011[81]	American Association of Blood Banking technical manual. Recommends antibody testing using plasma or serum from the infant or mother.
	Christensen, 2011[68]	10 VLBW infant pilot study.
	Baer, 2013[70]	91 VLBW infants. No paired samples. Outcome study.
	Alissa, 2021[82]	78 paired term samples compared ABO and Rh, DAT and antibody screen. Concordance demonstrated between cord and heel stick samples.
Newborn Metabolic Screen	Miller, 2008[82]	CLSI newborn screening guidelines. Recommends first newborn metabolic test be obtained upon admission of premature infants.
	Christensen, 2011[68]	10 VLBW infant pilot study.
	Baer, 2013[70]	91 VLBW infants. No paired samples. Outcome study.

ABO, A, B, and O Blood type; *APTT,* Activated Partial Thromboplastin Time; *CBC,* Complete Blood Count; *DAT,* Direct Antiglobulin Test; *I:T Ratio,* Immature to Total neutrophil Ratio; *mL,* Milliliters; *MPV,* Mean Platelet Volume; *PT,* Prothrombin Time; *Rh (D),* rhesus D antigen; *TEG,* Thromboelastogram; *TGA,* Thrombin Generation Assay; *VLBW,* Very Low Birth Weight; *WBC,* White Blood Cell.

sample (NBS) drawn directly from the neonate at birth. In 2004, Hansen et al. demonstrated that among term infants there was no difference in WBC, hematocrit, or platelet count between a CBS and NBS.[66] Subsequently this same finding was repeated and confirmed in premature infants and repeated in term infants.[67-73] Platelet count and platelet count function was specifically evaluated between CBS and NBS. Both the platelet count and the mean platelet volume (MPV) were equivalent.[74] Additionally, prothrombin time and activated partial thromboplastin time have been similar between CBS and NBS.[75]

There are varying recommendations for optimal blood volume for a neonatal blood culture. The Infectious Disease Society of America recommends a weight-based inoculant volume adapted from the work of Kellogg et al. that would result in blood culture volumes as high as 4.5% of the total blood volume of an infant,[76] as the accuracy of a blood culture is correlated with the blood culture volume. Obtaining blood cultures directly from the neonate often yields inadequate blood culture volumes.[77] Conversely, obtaining a blood culture from a CBS has been shown to yield higher blood culture volume.[73] The practice of using CBS (including samples from placental vessels) has been reported in several studies.[66,68,69-73,79-81] These include studies using 70% isopropyl alcohol, chlorhexidine, or betadine as a sterilizing agent. Contamination of blood cultures is a frequently raised concern when implementing CBS for blood cultures. Studies range from no contaminants to over 12% contamination rate, underscoring the importance of sterile technique when obtaining CBS for blood cultures.

Neonatal blood ABO and Rh typing can be successfully obtained from CBS as demonstrated in a recent study of paired samples.[82] This reinforces the common practice of obtaining blood type and Coombs test from cord blood.[83] Obtaining the newborn metabolic screen differs from region to region. In regions where at least two separate newborn metabolic panels are obtained it may be advised to obtain the first sample from cord blood. This is the recommended approach by the Clinical Laboratory Standards Institute.[84] Benefits of drawing the first newborn metabolic screen from CBS includes decreasing phlebotomy loss from the neonate and obtaining blood prior to total parenteral nutrition and antibiotics.

Outcomes

To date, one pilot study,[68] one multicenter with historical control,[70] one single-center randomized trial,[85] and one multicenter randomized trial[86] have evaluated outcomes of using CBS for admission studies in neonates. The initial pilot study of 10 VLBW neonates reported decreased phlebotomy loss in the first day of life, decreased transfusions, and a decrease in IVH.[68] The multicenter trial with historical controls enrolled 96 patients. This trial reported lower vasopressor use, increased hemoglobin in the first 12 to 24 hours of life, fewer transfusions per patient, and fewer patients requiring any transfusion in the CBS group. The incidence of IVH appeared lower in the CBS group but was not statistically significant.[70]

In a single-center trial, 80 ELBW infants were randomized to either CBS or NBS. Infants in the CBS were found to have a 56% lower probability of needing a pRBC transfusion.[85] Those in the CBS group received their first transfusion 30 days (interquartile range [IQR] 21–41) after birth and those in the NBS group received their first transfusion 14 days (IQR 7–26) after birth. There was no difference in IVH or chronic lung disease (CLD) rates between groups. Significant ROP requiring treatment was not different between groups, with 32% requiring treatment in the CBS group and 57% in the NBS group (p=0.057). This study may have been underpowered to detect this outcome.

Among VLBW randomized in a multicenter trial,[86] those in the CBS group were found to have a 1.5 g/dL higher hemoglobin at 12 to 24 hours of life. The median time to first transfusion was 7 days in the NBS group and 24 days in the CBS group. The CBS group had fewer RBC donor exposures (1.8 vs. 1.1; p=0.04). In this trial infants randomized to the CBS group had a lower rate of grade 3–4 IVH, with an IVH rate of 32% in the NBS group and 11% in the CBS group. BPD rates were lower in the CBS group (57% vs. 80%; p=0.04). Severe ROP was not statistically different in this trial with 28% severe ROP in the NMS group and 11% in the CBS group (p=0.08).

Implementation

Two methods have been described for obtaining CBS. The first is for the obstetrician to double clamp the umbilical cord at the proximal (placental) and distal (fetal) ends. Fetal blood can then be obtained from an isolated cord segment. The second method is to draw blood from a fetal vessel on the placental surface near the umbilical cord insertion site. One study[87] compared CBC indices at 2, 10, and 30 minutes via both methods. This study found that blood drawn from an isolated umbilical cord segment at 30 minutes was not different than the 2-minute results. This is in contrast to the samples obtained from the fetal vessel on the placental surface in which the 2- and 10-minute results were not different, but the 30-minute sample was different than the 2- and 10-minute samples.

Successfully obtaining fetal blood via CBS can be done at a high rate. In a recent trial, CBS were obtained in 95% of eligible neonates, including infants as young as 23 weeks of gestation, those undergoing DCC, twins/triplets, and in both vaginal and cesarean deliveries.[70] An implementation study whereby labor and delivery and NICU staff were trained to obtain CBS demonstrated samples were successfully collected on 64% of all high-risk infants between 22 and 42 weeks of gestation admitted to the NICU.[88] Similarly, a single-site trial on feasibility and accuracy of CBS reported collection was feasible for blood culture 90% of the time.[73]

TIMELY REMOVAL OF UMBILICAL ARTERY CATHETERS

The presence of an umbilical artery catheter (UAC) allows for reliable, nonpainful arterial sampling rather than a painful heel stick. It also allows for continuous blood pressure monitoring. However, umbilical arterial catheters are associated with risks and may lead to excess phlebotomy loss. Our group demonstrated that after correcting for gestational age and SNAPPE score at birth, each day the UAC was available for use was associated with a 2.2 (+0.7) mL increase in phlebotomy loss.[89]

ELIMINATE UNNECESSARY PHLEBOTOMY

Not every laboratory test that is sent is necessary. The challenge remains determining which are necessary and which are unnecessary. In 2019 Kazmi et al. evaluated whether a routine CBC or liver function test (LFT) resulted in an intervention for the neonate.[90] Among infants 32 to 34 weeks of gestation, 0% of CBC (n=70) and LFT (n=4) resulted in a clinical intervention. Among infants born less than 28 weeks

and 28 to 31 6/7 weeks of gestation, a routine CBC resulted in a clinical intervention only 8.4% and 4.6% of the time, respectively. Among the same gestational age groups LFTs resulted in clinical intervention only 4.2% and 5.7% of the time, respectively. King et al. developed a prioritization framework for improving the value of care of neonates following identification of significant interhospital variability of common laboratory tests.[91] Klunk et al. recently reported an initiative to decrease laboratory testing in a NICU,[92] resulting in a 27% decrease in laboratory tests within 24 months, including a 28% decrease in glucose tests.

Stimulate Red Cell Production

Erythropoiesis stimulating agents (ESAs) have been studied for over 30 years in preterm infants. Details of ESA use in neonates can be found in Chapter 9. Both erythropoietin (Epo) and darbepoetin (Darbe) have proven to stimulate red cell production and increase red cell mass in term and preterm infants. In some infants this results in an increase in hematocrit; in other infants, hematocrit can be maintained over weeks, reflecting an increased red cell mass as the infant grows. The red cell mass is calculated as hematocrit × estimated blood volume of 85 mL/kg × weight. In some growing infants, even a slight decrease in hematocrit may still reflect an increasing red cell mass, if the rate of growth exceeds the rate of decline in hematocrit.

Here is an example: An infant weighing 1 kg with a hematocrit of 40% begins receiving a red cell growth factor. The calculated red cell mass is 0.4 × 85 mL/kg × 1 kg = 34 mL. The infant's hematocrit declines over the next 4 weeks as the infant gains weight. After 4 weeks the infant now weighs 2 kg, and the hematocrit is slightly lower at 34%. Despite a lower hematocrit, the red cell mass has increased to 58 mL (0.34 × 85 mL/kg × 2 kg).

The result of increasing the red cell mass using ESAs, reported in study after study, is a decreased need for transfusions. ESAs unquestionably decrease transfusion requirements in neonates. In NICUs that apply restrictive transfusion guidelines and couple them with effective use of ESAs and iron supplementation, the number of transfusions ordered decreases significantly.[93] Moreover, the number of infants who remain transfusion free during their hospitalization increases markedly. These strategies result in improved care of ELBW infants.

Conclusion

Neonatal anemia and the administration of frequent red cell transfusions continues to be a common occurrence in neonatal care. Attention to three general strategies can improve anemia: starting with a higher hematocrit, decreasing phlebotomy, and stimulating RBC production. Combining these strategies with the implementation of current evidence-based transfusion guidelines will reduce the need for red cell transfusions and lead to improved long-term outcomes in preterm infants.

REFERENCES

1. Ohls RK. Why, when and how should we provide red cell transfusions to neonates? In: Ohls RK, Yoder MC, eds. *Hematology, Immunology and Infectious Disease: Neonatology Questions and Controversies*. Philadelphia, PA: Elsevier; 2008:294.
2. Kondo W. Canadian Red Cross found negligent. *Lancet*. 1997; 350:1154.
3. Hebert PC, Wells G, Blajchman MA, et al. A multicenter, randomized, controlled clinical trial of transfusion requirements in critical care. Transfusion Requirements in Critical Care Investigators, Canadian Critical Care Trials Group. *N Engl J Med*. 1999;340(6):409-417.
4. Lacroix J, Hebert PC, Hutchison JS, et al. Transfusion strategies for patients in pediatric intensive care units. *N Engl J Med*. 2007;356(16):1609-1619.
5. Bell EF, Strauss RG, Widness JA, et al. Randomized trial of liberal versus restrictive guidelines for red blood cell transfusion in preterm infants. *Pediatrics*. 2005;115:1685-1691.
6. McCoy TE, Conrad AL, Richman LC, et al. Neurocognitive profiles of preterm infants randomly assigned to lower or higher hematocrit thresholds for transfusion. *Child Neuropsychol*. 2011;17(4):347-367.
7. Nopoulos PC, Conrad AL, Bell EF, et al. Long-term outcome of brain structure in premature infants: effects of liberal vs restricted red blood cell transfusions. *Arch Pediatr Adolesc Med*. 2011;165(5):443-450.
8. Kirpalani H, Whyte RK, Andersen C, et al. The premature infants in need of transfusion (PINT) study: a randomized, controlled trial of a restrictive (low) versus liberal (high) transfusion threshold for extremely low birth weight infants. *J Pediatr*. 2006;149:301-307.
9. Whyte RK, Kirpalani H, Asztalos EV, et al. Neurodevelopmental outcome of extremely low birth weight infants randomly assigned to restrictive or liberal hemoglobin thresholds for blood transfusion. *Pediatrics*. 2009;123:207-213.
10. Whyte R, Kirpalani H. Low versus high haemoglobin concentration threshold for blood transfusion for preventing morbidity and mortality in very low birth weight infants. *Cochrane Database Syst Rev*. 2011;11:CD000512.
11. Venkatesh KK, Lynch CD, Costantine MM, et al. Trends in active treatment of live-born neonates between 22 weeks 0 days and 25 weeks 6 days by gestational age and maternal race and ethnicity in the US, 2014 to 2020. *JAMA*. 2022;328(7):652-662.
12. Kirpalani H, Bell EF, Hintz SR, et al. Higher or lower hemoglobin transfusion thresholds for preterm infants. *N Engl J Med*. 2020;383(27):2639-2651.
13. Franz AR, Engel C, Bassler D, et al. Effects of liberal vs restrictive transfusion thresholds on survival and neurocognitive outcomes in extremely low-birth-weight infants: the ETTNO Randomized Clinical Trial. *JAMA*. 2020;324(6):560-570.
14. Guillen U, Cummings JJ, Bell EF, et al. International survey of transfusion practices for extremely premature infants. *Semin Perinatol*. 2012;36(4):244-247.
15. ETTNO Investigators. The effects of transfusion thresholds on neurocognitive outcomes of extremely ow birth weight infants (ETTNO) study: background, aims and study protocol. *Neonatology*. 2012;101:301-305.
16. Dallman PR. Anemia of prematurity. *Annu Rev Med*. 1981;32: 143-160.
17. Jopling J, Henry E, Wiedmeier SE, et al. Reference ranges for hematocrit and blood hemoglobin concentration during the neonatal period: data from a multihospital health care system. *Pediatrics*. 2009;123(2):e333-e337.
18. Obladen M, Diepold K, Maier RF. Venous and arterial hematologic profiles of very low birth weight infants. European Multicenter rhEPO Study Group. *Pediatrics*. 2000;106(4):707-711.
19. Widness JA. Pathophysiology of anemia during the neonatal period, including anemia of prematurity. *Neoreviews*. 2008; 9(11):e520.
20. Hellstrom W, Forssell L, Morsing E, et al. Neonatal clinical blood sampling led to major blood loss and was associated with bronchopulmonary dysplasia. *Acta Paediatr*. 2020;109(4):679-687.
21. Obladen M, Sachsenweger M, Stahnke M. Blood sampling in very low birth weight infants receiving different levels of intensive care. *Eur J Pediatr*. 1988;147(4):399-404.
22. Shannon KM, Keith JF III, Mentzer WC, et al. Recombinant human erythropoietin stimulates erythropoiesis and reduces erythrocyte transfusions in very low birth weight preterm infants. *Pediatrics*. 1995;95(1):1-8.
23. Widness JA, Madan A, Grindeanu LA, et al. Reduction in red blood cell transfusions among preterm infants: results of a randomized trial with an in-line blood gas and chemistry monitor. *Pediatrics*. 2005;115(5):1299-1306.
24. Ringer SA, Richardson DK, Sacher RA, et al. Variations in transfusion practice in neonatal intensive care. *Pediatrics*. 1998; 101(2):194-200.
25. Nexo E, Christensen NC, Olesen H. Volume of blood removed for analytical purposes during hospitalization of low-birth-weight infants. *Clin Chem*. 1981;27(5):759-761.
26. Rosebraugh MR, Widness JA, Nalbant D, et al. A mathematical modeling approach to quantify the role of phlebotomy losses and need for transfusions in neonatal anemia. *Transfusion*. 2013;53(6):1353-1360.
27. Counsilman CE, Heeger LE, Tan R, et al. Iatrogenic blood loss in extreme preterm infants due to frequent laboratory tests and procedures. *J Matern Fetal Neonatal*. 2019:1-6.
28. Bowen JR, Patterson JA, Roberts CL, et al. Red cell and platelet transfusions in neonates: a population-based study. *Arch Dis Child Fetal Neonatal Ed*. 2015;100:F411-F415.
29. Keir AK, Yang J, Harrison A, et al. Temporal changes in blood product usage in preterm neonates born at less than 30 weeks' gestation in Canada. *Transfusion*. 2015;55(6):1340-1346.

30. Christensen RD, Baer VL, Del Vecchio A, et al. Unique risks of red blood cell transfusions in very-low-birth-weight neonates: associations between early transfusion and intraventricular hemorrhage and between late transfusion and necrotizing enterocolitis. *J Matern Fetal Neonatal.* 2013;26(2):S60-S63.

31. Christensen RD, Baer VL, Lambert DK, et al. Association, among very-low-birthweight neonates, between red blood cell transfusions in the week after birth and severe intraventricular hemorrhage. *Transfusion.* 2014;54(1):104-108.

32. La Gamma EF, Blau J. Transfusion-related acute gut injury: feeding, flora, flow, and barrier defense. *Semin Perinatol.* 2012; 36(4):294-305.

33. Patel RM, Knezevic A, Shenvi N, et al. Association of red blood cell transfusion, anemia, and necrotizing enterocolitis in very low-birth-weight infants. *JAMA.* 2016;315(9):889-897.

34. Zhang Z, Huang X, Lu H. Association between red blood cell transfusion and bronchopulmonary dysplasia in preterm infants. *Sci Rep.* 2014;4:4340.

35. Rayjada N, Barton L, Chan LS, et al. Decrease in incidence of bronchopulmonary dysplasia with erythropoietin administration in preterm infants: a retrospective study. *Neonatology.* 2012;102(4):287-292.

36. dos Santos AM, Guinsburg R, de Almeida MF, et al. Red blood cell transfusions are independently associated with intra-hospital mortality in very low birth weight preterm infants. *J Pediatr.* 2011;159(3):371-376.e1-e3.

37. Shah P, Cannon DC, Lowe JR, et al. Effect of blood transfusions on cognitive development in very low birth weight infants. *J Perinatol.* 2021;41(6):1412-1418.

38. Vu PT, Ohls RK, Mayock DE, et al. Transfusions and neurodevelopmental outcomes in extremely low gestation neonates enrolled in the PENUT trial: a randomized clinical trial. *Pediatr Res.* 2021;90(1):109-116.

39. Ohls RK, Kamath-Rayne BD, Christensen RD, et al. Cognitive outcomes of preterm infants randomized to darbepoetin, erythropoietin, or placebo. *Pediatrics.* 2014;133(6):1023-1030.

40. Ohls RK, Cannon DC, Phillips J, et al. Preschool assessment of preterm infants treated with darbepoetin and erythropoietin. *Pediatrics.* 2016;137(3):e20153859.

41. Katheria AC, Brown MK, Rich W, et al. Providing a placental transfusion in newborns who need resuscitation. *Front Pediatr.* 2017;5:1.

42. Rabe H, Gyte GM, Diaz-Rossello JL, et al. Effect of timing of umbilical cord clamping and other strategies to influence placental transfusion at preterm birth on maternal and infant outcomes. *Cochrane Database Syst Rev.* 2019;9:CD003248.

43. Rabe H, Diaz-Rossello JL, Duley L, et al. Effect of timing of umbilical cord clamping and other strategies to influence placental transfusion at preterm birth on maternal and infant outcomes. *Cochrane Database Syst Rev.* 2012;8:CD003248.

44. McDonald SJ, Middleton P, Dowswell T, et al. Effect of timing of umbilical cord clamping of term infants on maternal and neonatal outcomes. *Cochrane Database Syst Rev.* 2013;7:CD004074.

45. Al-Wassia H, Shah PS. Efficacy and safety of umbilical cord milking at birth: a systematic review and meta-analysis. *JAMA Pediatr.* 2015;169(1):18-25.

46. Yao AC, Lind J, Tiisala R, et al. Placental transfusion in the premature infant with observation on clinical course and outcome. *Acta Paediatr Scand.* 1969;58(6):561-566.

47. Yao AC, Lind J. Effect of gravity on placental transfusion. *Lancet.* 1969;2(7619):505-508.

48. Sisson TR, Knutson S, Kendall N. The blood volume of infants. IV. Infants born by cesarean section. *Am J Obstet Gynecol.* 1973;117(3):351-357.

49. Vain NE, Satragno DS, Gorenstein AN, et al. Effect of gravity on volume of placental transfusion: a multicentre, randomised, non-inferiority trial. *Lancet.* 2014;384(9939):235-240.

50. Katheria A, Reister F, Essers J, et al. Association of umbilical cord milking vs delayed umbilical cord clamping with death or severe intraventricular hemorrhage among preterm infants. *JAMA.* 2019;322(19):1877-1886.

51. Carroll PD, Christensen RD. New and underutilized uses of umbilical cord blood in neonatal care. *Matern Health Neonatol Perinatol.* 2015;1:16.

52. Smit M, Dawson JA, Ganzeboom A, et al. Pulse oximetry in newborns with delayed cord clamping and immediate skin-to-skin contact. *Arch Dis Child Fetal Neonatal Ed.* 2014;99(4): F309-F314.

53. Katheria AC, Leone TA, Woelkers D, et al. The effects of umbilical cord milking on hemodynamics and neonatal outcomes in premature neonates. *J Pediatr.* 2014;164(5):1045-1050.e1.

54. Hosono S, Mugishima H, Fujita H, et al. Umbilical cord milking reduces the need for red cell transfusions and improves neonatal adaptation in infants born at less than 29 weeks gestation: a randomised controlled trial. *Arch Dis Child.* 2008;93(1): F14-F19.

55. Hosono S, Mugishima H, Fujita H, et al. Blood pressure and urine output during the first 120 h of life in infants born at less than 29 weeks gestation related to umbilical cord milking. *Arch Dis Childhood Fetal Neonatal Ed.* 2009;94:F328-F331.

56. Jelin AC, Kuppermann M, Erickson K, et al. Obstetricians' attitudes and beliefs regarding umbilical cord clamping. *J Matern Fetal Neonatal.* 2014;27(14):1457-1461.

57. Boere I, Smit M, Roest AA, et al. Current practice of cord clamping in the Netherlands: a questionnaire study. *Neonatology.* 2015;107(1):50-55.

58. Rabe H, Diaz-Rossello JL, Duley L, et al. Effect of timing of umbilical cord clamping and other strategies to influence placental transfusion at preterm birth on maternal and infant outcomes. *Cochrane Database Syst Rev.* 2012;8:CD003248.

59. Tarnow-Mordi W, Morris J, Kirby A, et al. Delayed versus immediate cord clamping in preterm infants. *N Engl J Med.* 2017;377(25):2445-2455.

60. Backes CH, Rivera BK, Haque U, et al. Placental transfusion strategies in very preterm neonates: a systematic review and meta-analysis. *Obstet Gynecol.* 2014;124(1):47-56.

61. Patel S, Clark EA, Rodriguez CE, et al. Effect of umbilical cord milking on morbidity and survival in extremely low gestational age neonates. *Am J Obstet Gynecol.* 2014;211(5):519.e1-e7.

62. Mercer JS, Erickson-Owens DA, Vohr BR, et al. Effects of placental transfusion on neonatal and 18 month outcomes in preterm infants: a randomized controlled trial. *J Pediatr.* 2016;168:50-55.e1.

63. Rabe H, Sawyer A, Amess P, et al. Neurodevelopmental outcomes at 2 and 3.5 years for very preterm babies enrolled in a randomized trial of milking the umbilical cord versus delayed cord clamping. *Neonatology.* 2016;109(2):113-119.

64. Katheria A, Garey D, Truong G, et al. A randomized clinical trial of umbilical cord milking vs delayed cord clamping in preterm infants: neurodevelopmental outcomes at 22-26 months of corrected age. *J Pediatr.* 2018;194:76-80.

65. Aziz K, Lee HC, Escobedo MB, et al. Part 5: neonatal resuscitation: 2020 American Heart Association guidelines for cardiopulmonary resuscitation and emergency cardiovascular care. *Circulation.* 2020;142(16/2):S524-S550.

66. Hansen A, Forbes P, Buck R. Potential substitution of cord blood for infant blood in the neonatal sepsis evaluation. *Biol Neonate.* 2005;88:12-18.

67. Carroll PD, Nankervis CA, Iams J, et al. Umbilical cord blood as a replacement source for admission complete blood count in premature infants. *J Perinatol.* 2012;32(2):97-102.

68. Christensen RD, Lambert DK, Baer VL, et al. Postponing or eliminating red blood cell transfusions of very low birth weight neonates by obtaining all baseline laboratory blood tests from otherwise discarded fetal blood in the placenta. *Transfusion.* 2011;51(2):253-258.

69. Beeram MR, Loughran C, Cipriani C, et al. Utilization of umbilical cord blood for the evaluation of group B streptococcal sepsis screening. *Clin Pediatr (Phila).* 2012;51(5):447-453.

70. Baer VL, Lambert DK, Carroll PD, et al. Using umbilical cord blood for the initial blood tests of VLBW neonates results in higher hemoglobin and fewer RBC transfusions. *J Perinatol.* 2013;33(5):363-365.

71. Rotshenker-Olshinka K, Shinwell ES, Juster-Reicher A, et al. Comparison of hematologic indices and markers of infection in umbilical cord and neonatal blood. *J Matern Fetal Neonatal.* 2014;27(6):625-628.

72. Greer R, Safarulla A, Koeppel R, et al. Can fetal umbilical venous blood be a reliable source for admission complete blood count and culture in NICU patients? *Neonatology.* 2019;115(1):49-58.

73. Medeiros PB, Stark M, Long M, et al. Feasibility and accuracy of cord blood sampling for admission laboratory investigations: a pilot trial. *J Paediatr Child Health.* 2021;57(5):611-617.

74. Grevsen AK, Hviid CVB, Hansen AK, et al. Platelet count and function in umbilical cord blood versus peripheral blood in term neonates. *Platelets.* 2021;32(5):626-632.

75. Raffaeli G, Tripodi A, Manzoni F, et al. Is placental blood a reliable source for the evaluation of neonatal hemostasis at birth? *Transfusion.* 2020;60(5):1069-1077.

76. Kellogg JA, Manzella JP, Bankert DA. Frequency of low-level bacteremia in children from birth to fifteen years of age. *J Clin Microbiol.* 2000;38(6):2181-2185.

77. Woodford EC, Dhudasia MB, Puopolo KM, et al. Neonatal blood culture inoculant volume: feasibility and challenges. *Pediatr Res.* 2021;90(5):1086-1092.

78. Polin JI, Knox I, Baumgart S, et al. Use of umbilical cord blood culture for detection of neonatal bacteremia. *Obstet Gynecol.* 1981;57(2):233-237.

79. Herson VC, Block C, McLaughlin JC, et al. Placental blood sampling: an aid to the diagnosis of neonatal sepsis. *J Perinatol.* 1998;18(2):135-137.

80. American Academy of Pediatrics, Subcommittee on Hyperbilirubinemia. Management of hyperbilirubinemia in the newborn infant 35 or more weeks of gestation. *Pediatrics.* 2004:297-316.

81. Josephson C, Meyer E. Neonatal and pediatric transfusion practice. In: Fung M, ed. *American Association of Blood Banking Technical Manual.* 2011:645-70.

82. Alissa R, Williams PD, Baker EL, et al. Suitability of placental blood samples of newborns for pre-transfusion testing. *Front Pediatr.* 2021;9:661321.

83. Judd WJ. Practice guidelines for prenatal and perinatal immunohematology, revisited. *Transfusion.* 2001;41(11):1445-1452.

84. Miller JJT. Newborn Screening Guidelines for Premature and/or Sick Newborns; Proposed Guidelines. Wayne, PA: Clinical and Laboratory Standards Institute; 2008.

85. Balasubramanian H, Malpani P, Sindhur M, et al. Effect of umbilical cord blood sampling versus admission blood sampling on requirement of blood transfusion in extremely preterm infants: a randomized controlled trial. *J Pediatr.* 2019;211:39-45.e2.

86. Mu TS, Prescott AC, Haischer-Rollo GD, et al. Umbilical cord blood use for admission blood tests of VLBW preterm neonates: a randomized control trial. *Am J Perinatol.* 2021.

87. Carroll PD, Livingston E, Baer VL, et al. Evaluating otherwise-discarded umbilical cord blood as a source for a neonate's complete blood cell count at various time points. *Neonatology.* 2018;114(1):82-86.

88. George R. *Use of Cord Blood for Admission Lab Testing in High Risk Neonates.* School of Nursing. Baltimore: University of Maryland; 2019.

89. Carroll PD, Zimmerman MB, Nalbant D, et al. Neonatal umbilical arterial catheter removal is accompanied by a marked decline in phlebotomy blood loss. *Neonatology.* 2020;117(3):294-299.

90. Kazmi SH, Caprio M, Boolchandani H, et al. The value of routine laboratory screening in the neonatal intensive care unit. *J Neonatal Perinatal Med.* 2020;13(2):247-251.

91. King BC, Richardson T, Patel RM, et al. Prioritization framework for improving the value of care for very low birth weight and very preterm infants. *J Perinatol.* 2021;41(10):2463-2473.

92. Klunk CJ, Barrett RE, Peterec SM, et al. An initiative to decrease laboratory testing in a NICU. *Pediatrics.* 2021;148(1):e2020000570.

93. Henry E, Christensen RD, Sheffield MJ, et al. Why do four NICUs using identical RBC transfusion guidelines have different gestational age-adjusted RBC transfusion rates? *J Perinatol.* 2015;35(2):132-136.

Chapter 11

Neonatal Blood Banking and Transfusion: Current Questions and Controversies

Sarah M. Tweddell, MS, MD and Cassandra Josephson, MD

Chapter Outline

Introduction

Blood component transfusion is critical to modern neonatal medicine to support oxygen delivery, cardiac output, and maintain hemostasis, especially in the context of preventing bleeding or treating the bleeding neonate. Of all admissions to the neonatal intensive care unit (NICU) in the United States, approximately 1.6% receive any blood transfusion, with red blood cell (RBC) transfusion occurring most commonly.[1] Despite the relatively high frequency of transfusions, the indications, thresholds for transfusion, and blood component special processing are variable across institutions. This chapter will introduce the types of blood components transfused in the NICU and discuss important questions and controversies in modern neonatal transfusion medicine and blood banking.

Red Blood Cells

COMPONENT

RBCs are prepared from centrifugation of whole blood (WB) or by apheresis. In the case of WB, once the 450- to 500-mL unit is collected, it is centrifuged and then separated into components, one of which is packed RBCs. In the instance of apheresis collection, blood is collected on an apheresis instrument, which separates and removes the RBC component while returning the other parts of the donors' blood to them via a centrifugation process. Traditionally, WB is stored in anticoagulant preservative solutions containing different concentrations and combinations of citrate, phosphate, and dextrose (CPD), and an apheresis produced RBC component is stored in acid citrate dextrose (ACD); both have a maximum storage duration of 21 days (Table 11.1). A solution of CPD and adenine (CPDA-1) has a storage duration of up to 35 days and has been safely used and studied for large volume transfusions ($\geq$20 mL/kg) in neonates.[2] CPDA-1 is one of the most commonly used storage solutions for neonatal RBC transfusions and is often the standard by which other solutions are compared.[3,4] Newer alternatives are the additive solutions (AS), typically containing combinations of saline, dextrose, citrate, and sometimes mannitol to

TABLE 11.1	Transfusion Products and Expected Results			
Product	**Collection Method**	**Volume**	**Expected Increase**	**Storage Considerations**
Red cells	Whole blood–derived apheresis	10–20 mL/kg	2–3 g/dL rise in Hb	21 days (ACD, CPD, CP2D) 35 days (CPDA-1) 42 days (AS-1, AS-3, AS-5, AS-7)
Platelets	Whole blood–derived apheresis	5–10 mL/kg	50,000–100,000/μL rise in platelet count	5–7 days Room temperature Constant agitation
Plasma	Whole blood–derived apheresis	10–15 mL/kg	15–20% rise in factor level	Frozen: 1 yr Thawed: immediate
Cryoprecipitate	Whole blood–derived apheresis	2–5 mL/kg	60–100 mg/dL rise in fibrinogen	Frozen: 1 yr Thawed: immediate

ACD, anticoagulant citrate dextrose; *AS-1,* Additive solution-1 (Adsol); *AS-3,* Additive solution-3 (Nutricel); *AS-5,* Additive solution-5 (Optisol); *AS-7,* Additive solution-7 (SOLX); *CPD,* citrate-phosphate-dextrose; *CPD2,* citrate-phosphate-dextrose-dextrose; *CPDA-1,* Citrate-phosphate-dextrose-adenine.

stabilize the RBC membrane and prevent hemolysis, which increases the shelf life to 42 days.[2] The most commonly used AS in neonates is AS-3 since it does not contain mannitol. AS-3 stored units have not been studied thoroughly for large volume neonatal transfusions (≥20 mL/kg) but are becoming more common as CPDA-1 unit production is being phased out of many blood centers across the United States. A unit of RBCs will have a hematocrit of 55% to 75% depending on the storage solution, with higher hematocrits in CPDA-1 units and lower hematocrits in AS units due to the amount of storage solution added to the packed RBCs. Each 10 mL/kg RBC transfusion is expected to raise the neonate's hemoglobin by about 1 to 3 g/dL.[2]

INDICATIONS

RBCs are the most commonly transfused blood component, and neonates are among the most frequently transfused populations. NICU patients often require blood transfusions as a result of both inadequate erythropoietin production and phlebotomy losses, commonly referred to as anemia of prematurity. Approximately 64% of extremely low birth weight infants (birth weight <1000 g) will require at least one RBC transfusion during their NICU stay.[1] The decision to transfuse an infant must be weighed against the risks of adverse effects, including blood donor exposures, transfusion-transmitted infections (TTIs), and the effects of blood storage, among others. Common indications for transfusion of RBCs include anemia, bleeding, and acute need for

increased oxygen carrying capacity. The trend in recent years has been toward lower thresholds of anemia to trigger transfusion based on the results of large clinical trials, including the Effects of Transfusion Thresholds on Neurocognitive Outcome of Extremely Low Birth Weight Infants (ETTNO) trial in Europe and the Transfusion of Prematures (TOP) trial in the United States.

QUESTIONS AND CONTROVERSIES

Use of Hemoglobin for Transfusion Trigger

Hemoglobin and hematocrit levels are used as indications for transfusion across all patient populations and provide thresholds for RBC transfusion in clinical guidelines. Despite the intentions of these thresholds to provide a standard of treatment for patients, a single hemoglobin or hematocrit value may not be the best indicator for transfusion in all patients.[5] Clinical guidelines are based on large randomized controlled trials in adults, children, and neonates but may not be generalizable to individuals of differing clinical status. In neonates there have been three large clinical trials attempting to answer the question of appropriate RBC thresholds for preterm infants using hemoglobin or hematocrit thresholds.[6-8]

The TOP trial in the United States was a multicenter investigation of higher or lower transfusion thresholds for preterm infants and found no difference in survival, neurodevelopmental impairment, or other morbidities at 22 to 26 months of age for preterm infants in the lower threshold group (hemoglobin ~8 g/dL).[7] The ETTNO trial in Europe achieved a difference in hematocrit values of 3% and similarly found no difference in morbidity or mortality between groups at 24 months of age.[6] The Premature Infants in Need of Transfusion (PINT) trial reported a clinically (but not statistically) significant decrease in cognitive scores among infants in the lower threshold group at 18 to 21 months.[6-9] There were more protocol violations in the lower threshold groups for the ETTNO and TOP trials possibly due to both trials being unmasked and providers choosing to transfuse during acute illness in the face of anemia.[7,8] Observational studies have suggested a relationship between RBC transfusion and necrotizing enterocolitis (NEC), but these findings remain inconsistent across different studies.[10-13] In contrast, a prospective observational study supported the association of severe anemia (hemoglobin <8 g/dL) rather than transfusion with NEC.[10] There was no difference in the rate of NEC between infants in the high or low threshold groups of the ETTNO, TOP, or PINT trials, but the studies were admittedly not powered to detect differences in many of the secondary outcomes. The trend toward more conservative transfusion practices to limit RBC exposure is likely to continue in the neonatal population, although there remains significant variation in transfusion thresholds and guidelines across US centers.[1]

Near infrared spectroscopy (NIRS) is a noninvasive technology that provides information about regional tissue oxygenation and has been studied in term neonates undergoing cardiac and abdominal surgery, and may be an additional data point to help determine the need for transfusion. NIRS monitors are typically placed over the renal or cerebral tissue beds (back and forehead) and provide a weighted venous saturation value rather than the arterial saturation that pulse oximetry reflects. The NIRS value reflects the amount of oxygen extracted from the tissue with lower values indicating more oxygen extraction and increased metabolic demand.[14] Studies have attempted to evaluate the relationship between anemia, NIRS, and transfusion. Mintzer et al. provided preterm neonates 500 to 1250 g with an empiric RBC transfusion of 15 mL/kg in the first week of life if their phlebotomy losses totaled at least 10 mL/kg. All infants demonstrated increases in cerebral, renal, and splanchnic NIRS readings, which was not observed in the control group. There were no changes in other markers of tissue perfusion, including pH, lactate, base deficit, and creatinine.[15] While there is less evidence for the use of NIRS in premature infants, the data for term infants demonstrate that NIRS strongly correlates with invasive venous saturation monitoring and can detect hemodynamic changes compared to pulse oximetry.[14] This technology may be useful in stratifying neonates to receive RBC transfusion based on indices of tissue perfusion rather than a single hemoglobin value.

Irradiation

Gamma irradiation of RBCs, with either x-rays or cesium, is the recommended strategy to prevent transfusion-associated graft vs. host disease (TA-GVHD). Irradiation targets nucleic acids within T lymphocytes contaminating the RBC component, preventing donor lymphocyte proliferation in the recipient.[16,17] TA-GVHD is rare but can be fatal when competent donor T lymphocytes from the blood donor recognize patient human leukocyte antigens (HLAs) on hematopoietic, skin, liver, spleen, and thymus cells in an immunocompromised or immune-incompetent host.[18] Preterm infants are considered relatively immunocompromised due to an immature immune system, especially those weighing less than 1200 g, necessitating cellular product irradiation to prevent TA-GVHD.[19] Irradiation to prevent TA-GVHD is also recommended for infants receiving directed blood donation from biologic relatives, in utero fetal transfusions, and rarely used granulocyte transfusions.[20]

TA-GVHD has been reported as a complication of in utero transfusion for erythroblastosis fetalis, therefore irradiation is always recommended for this use.[18] When ordering blood for exchange transfusion to treat hemolytic disease of the newborn, irradiation may not always be possible. If irradiation results in delay of care for the infant, it may not be clinically indicated.[18] Unfortunately there are major effects to RBCs after irradiation, including lipid peroxidation, compromised integrity of the cell membrane leading to decreased deformability and elasticity, and leakage of potassium into the extracellular space.[17] These effects result in increased hemolysis and decreased survivability of RBCs after transfusion.[17,21] Irradiation can also have minimal effects on platelets, fibrinolysis, and coagulation.

Irradiation has been shown to alter metabolic properties of RBCs and accelerate the aging process.[19] Current US Food and Drug Administration (FDA) guidelines allow RBCs to be stored in CPDA-1 media up to 35 days following collection, but after the cells are irradiated, they must be used within 28 days, depending on the date the product was irradiated.[22] Patel et al. used metabolomics to demonstrate that irradiated RBCs exhibited elements of the storage lesion after only 10 days.[19]

There is variability in irradiation practice among US centers, including where the irradiation occurs (at the location of the supplier or in the hospital) and how long RBCs are considered safe following irradiation.[7,23] In the TOP trial, in which the appropriate threshold of hemoglobin for transfusion of premature infants was investigated, the 29 participating NICUs were surveyed for their irradiation practices. Ninety-three percent of centers reported irradiating blood with two-thirds performing irradiation on site.[24] In the American Association of Blood Banks (AABB) survey of 35 pediatric centers' blood banking practices, 88.6% of neonatal RBC transfusions were always irradiated and 11.4% were sometimes irradiated.[25] Seventy-one percent were irradiated on site, 37% were irradiated at the time the order was received, and 31% were irradiated at the time the blood was issued.[25] Irradiation is likely safest if performed immediately before transfusion so the effects of accelerated aging are not experienced by the recipient.[17,26,27]

Solutions and Modifications

Storage Solutions

During storage RBCs are known to undergo biochemical changes, referred to as the storage lesion. This includes development of oxygen free radicals that damage the cell membrane and cause brittleness and decreased flexibility.[27] Additional procedures, including irradiation, leukocyte reduction, washing, and AS, may exacerbate or contribute to the storage lesion.[28,29]

There are a variety of AS utilized in blood banking with a wide range of ingredients.[2] Traditionally solutions containing CPDA have been used for neonatal transfusions.[30] Historically, fresh blood was preferred for neonates.[31] However, during the 1980s, concerns over contamination occurred due to human immunodeficiency virus (HIV) and hepatitis C being discovered in the blood supply, and the risk of multiple donor

exposures increased. Clinical practice shifted toward a goal of decreased donor exposure.

A decrease in donor exposure was achieved by separating a dedicated parent RBC unit into multiple small aliquots for transfusion over the lifespan of the RBC unit and the infant's hospitalization. This required RBCs for neonatal patients to be stored for extended periods and led to research to determine the safety of stored blood and storage solutions for neonatal patients.[32,33] Dedicated donor units have become common, with 77% of TOP trial NICUs using a single unit until expiration, but this practice is not universal or a regulatory requirement.[23]

AS allow RBCs to be stored for longer than the traditional preservative solutions. Strauss et al. compared AS-1[34] and later AS-3,[30] both of which have an extended shelf life of 42 days, to the standard CPDA-1 solution (35-day storage). The results of these controlled trials indicated that donor exposure could be significantly and safely reduced by using either AS-1 or AS-3 for small volume transfusions (<20 mL/kg) in preterm neonates.[30,34] These solutions have not been studied for larger volume transfusions (>20 mL/kg). The risks associated with prolonged storage of RBCs in these AS include the accumulation of potassium, decreased pH, loss of 2,3-diphosphoglycerate (2,3-DPG), and the potentially toxic effects of mannitol and adenine. Storage of RBCs at refrigerator temperatures (4°C) results in inactivation of the sodium-potassium–adenosine triphosphatase (ATPase) pump, leading to potassium leakage out of cells and accumulation in the extracellular space.[35] For the neonates in Strauss's studies there were no significant differences in the concentrations of electrolytes (including potassium) between the AS-1 and CPDA-1 groups, or the AS-3 and CPDA-1 groups.[30,34] Additionally, when Strauss compared older (≥22 days) stored AS-3 units to newer (<22 days), there were no significant differences in pre- and posttransfusion electrolytes.[30] However, it should be noted that for infants requiring rapid or large volume (>20 mL/kg) RBC transfusions, blood should be selected from fresh packed units or those washed with saline to prevent potentially fatal electrolyte derangements.[36]

Among US NICUs participating in the TOP trial[7] (n=29) there was significant variation in RBC solutions used for neonates, with 41% of NICUs allowing a combination of anticoagulant or preservative solutions, 21% allowing AS only, and 38% allowing CPDA/CPD only.[23] Similarly, Reeves et al. reported 94% of pediatric and neonatal centers surveyed by the AABB used CPDA, AS-1, AS-3, or AS-5.[25]

Leukocyte Reduction

Leukocyte reduction is an RBC modification procedure that uses a filter, either after the product is collected or with an apheresis instrument, to reduce the leukocyte concentration of an RBC unit to less than 5×10^6 cells. The filters also remove other cellular elements that may be inadvertently collected along with RBCs. Indications for leukocyte reduction include reducing febrile nonhemolytic transfusion reactions, preventing cytomegalovirus (CMV) transmission, and decreasing the incidence of HLA alloimmunization.[2]

Washing

Washing blood components is important for removing plasma proteins, including antibodies and cytokines and any unwanted additive components such as glycerol and mannitol. Washed products are typically prepared using saline solutions and sometimes small volumes of dextrose. Once washed, the shelf life is reduced to 24 hours if refrigerated (1–6°C) or 4 hours at room temperature (20–24°C).[2]

Washing of RBCs is not universal but has been shown in neonatal, pediatric, and adult patients to be associated with a reduction in morbidity and mortality.[37-39] Washing may confer a benefit to patients by reducing the inflammation associated with transfusion.[40,41] In a Cochrane review in 2016 Keir et al. noted only one trial of washed vs. unwashed RBC transfusions in premature neonates younger than 32 weeks.[32,42] This small study did not demonstrate a detectable difference in morbidity and mortality outcomes for premature neonates.[32] Among the 29 NICUs participating in the TOP trial,[7] 34% had a policy for washing blood used for large volume transfusions and 17% had a policy specifying washing procedures after irradiation or storage.[23] Among 47 blood banks participating in the US University Health Consortium,[3] 82% had no washing policy, only 18% had a policy addressing the risk of hyperkalemia, and 9% had a policy specifying the number of days after radiation or storage.[23]

Storage Duration

Multiple studies have been undertaken to investigate the storage duration of RBCs and the effects on neonatal outcomes. Historical practices have been aimed at using fresh blood for neonates despite the risk of increased donor exposure, whereas modern practices aim to reduce donor exposure by using dedicated donor units. Multiple retrospective and observational adult studies have failed to show difference in mortality of patients receiving blood stored at the limits of FDA regulations compared to fresh blood.[43-45] Conversely, several observational studies argued that longer storage time was associated with increased risk of infection, organ failure, and death.[46-49]

One study has attempted to determine if storage time impacts morbidity and mortality for premature neonates.[50] The Age of Red Blood Cells in Premature Infants (ARIPI) trial was a randomized, double blind, controlled trial in six Canadian NICUs that randomized premature neonates weighing less than 1250 g to receive fresh (<7 days old) vs. standard RBCs, and found no improvement in major morbidity in neonates receiving fresh blood.[50] Despite these findings there were important limitations to the ARIPI trial. The group receiving "standard" storage duration RBCs received blood that had been stored for 14 days on average, compared to the group receiving fresh RBCs, which were stored for 5 days on average and therefore may not be a large enough difference to show clinically significant results.[50,51] Additionally, the average storage age of RBC in the United States is 18 days, so this study is likely not generalizable to all populations.[51] This study also did not address important variations in storage solutions or irradiation.

Transfusion-Transmitted Infections

An important and serious risk of blood transfusion includes acquiring TTIs. One recent example of this problem in neonates is with *Babesia microti,* an intraerythrocytic protozoan parasite transmitted by the deer tick (Ixodes scapularis), which also serves as a vector for Lyme disease (Borrelia burgdorferi) and human granulocytic anaplasmosis (Anaplasma phagocytophilum). *B. microti* is the most common cause of TTI in the United States, and babesiosis may cause subclinical symptoms or severe disease and mortality depending on the immune status of the host.[52,53] The parasite is endemic in the northeastern and upper midwestern United States and can be transmitted during transfusion, usually of RBC products, though there have been a few cases of platelet-transmitted babesiosis.[53] As of 2016 there were over 250 cases of transfusion-transmitted babesiosis (165 recipients tested positive; in 60 cases, the recipient did not test positive).[52] Half (56%) of the recipients who tested positive had underlying disease, and 10% were less than 1 year of age.[52] Of the neonates (n=16) who developed babesiosis, eight were symptomatic but had uncomplicated disease, two were symptomatic with complicated disease, two died, and four were unable to be categorized based on severity of illness.[52] In neonates, the elderly, and immunocompromised patients, babesiosis can be severe with mortality rates ranging from 10% to 28%.[54] Eighty-one percent of transfusion-transmitted babesiosis cases are attributed to RBC transfusion, 4% to platelets, and none to fresh frozen plasma (FFP). In 15% of transmitted infections the product was unspecified.[52] Unfortunately the parasite can survive typical storage conditions, including refrigeration, leukoreduction, irradiation, freezing, and long storage duration.[55] Pathogen reduction strategies have been successful for plasma and platelet components, but they are not available for RBCs. Strategies that include limiting blood donation in endemic areas during peak tick season, attempting to stratify recipients according to risk of severe disease and mortality, and using questionnaires for blood donors regarding prior infection with *B. microti* have not been successful in reducing disease transmission.[55]

The FDA has recently licensed nucleic acid testing (NAT) to identify *B. microti* in donor blood.[53] The American Red Cross has been testing for *B. microti* since 2012 in endemic areas, including Connecticut, Massachusetts, Minnesota, and Wisconsin, where most of the TTIs originate. Despite decreasing transmission of babesiosis in blood transfusions there were cases of neonatal transmission, including a 24-week infant who received multiple aliquots of *B. microti*–positive blood and two other premature infants, one of whom received blood from two distinct *B. microti*–positive donors.[53]

Despite increasing rates of reported babesiosis in endemic states, Connecticut saw no transfusion-transmitted babesiosis in 2017 or 2018, likely as a result of nearly universal (95–96%) screening of blood donors using the FDA licensed ultrasensitive NAT assay.[53] The FDA recommends testing blood donations from 14 endemic states and Washington (DC), which would be expected to dramatically reduce the rate of transfusion-transmitted babesiosis and improve the safety of the blood supply.[53]

Platelets

COMPONENT

Platelets are available as either WB-derived platelets or apheresis platelets (see Table 11.1). Each method of blood collection provides different concentrations of platelets, with WB platelets containing 5.5×10^{10} or more platelets in approximately 50 mL of plasma compared to apheresis platelets providing more than 3×10^{11} platelets in a total volume of 250 to 300 mL. Thus WB-derived platelets must be pooled from multiple donors to deliver similar concentration and volume of platelets to the recipient. Transfusion of platelets is aimed at providing sufficient quantities of functional platelets to prevent or stop bleeding.[2] Platelets have the shortest shelf life of the components discussed in this chapter at only 5 days and must be stored under constant gentle agitation at room temperature.

INDICATIONS

Platelets are often transfused at a volume of 10 to 15 mL/kg for bleeding prophylaxis in neonates with thrombocytopenia. Thrombocytopenia can be broadly defined as a platelet count of less than 150×10^9/L but is subcategorized as mild ($100–149 \times 10^9$/L), moderate ($50–99 \times 10^9$/L), and severe ($<50 \times 10^9$/L). It occurs in 1% to 5% of all neonates, 12% to 35% of all patients admitted to the NICU, and 70% to 90% of extremely low birth weight infants.[56,57] Thrombocytopenia occurring within the first 72 hours of life is termed early thrombocytopenia and is associated with intrauterine growth restriction (IUGR) likely as a consequence of fetal hypoxia. Late thrombocytopenia occurs after the first 72 hours of life and is more commonly associated with sepsis and NEC.[57] Christensen et al. collected data from thrombocytopenic infants who were small for gestational age (SGA). Ninety percent of SGA thrombocytopenic infants had no identifiable cause for thrombocytopenia and had a low mortality rate compared to those with an identifiable cause.[58]

It has been recognized that patients receiving more platelet transfusions experience higher mortality, but in observational studies it is impossible to determine a causal effect of platelet transfusion on mortality.[56] A recent large randomized clinical trial of premature infants (PLaNET-2) was conducted showing those patients in the liberal threshold group (platelets maintained $>50 \times 10^9$/L) had an increased risk of death or severe bleeding and bronchopulmonary dysplasia compared to patients in the restrictive threshold group (platelets maintained $>25 \times 10^9$/L).[59]

QUESTIONS AND CONTROVERSIES

Pathogen Reduction

Platelets are particularly vulnerable to bacterial contamination because they require storage at room temperature (22–24°C). The storage duration is limited to 5 days due to increasing risk for bacterial contamination at longer lengths of storage, not due to hemostatic efficacy.[60] About 1 in 1500 platelet units is contaminated with bacteria, and clinical sepsis occurs in 1 in 100,000 platelet transfusions.[61-63] The first identified TTI was syphilis in 1915,[64] and while the blood supply is now safer than ever before, the risk of pathogen transmission has not been completely eliminated. The prevention of TTIs is an important aspect of blood banking and relies on donor questionnaires to risk stratify, a voluntary donation system, and screening of pooled blood for known infectious organisms. Bacterial screening of pathogens is universal and typically accomplished with continuous culture methods or direct detection using polymerase chain reaction technology.[65]

Unfortunately these systems cannot eliminate the risk of TTI due to pathogens that can escape detection, or emerging diseases for which there are no tests available or which are not yet recognized. Important examples include HIV and hepatitis C transmission during the 1980s and Zika transmission in 2016.[66,67] These emerging diseases highlight the need for a proactive approach to blood banking safety and have inspired technologies to universally neutralize many diverse pathogens in the blood supply. Since the 1990s pathogen inactivation or pathogen reduction technologies (PRT) have been used to reduce the transmission of pathogens in plasma.[66,68] These technologies have been applied to platelet concentrates in Europe for the past few decades[61,67] but have remained controversial and slow to be adopted in the United States.[66]

The benefits of PRTs include protecting recipients from many known and unknown pathogens, prevention of TA-GVHD, transfusion-transmitted CMV, and increased storage time from 5 to 7 days.[68-71] The primary safety concerns of PRTs include the clinical efficacy of the treated blood products.[72] Platelets are activated when stimulated to undergo changes needed to induce hemostasis. This can be a challenge for storage and treatment with PRTs because platelet survival and recovery are crucial to provide functional platelets to infants.

Most PRTs use ultraviolet irradiation with or without a photosensitizer such as psoralen to cause crosslinking of pathogen nucleotides and to prevent replication.[73] These technologies are capable of inactivating a wide variety of pathogens, including bacteria, parasites, and many viruses, but are not effective against nonenveloped viruses such as hepatitis A and E or prions.[73-75] They also have the advantage of inactivating donor leukocytes and reducing the risk of TA-GVHD.[73]

There are three pathogen inactivation methods approved for use in Europe: INTERCEPT, Mirasol, and Theraflex UVC. INTERCEPT is currently used in Europe and is the only one of these technologies that is approved for use in the United States for platelets and plasma.[66] It uses amotosalen, a psoralen derivative compound found naturally in foods and plants, to bind nucleic acids. After activation by ultraviolet A (UVA) radiation, it crosslinks nucleic acids preventing replication of pathogens that may be present in the platelet concentrate.[67] Before transfusion, an adsorption device is required to remove excess amotosalen from the media. The INTERCEPT technology is contraindicated in neonates receiving phototherapy due to the risk of skin erythema following a reaction from psoralen and UV light at certain wavelengths.[76]

Mirasol uses riboflavin (vitamin B2) to bind to nucleic acids resulting in DNA and RNA damage after exposure to UV light, preventing pathogen replication.[67] Unlike INTERCEPT, the residual riboflavin does not require removal from the platelet media since it is "generally regarded as safe" by the FDA.[73] Theraflex uses UVC radiation alone without additive chemicals to cause direct DNA damage to any pathogens and requires constant platelet agitation to ensure that the platelets are fully exposed.[77]

Preclinical studies have demonstrated exaggeration of the storage lesion on pathogen reduced platelets,[73,78,79] but clinical studies were overall reassuring.[80] Ten randomized clinical trials were conducted evaluating the safety and efficacy of Intercept, Mirasol, or UVC treated platelets in adults.[81-90] All but one of these trials found no difference in bleeding risk from the pathogen reduced platelets. Only the HOVON trial (amotosalen/UVA-treated platelets) reported an increase in the odds of bleeding for the pathogen reduced platelets compared to the control group (odds ratio [OR] = 2.66; 95% confidence interval 1.28–5.51).[85] The platelet recovery after PRT, and the 1-hour and 24-hour platelet survival after transfusion, tended to be lower in the groups receiving pathogen reduced platelets, resulting in more frequent transfusions.[80,91] However, the reduced recovery of platelets after pathogen reduction resulted in a lower platelet count in the transfused product, and overall a similar number of platelets were transfused into the pathogen-reduced and control groups, indicating that perhaps a larger volume transfusion might provide an equivalent amount of functional platelets.[91] In the most recent clinical trial evaluating the efficacy of UVC-treated platelets, the authors did not report bleeding but suggested that the hemostatic function of platelets was acceptable because RBC transfusions did not differ between groups.[89]

There are few studies evaluating pediatric and neonatal patients treated with pathogen reduced platelets. From 2017 to 2018 the AABB reported on variation in practices among pediatric and neonatal units in the United States. Of the 15 centers responding, seven reported using pathogen reduced platelets for pediatric and neonatal patients.[25] In 2019 Schulz et al. published a retrospective, observational study describing the safety and efficacy of pathogen reduced platelets in pediatric and neonatal patients using the INTERCEPT technology.[76] Pediatric patients in this study had a higher platelet transfusion requirement in those receiving pathogen reduced platelets compared to standard platelets (1.4 vs. 0.9 [p<.001]).[76] This increased transfusion burden was not observed in neonatal patients who showed similar transfusion rates (1.2 vs. 1.0 [p=0.29]).[76] Additionally, both groups had similar rates of RBC transfusions, used as a surrogate indicator of acceptable hemostasis.[76] Finally, no instances of rashes were noted for patients receiving phototherapy.[76] Jimenez et al. published a study in Spain evaluating the efficacy of riboflavin/UVA-treated platelets in 132 neonates compared to a retrospective group of neonates treated with standard platelets.[92] In contrast to the findings of Schulz et al., Jimenez reported a higher platelet transfusion requirement in neonates receiving the pathogen reduced platelets compared to the retrospective control group (3.6 vs. 1.8 [p=0.03]).[92] The potential for PRT to decrease platelet efficacy and increase transfusion requirements should not be overlooked considering there have been multiple observational studies associating increased platelet transfusion with increased rates of mortality, as reported in the PLaNeT-2 study.[93-96] Therefore if PRT leads to increased transfusion requirements, the risks of increased morbidity and mortality must be weighed against the benefits of reduced pathogen transmission.

Matched vs. ABO Incompatible Platelets

The ABO blood group system was first discovered by Karl Landsteiner in 1909, but it was not until the 1950s that researchers confirmed platelets also express the ABO antigens.[97] Platelets express ABO antigens on their surface, just like RBCs, although they are only strongly expressed in 4% to 7% of patients.[98] It was previously understood that although the antigens were expressed on platelets, the low detectable quantities of antigens on platelets meant that ABO-incompatible platelets could be transfused without affecting the survival of platelets in the recipient.[98] Platelets are collected in plasma containing ABO antibodies. Ideally, platelet products are selected as ABO compatible or identical to decrease the transfer of incompatible plasma (containing anti-A, anti-B, or anti-A,B antibodies), which can result in hemolysis of recipient RBCs and morbidity and mortality in recipients.[99,100] Patients with blood type O produce anti-A and anti-B IgG antibodies, which are contained in the donor plasma. Transfusing platelets from O donors into A, B, or AB recipients may cause hemolysis of RBCs of the recipient and an acute hemolytic transfusion reaction. Plasma from platelets can also transfer small numbers of RBCs, which may contain RhD antigens (RhD-positive to RhD-negative recipient) on their surface and be immunogenic, leading to RhD hemolytic disease of the newborn. The passive transfer of antibodies in plasma from platelets can also lead to alloimmunization in platelet transfusion recipients.[101] Research has demonstrated improved platelet recovery when ABO-matched and ABO-identical platelets are transfused compared to ABO-mismatched platelets.[102-105] Most authors agree that platelet transfusions should be ABO identical to the recipient, including Rh antigen.[101] However, the short storage time and limited supply of blood products make ABO-identical platelet transfusion logistically challenging and have been associated with increased platelet waste.[106] Unlike other blood products that have longer shelf lives (35–42 days for RBCs, 1 year for FFP and cryoprecipitate), platelets are only shelf stable for 5 days.

While hemolytic reactions to ABO-incompatible platelets are rare, there are important benefits achieved in matching or transfusing identical platelet products.[107] Several randomized and observational studies have demonstrated that non–ABO-matched platelets resulted in a smaller improvement in platelet count compared with ABO-matched platelets.[102] Additionally, patients receiving ABO-matched platelets showed improved clotting.[102-105] In trials of adult patients undergoing cardiac surgery, those who received ABO-mismatched platelets had longer hospital days and required more RBC transfusions. In contrast, patients receiving ABO-identical platelets had lower mortality, fewer days of antibiotics, and shorter ICU stays.[108] Other studies failed to find important clinical benefits, including survival, bleeding, or transfusion reactions, but did confirm an increase in platelet count when ABO-identical transfusions were used.[109]

The recommendation in pediatric patients is to transfuse ABO-compatible or -identical platelet products; however, as mentioned previously, due to lack of available donors or rapid expiration this is not always feasible.[106,110] In pediatric patients there have been case reports of death in three patients who received ABO-incompatible platelet transfusions.[111-113] There have also been reports of morbidity in pediatric patients receiving ABO-incompatible blood transfusions from O donors into A recipients with varying anti-A titers.[99,110] In adult patients the plasma volume associated with

platelet transfusions may be diluted to reduce the quantity of incompatible antibodies transferred. In pediatric patients and neonates this practice is not appropriate because it would make the transfused volume too large.[110] Similar to adults, pediatric studies have demonstrated improved platelet recovery, decreased transfusion reactions, and decreased alloimmunization when platelets were ABO matched.[102,104,111,114,115] Additionally, in patients receiving multiple platelet transfusions, platelet refractoriness is increased with multiple ABO-incompatible transfusions.[116] As mentioned previously, more platelet transfusions are associated with increased morbidity and mortality in neonates,[59] thus strategies to reduce unnecessary transfusions, including providing ABO-identical or ABO-matched platelet products, should be prioritized.

Plasma (Fresh Frozen/Cryoprecipitate)

COMPONENT

Plasma is the aqueous portion of blood that contains albumin, coagulation factors, fibrinolytic proteins, immunoglobulins, and many other proteins. It is derived from whole blood or apheresis (see Table 11.1). FFP is frozen at -18°C within 6 to 8 hours of collection and contains all the coagulation factors, including the labile factors (F) V and VIII. Once thawed, FFP must be used immediately or stored at 1° to 6°C. Plasma frozen within 24 hours after phlebotomy (FP24) is a source of nonlabile plasma proteins, including albumin, ADAMTS13, fibrinogen, and factors II, VII, IX, X, and XI, which are present in similar concentrations compared to FFP. In FP24 the levels of FVIII and protein C are reduced, while the levels of FV are variable compared to FFP. FP24 and FFP may be used interchangeably, and neither product is indicated in situations where a specific factor may be replaced.

Cryoprecipitate is obtained by thawing FFP between 1°C and 6°C, and isolating the precipitate, which contains all of the high molecular weight proteins. The cold-insoluble precipitate must be placed in the freezer within 1 hour of the initial thaw and can be stored at a temperature of -18°C or lower for up to 1 year.[2] Cryoprecipitate has the highest concentrations of FVIII, FXIII, von Willebrand factor (vWF), fibrinogen, and fibronectin.[117]

INDICATIONS

FFP is administered to 6% to 12% of neonates in the NICU.[118-120] Reasons for FFP transfusion in neonatal patients have included preventing intraventricular hemorrhage (IVH), treating disseminated intravascular coagulation (DIC), providing volume expansion, and correcting abnormal coagulation tests.[118,121] Despite the relatively common use of FFP, the majority of transfusions are noncompliant with clinical guidelines or are not aligned with evidence-based practices.[118] Unlike the cellular components of blood (platelets, RBCs) there are less robust data to guide the use of FFP in neonates, thus most of the recommendations and guidelines are based on expert opinion.[118,122,123]

Indications for FFP transfusion include coagulopathy with active bleeding, coagulopathy in a neonate undergoing an invasive procedure, and congenital deficiency of clotting factors when the specific clotting factor is not available.[124] The transfusion of FFP to neonates as a volume expander, for sepsis, or for prevention of IVH is not appropriate.[118,124] Neonates often receive FFP transfusions based on abnormal coagulation testing in the absence of bleeding. While this may be appropriate in some circumstances, it should be noted that the reference ranges for prothrombin time (PT) and activated partial thromboplastin time (aPTT) in preterm neonates are higher compared to term neonates.[124-126]

Cryoprecipitate is used to prevent or treat bleeding in neonates with hypofibrinogenemia, which is defined as a fibrinogen level less than 100 or 150 mg/dL. A single unit of cryoprecipitate contains at least 80 IU of factor VIII and 150 mg of fibrinogen, and it raises the plasma fibrinogen level by 100 mg/dL (see Table 11.1). Cryoprecipitate is used to prevent or treat bleeding in critically ill patients with low fibrinogen levels.[127] Guidelines for the use of plasma products in the NICU have been published but lack adequate evidence for treatment of acquired bleeding disorders and recommendations for prophylactic use.[128] Small trials and single patient reports have supported the use of cryoprecipitate and FFP together to stabilize patients with DIC.[117] A larger study determined that maintaining normal coagulation, by correcting coagulopathy early in critically ill neonates, conferred a greater chance of survival compared to infants who were coagulopathic.[129] However, this study was published in the 1980s before the advent of surfactant and therapeutic hypothermia, thus may not be applicable in the modern era. More robust clinical trials are needed to understand the benefit of cryoprecipitate and the target range for fibrinogen in selected conditions.[117]

QUESTIONS AND CONTROVERSIES

Fresh Frozen Plasma Use in Patients With Hypoxic Ischemic Encephalopathy

One important group of patients likely to receive FFP transfusion is the neonate with hypoxic ischemic encephalopathy (HIE). RBC transfusions are the most commonly prescribed blood product in the NICU, but in infants receiving therapeutic hypothermia for HIE the rate of plasma transfusion is twice the rate of RBC and platelet transfusion.[1] The only patients more likely to receive FFP in a large multicenter observational study were those with conditions requiring extracorporeal membrane oxygenation (ECMO)/cardiopulmonary bypass or with acute kidney failure.[1] Following the perinatal insult, lack of oxygen and blood flow to the infant commonly results in multiorgan dysfunction. In fact, the most common complication observed in patients with moderate or severe HIE was coagulopathy (85.1% and 96.6%, respectively).[130] Bone marrow dysfunction is also evident, with thrombocytopenia occurring in 29.6% of infants with moderate HIE and 70% of infants with severe HIE.[130] Therapeutic hypothermia is the standard treatment for infants with moderate to severe HIE and has been shown to reduce the effects of reperfusion injury if initiated within 6 hours of birth and maintained for 72 hours. A common side effect of therapeutic hyperthermia is slowed activity of enzymes involved in the clotting cascade,[131,132] and as a result infants undergoing cooling will universally demonstrate abnormal coagulation tests.[131]

Hemostatic dysfunction may result from hemorrhage, DIC, and ischemic injury.[131-135] The incidence of bleeding has ranged widely (depending on the study) from 3% to 54%, likely due to differences in bleeding scales utilized.[131,136,137] Prior to initiation of therapeutic hyperthermia as the standard of care, one retrospective study evaluated the differences in IVH among neonates receiving therapeutic hyperthermia vs. those who did not and found no statistically significant difference in rates of IVH.[138] Similarly, other studies have reported no major hemorrhage in patients receiving therapeutic hyperthermia.[131,139]

An important question to consider is how to predict which patients with HIE will experience clinically significant bleeding. Two studies have attempted to identify clinical and laboratory characteristics of infants with bleeding while undergoing therapeutic hyperthermia for HIE.[131,135] Both reported a high incidence of bleeding in patients with moderate to severe HIE (54–69%), with thrombocytopenia and hypofibrinogenemia as risk factors for clinical bleeding.[131,135] Both studies reported high rates of blood transfusions among bleeding and nonbleeding patients.[131,135] Pakvasa et al. reported statistically significantly higher rates of almost all blood product use in the bleeding group with the exception of cryoprecipitate.[135] It is understood that coagulation indices, including PT and aPTT, may be more prolonged at temperatures of 33.5°C, and therefore when performed at a temperature of 37°C in the lab the test may underestimate the risk of bleeding.[131] Perhaps for this reason, Pakvasa et al. attempted to use the initial coagulopathy and hematologic indices with the first 12 hours of life to predict the bleeding risk in neonates undergoing therapeutic hyperthermia.[135] The authors of both studies found a strong correlation between hemostatic dysfunction and bleeding risk, as well as a high utilization of blood products, indicating a need for specific protocols to address transfusion in neonates treated with therapeutic hyperthermia for HIE.[131,135]

Cryoprecipitate Use and Misuse in the NICU

Cryoprecipitate is most commonly administered prophylactically to restore fibrinogen levels in critically ill patients and those undergoing cardiac surgery.[140] The etiology of hypofibrinogenemia includes reduced synthesis, fibrinogen loss, and increased fibrinolysis. Reduced fibrinogen synthesis is observed in severe liver disease, fibrinogen loss is observed in cases of massive hemorrhage, and increased fibrinolysis is common in neonates on ECMO or with DIC.[127]

Pediatric and adult guidelines differ in their recommendations for the appropriate fibrinogen threshold requiring cryoprecipitate transfusion (100 or 150 mg/dL), but bleeding has rarely been observed at fibrinogen levels greater than 100 mg/dL.[141] Without robust evidence, neonatal transfusion guidelines for cryoprecipitate vary

in both the thresholds and indications for transfusion with most recommending against prophylactic transfusion to correct coagulation abnormalities. The target fibrinogen levels and dosage for transfusion also differ, with some guidelines recommending prophylactic use of cryoprecipitate for the most critically ill infants, especially those requiring surgery or ECMO.[127]

Most guidelines recommend a volume of 2 to 3 mL/kg for preterm infants or 0.5 unit of cryoprecipitate for term infants, which should increase the fibrinogen levels by 60 to 100 mg/dL; however, others recommend doses up to 5 to 15 mL/kg of cryoprecipitate.[140] FFP contains fibrinogen in lower concentrations and should not be used to correct hypofibrinogenemia, especially in neonates in whom volume overload can occur quickly.

Given the variation among guidelines and their limited specificity, it is not surprising that there is considerable variability in transfusion practice among clinicians. For example, a single institutional study in the United States found that critically ill children were likely to receive cryoprecipitate transfusions for cardiac surgery, DIC, and sepsis, and 60% of the transfusions were noncompliant with local guidelines.[142] In an Australian neonatal audit, only 57% had appropriate pretransfusion laboratory testing and received guideline compliant transfusions.[127] A study of multiple National Health Service Trusts in the United Kingdom noted a wide variation in practice of cryoprecipitate use and dose among adult and pediatric patients, with half of infants receiving cryoprecipitate during cardiac surgery and 75% of NICU patients receiving prophylactic cryoprecipitate transfusions.[143] Pretransfusion fibrinogen was recorded in 82% of neonatal and pediatric cases, and the mean pretransfusion fibrinogen was 80 mg/dL in cases of prophylaxis and 100 mg/dL in cases of bleeding.[143]

Tkach et al. instituted a policy to limit donor exposure to cryoprecipitate in the NICU by limiting the transfusion volume to 1 unit. This change was successful in reducing donor exposure while comparably increasing fibrinogen levels to similar values as were observed before the policy change.[140] Compared to the previous policy, which recommended a volume of 10 mL/kg of cryoprecipitate and required pooling the blood product from more than one donor, this change prevented term infants from receiving cryoprecipitate from more than one donor.[140]

As mentioned previously, the neonatal patient with moderate to severe HIE is likely to experience DIC and hypofibrinogenemia. Interestingly, the transfusion of these patients with cryoprecipitate is inconsistent between studies. One multicenter study reported only 11% of bleeding neonates received any cryoprecipitate, and the other study reported 32% of bleeding neonates received cryoprecipitate transfusion. This occurred in the setting of hypofibrinogenemia (fibrinogen <150 mg/dL) found in 77% of bleeding neonates.[135] Cryoprecipitate is expected to improve the fibrinogen level more robustly than an FFP transfusion, which only has 30% to 50% of the fibrinogen concentration per volume. It is likely that many adult and neonatal physicians inappropriately use FFP to treat hypofibrinogenemia or fail to monitor fibrinogen levels in patients with coagulopathy, putting them at risk for volume overload and administering subtherapeutic doses of fibrinogen.[144]

Conclusion

Neonatal transfusion medicine is an emerging field of study with limited evidence base to support many of the transfusion strategies adapted from pediatric and adult medicine. Nevertheless, nearly all extremely low birth weight infants and critically ill infants will not leave the NICU without at least one blood component transfusion. This life-saving therapy should be considered distinct from pharmacologic intervention because it is a biologic product with variations in the constituents and interactions with the host based on qualities of the donor, storage conditions, processing, and additives. Acute transfusion reactions are clearly defined and monitored in adult transfusion but do not have uniform definitions in neonatal medicine. The diagnosis of transfusion reactions is therefore poorly recognized and likely underreported. For example, transfusion-related acute lung injury (TRALI) and transfusion-related circulatory overload (TACO) are monitored in adult hemovigilance databases, but they are limited to case reports in neonates. Large multicenter studies have improved our understanding of RBC and platelet transfusion in neonates, but the data on plasma transfusion are limited. This population of patients has the longest life expectancy after transfusion, is highly transfused, and at risk for both short- and long-term effects from transfusion. It is imperative that we continue to improve our understanding of neonatal transfusions to provide the maximum benefit and minimum harm to these vulnerable patients.

REFERENCES

1. Patel RM, Hendrickson JE, Nellis ME, et al. Variation in neonatal transfusion practice. *J Pediatr.* 2021;235:92-99.e4.
2. American Association of Blood Banks, American Red Cross. *Circular of Information for the Use of Human Blood and Blood Components.* Authors; 2017.
3. Fung MK, Roseff SD, Vermoch KL. Blood component preferences of transfusion services supporting infant transfusions: a University HealthSystem Consortium benchmarking study. *Transfusion.* 2010;50(9):1921-1925.
4. Josephson CF, Pizzini DS, Higgins HNRD, et al. *Variability in Preparation, Storage, and Processing of Red Blood Cell Products for Extremely Low Birth Weight Infants: A Blood Bank Survey for the Transfusion of Prematures (TOP) Trial.* San Diego: Pediatric Academic Society; 2015.
5. Klein HG, Flegel WA, Natanson C. Red blood cell transfusion. *JAMA.* 2015;314(15):1557.
6. Franz AR, Engel C, Bassler D, et al. Effects of liberal vs restrictive transfusion thresholds on survival and neurocognitive outcomes in extremely low-birth-weight infants. *JAMA.* 2020;324(6):560.
7. Kirpalani H, Bell EF, Hintz SR, et al. Higher or lower hemoglobin transfusion thresholds for preterm infants. *N Engl J Med.* 2020;383(27):2639-2651.
8. Kirpalani H, Whyte RK, Andersen C, et al. The premature infants in need of transfusion (PINT) study: a randomized, controlled trial of a restrictive (LOW) versus liberal (HIGH) transfusion threshold for extremely low birth weight infants. *J Pediatr.* 2006;149(3):301-307.
9. Whyte R, Kirpalani H. Low versus high haemoglobin concentration threshold for blood transfusion for preventing morbidity and mortality in very low birth weight infants. *Cochrane Database Syst Rev.* 2011;(11):CD000512.
10. Patel RM, Knezevic A, Shenvi N, et al. Association of red blood cell transfusion, anemia, and necrotizing enterocolitis in very low-birth-weight infants. *JAMA.* 2016;315(9):889.
11. McGrady GA, Rettig PJ, Istre GR, et al. An outbreak of necrotizing enterocolitis. Association with transfusions of packed red blood cells. *Am J Epidemiol.* 1987;126(6):1165-1172.
12. Kirpalani H, Zupancic JA. Do transfusions cause necrotizing enterocolitis? The complementary role of randomized trials and observational studies. *Semin Perinatol.* 2012;36(4):269-276.
13. Mohamed A, Shah PS. Transfusion associated necrotizing enterocolitis: a meta-analysis of observational data. *Pediatrics.* 2012;129(3):529-540.
14. Marin T, Williams BL. Renal oxygenation measured by near-infrared spectroscopy in neonates. *Adv Neonatal Care.* 2021; 21(4):256-266.
15. Mintzer JP, Parvez B, Chelala M, et al. Monitoring regional tissue oxygen extraction in neonates <1250 g helps identify transfusion thresholds independent of hematocrit. *J Neonatal Perinatal Med.* 2014;7(2):89-100.
16. El Kenz H, Corazza F, Van Der Linden P, et al. Potassium content of irradiated packed red blood cells in different storage media: is there a need for additive solution-dependent recommendations for infant transfusion? *Transfus Apher Sci.* 2013;49(2):249-253.

17. Zimmermann R, Wintzheimer S, Weisbach V, et al. Influence of prestorage leukoreduction and subsequent irradiation on in vitro red blood cell (RBC) storage variables of RBCs in additive solution saline-adenine-glucose-mannitol. *Transfusion.* 2009;49(1):75-80.

18. Schroeder ML. Transfusion-associated graft-versus-host disease. *Br J Haematol.* 2002;117(2):275-287.

19. Patel RM, Roback JD, Uppal K, et al. Metabolomics profile comparisons of irradiated and nonirradiated stored donor red blood cells. *Transfusion.* 2015;55(3):544-552.

20. Leitman S, Holland P. Irradiation of blood products. Indications and guidelines. *Transfusion.* 1985;25(4):293-303.

21. Brugnara C, Churchill W. Effect of irradiation on red cell cation content and transport. *Transfusion.* 1992;32(3):246-252.

22. Williamson LM, Warwick RM. Transfusion-associated graft-versus-host disease and its prevention. *Blood Rev.* 1995;9(4): 251-261.

23. Patel RM, Meyer EK, Widness JA. Research opportunities to improve neonatal red blood cell transfusion. *Transf Med Rev.* 2016;30(4):165-173.

24. Kirpalani H, Bell EF, Hintz SR, et al. Higher or lower hemoglobin transfusion thresholds for preterm infants. *N Engl J Med.* 2020;383(27):2639-2651.

25. Reeves HM, Goodhue Meyer E, Harm SK, et al. Neonatal and pediatric blood bank practice in the United States: results from the AABB pediatric transfusion medicine subsection survey. *Transfusion.* 2021;61(8):2265-2276.

26. Reverberi R, Govoni M, Verenini M. Deformability and viability of irradiated red cells. *Ann Ist Super Sanita.* 2007;43(2): 176-185.

27. Ran Q, Hao P, Xiao Y, et al. Effect of irradiation and/or leucocyte filtration on RBC storage lesions. *PLoS One.* 2011;6(3):e18328.

28. Tinmouth A, Chin-Yee I. The clinical consequences of the red cell storage lesion. *Transfus Med Rev.* 2001;15(2):91-107.

29. Tinmouth A, Fergusson D, Yee IC, et al. Clinical consequences of red cell storage in the critically ill. *Transfusion.* 2006;46(11): 2014-2027.

30. Strauss RG, Burmeister LF, Johnson K, et al. Feasibility and safety of AS-3 red blood cells for neonatal transfusions. *J Pediatr.* 2000;136(2):215-219.

31. Levy GJ, Strauss RG, Hume H, et al. National survey of neonatal transfusion practices: I. Red blood cell therapy. *Pediatrics.* 1993;91(3):523-529.

32. Lee DA, Slagle TA, Jackson TM, et al. Reducing blood donor exposures in low birth weight infants by the use of older, unwashed packed red blood cells. *J Pediatr.* 1995;126(2):280-286.

33. Liu EA, Mannino FL, Lane TA. Prospective, randomized trial of the safety and efficacy of a limited donor exposure transfusion program for premature neonates. *J Pediatr.* 1994;125(1): 92-96.

34. Strauss R, Burmeister L, Johnson K, et al. AS-1 red cells for neonatal transfusions: a randomized trial assessing donor exposure and safety. *Transfusion.* 1996;36(10):873-878.

35. Wood L, Beutler E. Temperature dependence of sodium-potassium activated erythrocyte adenosine triphosphatase. *J Lab Clin Med.* 1967;70(2):287-294.

36. Hall TL, Barnes A, Miller JR, et al. Neonatal mortality following transfusion of red cells with high plasma potassium levels. *Transfusion.* 1993;33(7):606-609.

37. Cholette JM, Henrichs KF, Alfieris GM, et al. Washing red blood cells and platelets transfused in cardiac surgery reduces postoperative inflammation and number of transfusions. *Pediatr Crit Care Med.* 2012;13(3):290-299.

38. Blumberg N, Heal JM, Gettings KF, et al. An association between decreased cardiopulmonary complications (transfusion-related acute lung injury and transfusion-associated circulatory overload) and implementation of universal leukoreduction of blood transfusions. *Transfusion.* 2010;50(12):2738-2744.

39. Blumberg N, Heal JM, Rowe JM. A randomized trial of washed red blood cell and platelet transfusions in adult acute leukemia [ISRCTN76536440]. *BMC Blood Disord.* 2004;4(1):6.

40. Belizaire RM, Makley AT, Campion EM, et al. Resuscitation with washed aged packed red blood cell units decreases the proinflammatory response in mice after hemorrhage. *J Trauma Acute Care Surg.* 2012;73(2):S128-S133.

41. Crawford TM, Andersen CC, Hodyl NA, et al. Effect of washed versus unwashed red blood cells on transfusion-related immune responses in preterm newborns. *Clin Transl Immunol.* 2022; 11(3):e1377.

42. Keir AK, Wilkinson D, Andersen C, et al. Washed versus unwashed red blood cells for transfusion for the prevention of morbidity and mortality in preterm infants. *Cochrane Database Syst Rev.* 2016(1):CD011484.

43. Lacroix J, Hébert PC, Fergusson DA, et al. Age of transfused blood in critically ill adults. *N Engl J Med.* 2015;372(15): 1410-1418.

44. Heddle NM, Cook RJ, Arnold DM, et al. Effect of short-term vs. long-term blood storage on mortality after transfusion. *N Engl J Med.* 2016;375(20):1937-1945.

45. Dhabangi A, Ainomugisha B, Cserti-Gazdewich C, et al. Effect of transfusion of red blood cells with longer vs shorter storage duration on elevated blood lactate levels in children with severe anemia. *JAMA.* 2015;314(23):2514.

46. Koch CG, Li L, Sessler DI, et al. Duration of red-cell storage and complications after cardiac surgery. *N Engl J Med.* 2008;358(12): 1229-1239.

47. Pettilä V, Westbrook AJ, Nichol AD, et al. Age of red blood cells and mortality in the critically ill. *Crit Care.* 2011;15(2):R116.

48. Eikelboom JW, Cook RJ, Liu Y, et al. Duration of red cell storage before transfusion and in-hospital mortality. *Am Heart J.* 2010;159(5):737-743.e1.

49. Gauvin F, Spinella PC, Lacroix J, et al. Association between length of storage of transfused red blood cells and multiple organ dysfunction syndrome in pediatric intensive care patients. *Transfusion.* 2010;50(9):1902-1913.

50. Fergusson DA, Hébert P, Hogan DL, et al. Effect of fresh red blood cell transfusions on clinical outcomes in premature, very low-birth-weight infants. *JAMA.* 2012;308(14):1443.

51. Patel RM, Josephson CD. Storage age of red blood cells for transfusion of premature infants. *JAMA.* 2013;309(6):544.

52. Fang DC, McCullough J. Transfusion-transmitted *Babesia microti.* *Transfus Med Rev.* 2016;30(3):132-138.

53. Tonnetti L, Townsend RL, Dodd RY, et al. Characteristics of transfusion-transmitted *Babesia microti,* American Red Cross 2010-2017. *Transfusion.* 2019;59(9):2908-2912.

54. Young C, Chawla A, Berardi V, et al. Preventing transfusion-transmitted babesiosis: preliminary experience of the first laboratory-based blood donor screening program. *Transfusion.* 2012; 52(7):1523-1529.

55. Tonnetti L, Eder AF, Dy B, et al. Transfusion complications: transfusion-transmitted *Babesia microti* identified through hemovigilance. *Transfusion.* 2009;49(12):2557-2563.

56. Sparger KA, Assmann SF, Granger S, et al. Platelet transfusion practices among very-low-birth-weight infants. *JAMA Pediatr.* 2016;170(7):687.

57. Gunnink SF, Vlug R, Fijnvandraat K, et al. Neonatal thrombocytopenia: etiology, management and outcome. *Expert Rev Hematol.* 2014;7(3):387-395.

58. Christensen RD, Baer VL, Henry E, et al. Thrombocytopenia in small-for-gestational-age infants. *Pediatrics.* 2015;136(2):e361-e370.

59. Curley A, Stanworth SJ, Willoughby K, et al. Randomized trial of platelet-transfusion thresholds in neonates. *N Engl J Med.* 2019;380(3):242-251.

60. Braine HG, Kickler TS, Charache P, et al. Bacterial sepsis secondary to platelet transfusion: an adverse effect of extended storage at room temperature. *Transfusion.* 1986;26(4):391-393.

61. Snyder EL, Stramer SL, Benjamin RJ. The safety of the blood supply—time to raise the bar. *N Engl J Med.* 2015;373(9):882.

62. Schrezenmeier H, Walther-Wenke G, Müller TH, et al. Bacterial contamination of platelet concentrates: results of a prospective multicenter study comparing pooled whole blood-derived platelets and apheresis platelets. *Transfusion.* 2007;47(4):644-652.

63. Kleinman S, Reed W, Stassinopoulos A. A patient-oriented risk-benefit analysis of pathogen-inactivated blood components: application to apheresis platelets in the United States. *Transfusion.* 2013;53(7):1603-1618.

64. Orton S. Syphilis and blood donors: what we know, what we do not know, and what we need to know. *Transfus Med Rev.* 2001;15(4):282-291.

65. Störmer M, Vollmer T. Diagnostic methods for platelet bacteria screening: current status and developments. *Transfus Med Hemother.* 2014;41(1):19-27.

66. Dean CL, Wade J, Roback JD. Transfusion-transmitted infections: an update on product screening, diagnostic techniques, and the path ahead. *J Clin Microbiol.* 2018;56(7):e00352-18.

67. Gehrie EA, Rutter SJ, Snyder EL. Pathogen reduction: the state of the science in 2019. *Hematol Oncol Clin North Am.* 2019;33(5):749-766.

68. Lozano M, Cid J. Pathogen inactivation: coming of age. *Curr Opin Hematol.* 2013;20(6):540-545.

69. Keil SD, Saakadze N, Bowen R, et al. Riboflavin and ultraviolet light for pathogen reduction of murine cytomegalovirus in blood products. *Transfusion.* 2015;55(4):858-863.

70. Cid J. Prevention of transfusion-associated graft-versus-host disease with pathogen-reduced platelets with amotosalen and ultraviolet A light: a review. *Vox Sang.* 2017;112(7):607-613.

71. Girona-Llobera E, Jimenez-Marco T, Galmes-Trueba A, et al. Reducing the financial impact of pathogen inactivation technology for platelet components: our experience. *Transfusion.* 2014;54(1):158-168.

72. Lozano M, Cid J. Analysis of reasons for not implementing pathogen inactivation for platelet concentrates. *Transfus Clin Biol.* 2013;20(2):158-164.

73. Magron A, Laugier J, Provost P, et al. Pathogen reduction technologies: the pros and cons for platelet transfusion. *Platelets.* 2018;29(1):2-8.

74. Singh Y, Sawyer LS, Pinkoski LS, et al. Photochemical treatment of plasma with amotosalen and long-wavelength ultraviolet light inactivates pathogens while retaining coagulation function. *Transfusion.* 2006;46(7):1168-1177.

75. Kwon SY, Kim IS, Bae JE, et al. Pathogen inactivation efficacy of mirasol PRT system and intercept blood system for non-leucoreduced platelet-rich plasma-derived platelets suspended in plasma. *Vox Sang.* 2014;107(3):254-260.

76. Schulz WL, McPadden J, Gehrie EA, et al. Blood utilization and transfusion reactions in pediatric patients transfused with conventional or pathogen reduced platelets. *J Pediatr.* 2019;209:220-225.

77. Thiele T, Pohler P, Kohlmann T, et al. Tolerance of platelet concentrates treated with UVC-light only for pathogen reduction—a phase I clinical trial. *Vox Sang.* 2015;109(1):44-51.

78. Li J, de Korte D, Woolum MD, et al. Pathogen reduction of buffy coat platelet concentrates using riboflavin and light: comparisons with pathogen-reduction technology-treated apheresis platelet products. *Vox Sang.* 2004;87(2):82-90.

79. Perez-Pujol S, Tonda R, Lozano M, et al. Effects of a new pathogen-reduction technology (mirasol PRT) on functional aspects of platelet concentrates. *Transfusion.* 2005;45(6):911-919.

80. Cid J, Lozano M. Pathogen inactivation of platelets for transfusion. *Platelets.* 2022;33(1):23-26.

81. Lozano M, Knutson F, Tardivel R, et al. A multi-centre study of therapeutic efficacy and safety of platelet components treated with amotosalen and ultraviolet A pathogen inactivation stored for 6 or 7 d prior to transfusion. *Br J Haematol.* 2011;153(3):393-401.

82. van der Meer PF, Ypma PF, van Geloven N, et al. Hemostatic efficacy of pathogen-inactivated vs untreated platelets: a randomized controlled trial. *Blood.* 2018;132(2):223-231.

83. Garban F, Guyard A, Labussière H, et al. Comparison of the hemostatic efficacy of pathogen-reduced platelets vs untreated platelets in patients with thrombocytopenia and malignant hematologic diseases. *JAMA Oncol.* 2018;4(4):468.

84. Rebulla P, Vaglio S, Beccaria F, et al. Clinical effectiveness of platelets in additive solution treated with two commercial pathogen-reduction technologies. *Transfusion.* 2017;57(5):1171-1183.

85. Kerkhoffs JL, van Putten WL, Novotny VM, et al. Clinical effectiveness of leucoreduced, pooled donor platelet concentrates, stored in plasma or additive solution with and without pathogen reduction. *Br J Haematol.* 2010;150(2):209-217.

86. Janetzko K, Cazenave JP, Klüter H, et al. Therapeutic efficacy and safety of photochemically treated apheresis platelets processed with an optimized integrated set. *Transfusion.* 2005;45(9):1443-1452.

87. McCullough J, Vesole DH, Benjamin RJ, et al. Therapeutic efficacy and safety of platelets treated with a photochemical process for pathogen inactivation: the SPRINT Trial. *Blood.* 2004;104(5):1534-1541.

88. van Rhenen D, Gulliksson H, Cazenave JP, et al. Transfusion of pooled buffy coat platelet components prepared with photochemical pathogen inactivation treatment: the euroSPRITE trial. *Blood.* 2003;101(6):2426-2433.

89. Brixner V, Bug G, Pohler P, et al. Efficacy of UVC-treated, pathogen-reduced platelets versus untreated platelets: a randomized controlled non-inferiority trial. *Haematologica.* 2021;106(4):1086-1096.

90. A randomized controlled clinical trial evaluating the performance and safety of platelets treated with MIRASOL pathogen reduction technology. *Transfusion.* 2010;50(11):2362-2375.

91. Rebulla P, Garban F, Meer PF, et al. A crosswalk tabular review on methods and outcomes from randomized clinical trials using pathogen reduced platelets. *Transfusion.* 2020;60(6):1267-1277.

92. Jimenez-Marco T, Garcia-Recio M, Girona-Llobera E. Use and safety of riboflavin and UV light-treated platelet transfusions in children over a five-year period: focusing on neonates. *Transfusion.* 2019;59(12):3580-3588.

93. Del Vecchio A, Sola MC, Theriaque DW, et al. Platelet transfusions in the neonatal intensive care unit: factors predicting which patients will require multiple transfusions. *Transfusion.* 2001;41(6):803-808.

94. Keene SD, Patel RM, Stansfield BK, et al. Blood product transfusion and mortality in neonatal extracorporeal membrane oxygenation. *Transfusion.* 2020;60(2):262-268.

95. Elgendy MM, Durgham R, Othman HF, et al. Platelet transfusion and outcomes of preterm infants: a cross-sectional study. *Neonatology.* 2021;118(4):425-433.

96. Moore CM, Curley A. Platelet transfusion thresholds in neonatal medicine. *Early Hum Dev.* 2019;138:104845.

97. Stolla M, Refaai MA, Heal JM, et al. Platelet transfusion—the new immunology of an old therapy. *Front Immunol.* 2015;6:28.

98. Curtis BR, Edwards JT, Hessner MJ, et al. Blood group A and B antigens are strongly expressed on platelets of some individuals. *Blood.* 2000;96(4):1574-1581.

99. Josephson CD, Castillejo MI, Grima K, et al. ABO-mismatched platelet transfusions: strategies to mitigate patient exposure to naturally occurring hemolytic antibodies. *Transfus Apher Sci.* 2010;42(1):83-88.

100. Harris SB, Josephson CD, Kost CB, et al. Nonfatal intravascular hemolysis in a pediatric patient after transfusion of a platelet unit with high-titer anti-A. *Transfusion.* 2007;47(8):1412-1417.

101. Dunbar NM. Does ABO and RhD matching matter for platelet transfusion? *Hematology.* 2020;2020(1):512-517.

102. Aster RH. Effect of anticoagulant and ABO incompatibility on recovery of transfused human platelets. *Blood.* 1965;26(6):732-743.

103. Pavenski K, Warkentin TE, Shen H, et al. Posttransfusion platelet count increments after ABO-compatible versus ABO-incompatible platelet transfusions in noncancer patients: an observational study. *Transfusion.* 2010;50(7):1552-1560.

104. Slichter SJ. Factors affecting posttransfusion platelet increments, platelet refractoriness, and platelet transfusion intervals in thrombocytopenic patients. *Blood.* 2005;105(10):4106-4114.

105. Heal JM, Rowe JM, McMican A, et al. The role of ABO matching in platelet transfusion. *Eur J Haematol.* 2009;50(2):110-117.

106. Henrichs KF, Howk N, Masel DS, et al. Providing ABO-identical platelets and cryoprecipitate to (almost) all patients: approach, logistics, and associated decreases in transfusion reaction and red blood cell alloimmunization incidence. *Transfusion.* 2012;52(3):635-640.

107. Cid J, Harm SK, Yazer MH. Platelet transfusion—the art and science of compromise. *Transf Med Hemother.* 2013;40(3):160-171.

108. Blumberg N, Heal JM, Hicks GL, et al. Association of ABO-mismatched platelet transfusions with morbidity and mortality in cardiac surgery. *Transfusion.* 2001;41(6):790-793.

109. Shehata N, Tinmouth A, Naglie G, et al. ABO-identical versus nonidentical platelet transfusion: a systematic review. *Transfusion.* 2009;49(11):2442-2453.

110. Patel RM, Josephson C. Neonatal and pediatric platelet transfusions. *Curr Opin Hematol.* 2019;26(6):466-472.

111. Conway LT, Scott EP. Acute hemolytic transfusion reaction due to ABO incompatible plasma in a plateletapheresis concentrate. *Transfusion.* 1984;24(5):413-414.

112. Valbonesi M, De Luigi MC, Lercari G, et al. Acute intravascular hemolysis in two patients transfused with dry-platelet units obtained from the same ABO incompatible donor. *Int J Artif Organs.* 2000;23(9):642-646.

113. Angiolillo A, Luban NL. Hemolysis following an out-of-group platelet transfusion in an 8-month-old with Langerhans cell histiocytosis. *J Pediatr Hematol Oncol.* 2004;26(4):267-269.

114. Duguesnoy R, Anderson A, Tomasulo P, et al. ABO compatibility and platelet transfusions of alloimmunized thrombocytopenic patients. *Blood.* 1979;54(3):595-599.

115. Heal J, Blumberg N, Masel D. An evaluation of crossmatching, HLA, and ABO matching for platelet transfusions to refractory patients. *Blood.* 1987;70(1):23-30.

116. Carr R, Hutton JL, Jenkins JA, et al. Transfusion of ABO-mismatched platelets leads to early platelet refractoriness. *Br J Haematol.* 1990;75(3):408-413.

117. Poterjoy BS, Josephson CD. Platelets, frozen plasma, and cryoprecipitate: what is the clinical evidence for their use in the neonatal intensive care unit? *Semin Perinatol.* 2009;33(1):66-74.

118. Motta M, Del Vecchio A, Perrone B, et al. Fresh frozen plasma use in the NICU: a prospective, observational, multicentred study. *Arch Dis Child Fetal Neonatal Ed.* 2014;99(4):F303-F308.

119. Puetz J, Darling G, McCormick KA, et al. Fresh frozen plasma and recombinant factor VIIa use in neonates. *J Pediatr Hematol Oncol.* 2009;31(12):901-906.

120. Baer VL, Henry E, Lambert DK, et al. Implementing a program to improve compliance with neonatal intensive care unit transfusion guidelines was accompanied by a reduction in transfusion rate: a pre-post analysis within a multihospital health care system. *Transfusion.* 2011;51(2):264-269.

121. Keir AK, Stanworth SJ. Neonatal plasma transfusion: an evidence-based review. *Transfus Med Rev.* 2016;30(4):174-182.

122. Puetz J, Witmer C, Huang YS, et al. Widespread use of fresh frozen plasma in US children's hospitals despite limited evidence demonstrating a beneficial effect. *J Pediatr.* 2012;160(2):210-215.e1.

123. Goel R, Josephson CD. Recent advances in transfusions in neonates/infants. *F1000Res.* 2018;7.

124. Girelli G, Antoncecchi S, Casadei AM, et al. Recommendations for transfusion therapy in neonatology. *Blood Transf.* 2015;13(3):484-497.

125. Christensen RD, Baer VL, Lambert DK, et al. Reference intervals for common coagulation tests of preterm infants (CME). *Transfusion.* 2014;54(3):627-632, quiz 626.

126. Andrew M, Paes B, Milner R, et al. Development of the human coagulation system in the healthy premature infant. *Blood.* 1988;72(5):1651-1657.

127. Crighton GL, Huisman EJ. Pediatric fibrinogen part II—overview of indications for fibrinogen use in critically ill children. *Front Pediatr.* 2021;9:647680.

128. Motta M, Del Vecchio A, Radicioni M. Clinical use of fresh-frozen plasma and cryoprecipitate in neonatal intensive care unit. *J Matern Fetal Neonatal Med.* 2011;24(1):S129-S131.

129. Turner T, Prowse CV, Prescott RJ, et al. A clinical trial on the early detection and correction of haemostatic defects in selected high-risk neonates. *Br J Haematol.* 1981;47(1):65-75.

130. Michniewicz B, Al Saad SR, Karbowski LM, et al. Organ complications of infants with hypoxic ischemic encephalopathy before therapeutic hypothermia. *Ther Hypothermia Temp Manag.* 2021;11(1):58-63.

131. Forman KR, Diab Y, Wong EC, et al. Coagulopathy in newborns with hypoxic ischemic encephalopathy (HIE) treated with therapeutic hypothermia: a retrospective case-control study. *BMC Pediatr.* 2014;14(1):277.

132. Bauman ME, Cheung PY, Massicotte MP. Hemostasis and platelet dysfunction in asphyxiated neonates. *J Pediatr.* 2011;158(2):Se35-Se39.

133. Suzuki S, Morishita S. Hypercoagulability and DIC in high-risk infants. *Semin Thromb Hemost.* 1998;24(05):463-466.

134. Shah P. Multiorgan dysfunction in infants with post-asphyxial hypoxic-ischaemic encephalopathy. *Arch Dis Child Fetal Neonatal Ed.* 2004;89(2):152F-155F.

135. Pakvasa MA, Winkler AM, Hamrick SE, et al. Observational study of haemostatic dysfunction and bleeding in neonates with hypoxic–ischaemic encephalopathy. *BMJ Open.* 2017;7(2):e013787.

136. Gluckman PD, Wyatt JS, Azzopardi D, et al. Selective head cooling with mild systemic hypothermia after neonatal encephalopathy: multicentre randomised trial. *Lancet.* 2005; 365(9460):663-670.

137. Shankaran S, Laptook AR, Ehrenkranz RA, et al. Whole-body hypothermia for neonates with hypoxic–ischemic encephalopathy. *N Engl J Med.* 2005;353(15):1574-1584.

138. Gorelik N, Faingold R, Daneman A, et al. Intraventricular hemorrhage in term neonates with hypoxic-ischemic encephalopathy: a comparison study between neonates treated with and without hypothermia. *Quant Imag Med Surg.* 2016;6(5):504-509.

139. Shankaran S, Pappas A, Laptook AR, et al. Outcomes of safety and effectiveness in a multicenter randomized, controlled trial of whole-body hypothermia for neonatal hypoxic-ischemic encephalopathy. *Pediatrics.* 2008;122(4):e791-e798.

140. Tkach EK, Mackley A, Brooks A, et al. Cryoprecipitate transfusions in the neonatal intensive care unit: a performance improvement study to decrease donor exposure. *Transfusion.* 2018;58(5):1206-1209.

141. Peyvandi F, Palla R, Menegatti M, et al. Coagulation factor activity and clinical bleeding severity in rare bleeding disorders: results from the European Network of Rare Bleeding Disorders. *J Thromb Haemost.* 2012;10(4):615-621.

142. DeSimone RA, Nellis ME, Goel R, et al. Cryoprecipitate indications and patterns of use in the pediatric intensive care unit: inappropriate transfusions and lack of standardization. *Transfusion.* 2016;56(8):1960-1964.

143. Tinegate H, Allard S, Grant-Casey J, et al. Cryoprecipitate for transfusion: which patients receive it and why? A study of patterns of use across three regions in England. *Transf Med.* 2012;22(5):356-361.

144. Levy JH, Goodnough LT. How I use fibrinogen replacement therapy in acquired bleeding. *Blood.* 2015;125(9):1387-1393.

Chapter 12

Recent Advances in NICU Platelet Transfusions

Patricia Davenport, MD and Martha C. Sola-Visner, MD

Chapter Outline

Introduction

Thrombocytopenia (defined as a platelet count $<150 \times 10^9/L$) is the second most common hematologic problem among neonates admitted to the neonatal intensive care unit (NICU), affecting 20% to 25% of this patient population.[1] The incidence of thrombocytopenia increases with decreasing gestational age and birth weight, reaching ~70% among extremely low birth weight (ELBW) neonates (born with a weight <1000 g).[2] The incidence of bleeding, particularly intracranial bleeding, is also highest among the most preterm neonates, with approximately 20% to 25% of neonates born at less than 1500 g developing an intraventricular hemorrhage (IVH) during the first week of life.

Consistent with the high frequency of thrombocytopenia and bleeding in this population, platelets are the second most common blood product (after red blood cells) transfused to NICU patients, with most platelet transfusions being given prophylactically to nonbleeding patients.[3] However, the platelet count below which the bleeding risk increases to the point of justifying a transfusion was (until recently) unknown, and this led to substantial worldwide variability in platelet count thresholds used to transfuse NICU patients. This was first evident in survey studies conducted among North American neonatologists, in which the platelet transfusion thresholds selected ranged from less than 10 to less than $100 \times 10^9/L$ in every one of the 15 clinical scenarios presented, with less than $50 \times 10^9/L$ being the most commonly chosen threshold throughout.[4] Interestingly, when the same survey was translated into German and sent to European neonatologists in German-speaking countries (Germany, Austria, and Switzerland), the most commonly selected transfusion threshold was lower ($<25 \times 10^9/L$) in most clinical vignettes, although similar overall variability was observed.[5] Statistical analysis comparing the transatlantic responses to the same survey suggested that North American neonatologists give 2.3-fold more platelet transfusions to NICU patients, based on practice variability alone.[5] Subsequent observational multicenter studies conducted in the United States and Europe further supported this conclusion: In a recent study of neonatal transfusion practices in seven US hospitals from 2013 and 2016, the median platelet count prior to over 1000 platelet transfusions was 71×10^9/L for neonates in general, and it was greater than 45×10^9/L in all gestational and postnatal age groups examined.[3] In an observational multicenter study from the United Kingdom, in contrast, the mean platelet count prior to transfusion was 27×10^9/L.[6]

Platelet Transfusions and Prevention of Bleeding

CORRELATION BETWEEN PLATELET COUNT AND BLEEDING RISK

Prophylactic platelet transfusions are given to NICU patients with the goal of decreasing their bleeding risk. This assumes that as the platelet count decreases, the bleeding risk increases, and therefore increasing the platelet count with a transfusion will reduce this risk. However, the available evidence offers little support for this premise. While studies have shown that thrombocytopenic neonates have a higher incidence of IVH than nonthrombocytopenic neonates,[7,8] several observational studies failed to show a correlation between the degree of thrombocytopenia and the incidence of clinically significant bleeding.[6,7,9,10] As an example, in a study by Sparger et al., neonates with thrombocytopenia in the first week of life (platelet count $<150 \times 10^9$/L) had a 2.3-fold higher risk of IVH compared to nonthrombocytopenic neonates.[7] However, the risk was the same at a platelet count of 10 to 30 or 80 to 90×10^9/L. This observation is not unique to neonates since studies correlating the morning platelet count with the incidence of grade II or higher bleeding in adult and pediatric patients with chemotherapy-induced thrombocytopenia have shown the same risk with platelet counts between 10 and 100×10^9/L.[11,12]

EFFECTS OF PLATELET TRANSFUSIONS: OBSERVATIONAL STUDIES

Given the lack of correlation between platelet count and bleeding risk, it is perhaps not surprising that a number of observational studies found no effect of platelet transfusions on the incidence of bleeding. A study comparing two NICUs with very different platelet transfusion practices (one liberal and one very restrictive) found no difference in the incidence of IVH

between the two.[13] Another study used logistic regression to examine the effects of platelet transfusions on the incidence of IVH in a large cohort of very low birth weight (VLBW) infants, also finding that transfusions had no effect after adjusting for other clinical factors, particularly the presence of thrombocytopenia.[7] More recently, a study evaluated the effects of platelet transfusions on platelet counts, primary hemostasis (using platelet function analyzer-closure times), and clinical bleeding. These investigators found that platelet transfusions significantly increased platelet counts but had a small effect on primary hemostasis and no effect on bleeding severity.[14] Taken together, these findings support the hypothesis that bleeding in preterm neonates is multifactorial and that factors other than the platelet count are more important determinants of their bleeding risk.

In addition to the lack of effectiveness of platelet transfusions in reducing bleeding, several observational studies over the last 2 decades reported concerning associations between the number of platelet transfusions and neonatal mortality.[15-19] However, in the setting of observational studies, it was impossible to determine whether this association simply reflected a higher severity of illness among neonates receiving the most transfusions. Baer et al. attempted to address this question using statistical sensitivity analysis, which suggested that at least some of the increased mortality was due to the platelet transfusions per se.[18] Two studies assessed the effects of platelet transfusions specifically in neonates with necrotizing enterocolitis (NEC). One found a higher incidence of complications (short gut and cholestasis) among neonates who received more platelet transfusions,[20] and the second found a higher mortality among those more heavily transfused, although the strength of this association decreased, and significance was lost after adjusting for birth weight and severity of illness.[21]

EFFECTS OF PLATELET TRANSFUSIONS: RANDOMIZED CONTROLLED TRIALS

Only three randomized controlled trials (RCTs) of neonatal platelet transfusion thresholds have been published to date, and their design and findings are summarized in Table 12.1. The first RCT, published in 1993, investigated if IVH could be prevented in preterm infants by maintaining a platelet count greater

TABLE 12.1 Characteristics of the Three Randomized Controlled Trials of Neonatal Platelet Transfusion Thresholds Published to Date

	Andrew et al., 1993 (n=152)	Kumar et al., 2019 (n=44)	Curley et al., 2019 (n=660)
Population	GA <33 wk and BW 500–1500 g	GA <34 6/7 wk and <14 days	GA <34 wk
Intervention	PLT Tx when PC <150 × 10⁹/L	PLT Tx when PC <100 × 10⁹/L	PLT Tx when PC <25 × 10⁹/L
Comparison	PLT Tx when PC <50 × 10⁹/L	PLT Tx when PC <20 × 10⁹/L	PLT Tx when PC <50 × 10⁹/L
Measured Outcome	ICH on DOL 7–10 HUS	Time to PDA closure Secondary: new onset IVH	Composite of death or major bleeding up to and including day 28
Key Findings	No difference in ICH between study groups	No difference in time to PDA closure but higher incidence of new IVH in intervention group	Higher rate of death or major bleeding in liberal transfusion (comparison) group

BW, Birth weight; *DOL,* day of life; *GA,* gestational age; *HUS,* head ultrasound; *ICH,* intracranial hemorrhage; *IVH,* intraventricular hemorrhage; *PC,* platelet count; *PDA,* patent ductus arteriosus; *PLT Tx,* platelet transfusion.

than 150×10^9/L (i.e., in the normal range) for the first 7 days of life.[22] In this study, 152 infants with gestational age less than 33 weeks and birth weight of 500 to 1500 g were randomized within 72 hours of birth to receive a platelet transfusion either when the platelet count fell below 150×10^9/L (treatment) or below 50×10^9/L (controls). This study found no difference in the incidence or severity of IVH between the groups, with 28% of infants in the treatment group and 26% in the control group showing an IVH on day of life 7 to 10 head ultrasound (HUS). In a subgroup analysis of the control neonates, the authors also compared outcomes in infants who had one or more platelet counts less than 60×10^9/L (i.e., more severe thrombocytopenia) to those who did not. Once again, there was no difference in the incidence of IVH between the two groups, although infants with a platelet count less than 60×10^9/L received significantly more platelet transfusions than infants with platelet counts consistently above this threshold. This landmark study demonstrated that a platelet count between 50 and 150×10^9/L is safe in preterm neonates during the first week of life but did not provide information on the safety of platelet counts below 50×10^9/L.

Over 20 years passed before another RCT of neonatal platelet transfusion thresholds was published. In 2019 two trials comparing liberal vs. restrictive platelet transfusion thresholds were reported, although they had very different patient numbers, transfusion thresholds, and primary outcomes (see Table 12.1). The smaller of the two studies was a single-center randomized trial designed to determine if thrombocytopenic preterm neonates transfused at a liberal platelet transfusion threshold ($<100 \times 10^9$/L) had earlier closure of a hemodynamically significant patent ductus arteriosus (PDA) compared to neonates transfused at a restrictive threshold ($<20 \times 10^9$/L), while undergoing standard medical treatment for the PDA.[23] The study enrolled a total of 44 preterm neonates and found no difference in the primary outcome of time to PDA closure, with a median of 72 hours in both groups. However, in an analysis of secondary outcomes, 40.9% of infants in the liberal transfusion group were found to have new onset IVH (of any grade) following randomization, compared to only 9.1% in the restrictive group (p=0.034). In multivariate analysis, the investigators found the cumulative volume of platelet concentrate transfused to be an independent predictor of IVH (p=0.019), with a 4.5% increase in odds of IVH for every mL/kg of platelets transfused. It is unclear if the higher incidence of IVH was due to the increased volume administered in the liberal transfusion group (median of 30 mL/kg vs. 0 mL/kg), the biologic interactions of the transfused platelets, or a combination of both. Nevertheless, these findings added to the growing body of evidence supporting a lack of benefit of liberal platelet transfusions and a possible association with harm.

Around the same time, the results of the much larger platelet transfusion thresholds in premature neonates (PlaNet-2) trial were also published. This multicenter RCT enrolled 660 preterm infants (gestational age <34 weeks) with severe thrombocytopenia admitted to NICUs in the United Kingdom, Ireland, and the Netherlands.[24] Infants were randomized to receive a platelet transfusion for platelet counts below 50×10^9/L (liberal group) or below 25×10^9/L (restrictive group), and were followed for 28 days to assess the primary composite outcome of death or major bleeding. Unexpectedly, infants in the liberal transfusion group had a significantly higher incidence of death or major bleeding compared to those in the restrictive group (26% vs. 19%, respectively; odds ratio [OR] 1.57; 95% confidence interval [CI] 1.06–2.32; p=0.02), with both components of the composite outcome favoring the restrictive approach. Among secondary outcomes, the incidence of bronchopulmonary dysplasia at 36 weeks corrected age was also higher in the liberal transfusion group (63% vs. 54%, OR 1.54; 95% CI 1.03–2.30). This landmark study, the largest to date, concluded that the use of a restrictive platelet transfusion threshold in neonates is not only safe but may also reduce harm by preventing death or major bleeding in 7 of 100 premature neonates with severe thrombocytopenia.

Despite the significant impact of the PlaNet-2 trial, there remained some hesitancy to lower the platelet transfusion threshold in the smallest, most premature infants at the highest risk of severe bleeding in the first week of life. While this high-risk population was represented in the PlaNet-2 trial (37% of infants were randomized in first 5 days of life and 55% in the first 10 days of life), all infants received a point of care HUS immediately prior to randomization to confirm the absence of a major bleed, which would have excluded them from the study. In many parts of the world, point-of-care HUS is not available, making it difficult for neonatologists to assess for a major bleed at the time of clinical decisions. Additionally, 39% of

infants in the study received at least one platelet transfusion prior to randomization, and it is unknown if most/some of these transfusions were administered to the most premature infants during this critical window when bleeding risk is the highest.

To address the question of whether the restrictive transfusion thresholds are only beneficial for stable, low-risk neonates, the investigators performed a secondary analysis of the PlaNeT-2 data using a mathematical model to examine whether the effects of a restrictive transfusion threshold varied depending on the neonate's baseline risk of bleeding/mortality (calculated based on known clinical factors, such as gestational age, postnatal age, underlying diagnosis, etc.).[25] This analysis found that neonates with the highest baseline risk of bleeding/mortality benefitted as much (or more) from the restrictive transfusion threshold as the lower-risk infants. While these findings strongly suggest that the findings from the PlaNet-2 trial can (and likely should) be applied to even the most vulnerable neonates, some uncertainty remains around the appropriate platelet transfusion threshold in extremely preterm neonates in the first few days of life who either do not have a HUS at the time of decision making or have a known significant IVH, since these infants were excluded from the PlaNeT-2 study.

Potential Mechanisms Underlying the Effects of Platelet Transfusions in Neonates

The mechanisms underlying the increased morbidity and mortality associated with liberal neonatal platelet transfusion practices remain unknown. Two RCTs[23,24] found that neonatal platelet transfusions paradoxically increased bleeding risk, specifically IVH. The mechanisms responsible for IVH in preterm neonates are multifactorial, with vascular, hemodynamic, and hemostatic factors playing important roles. In premature infants, most intracranial hemorrhages occur during the first few days of life and originate in the germinal matrix, a highly vascularized collection of neuronal and glial cells that lines the lateral ventricles. During this early period the germinal matrix is characterized by a paucity of pericytes, an immature basal lamina, and a deficiency of glial fibrillary acidic protein,[26] making it intrinsically fragile. When the germinal matrix vasculature encounters disturbances in cerebral blood flow (due to the impaired cerebral autoregulation of premature infants), the fragile blood vessels can rupture and bleed into the ventricles. Platelet transfusions are usually administered to neonates at a dose of 10 to 15 mL/kg (15 mL/kg in the PlaNet-2 trial and between 10 and 20 mL/kg in the study by Kumar et al.), given over 30 to 60 minutes. This contrasts with pediatric or adult platelet transfusions, which are usually given at a dose of 3 to 5 mL/kg. Thus it is possible that the rapid volume expansion caused by platelet transfusions given at these doses over a short period of time could contribute to the pathogenesis of IVH.

Alternatively, it has been hypothesized that there is a developmental mismatch that occurs when adult platelets are transfused into the physiologic environment of a preterm neonate, which could cause harm. Neonatal and adult platelets are morphologically identical but differ in both hemostatic and nonhemostatic functions. In regard to hemostasis, multiple studies have shown that neonatal platelets are hyporeactive compared to adult platelets,[27] but developmental differences in their nonhemostatic functions are just beginning to be explored. Over the last decade, it has become clear that platelets participate in several nonhemostatic processes, including angiogenesis, vascular development, blood/lymphatic separation, immune responses, and inflammatory reactions (Fig. 12.1).[28-30] A large body of work has described the extensive interactions between platelets and immune cells. P-selectin is a protein normally located in the alpha granules of platelets. Upon platelet activation, P-selectin translocates to the cell surface, where it is available to bind to its receptor (PSGL-1) found on multiple cells, including neutrophils and monocytes. These platelet-immune cell interactions can

regulate immune cell activation, the release of cytokines/chemokines, immune cell migration into tissues, and the release of neutrophil extracellular traps (NETs).[31-33] Importantly, activated neonatal platelets exhibit significantly less P-selectin on their surface compared to activated adult platelets, a deficiency that is more pronounced among preterm neonates.[34] The decreased P-selectin surface expression in both term and preterm neonatal platelets is a result of both their overall hyporeactivity and a defect in degranulation, and suggests that they may have a decreased ability to interact with immune cells compared to adult platelets.[34,35] Indeed, premature neonates form significantly less platelet-neutrophil aggregates following stimulation compared to term infants,[36] and neonates overall have a reduced ability to form NETs compared to adults, although this is due to the presence of a NET inhibitory factor produced by the placenta.[37] Additionally, a study comparing the proteome of neonatal (cord blood) and adult platelets found a downregulation of proteins related to the inflammatory response and complement activation in neonatal platelets.[38]

As our understanding of the hemostatic and immunologic differences between neonatal and adult platelets continues to grow, it is important to consider how the transfusion of comparatively hyperreactive adult platelets affects the neonatal hemostatic and immune balance. To investigate the potential hemostatic consequences of this, in vitro studies were performed mixing adult platelets with neonatal (cord) blood (in which the platelet count had been reduced to ~50 × 10^9/L), thus simulating platelet transfusions into thrombocytopenic neonates.[39] This study found that addition of adult platelets, but not endogenous neonatal platelets, to neonatal blood resulted in a significant shortening of the PFA-100 closure time in response to collagen and epinephrine (a measure of primary hemostasis), to levels that have been associated with cardiovascular risk. This finding provided the first proof of concept in support of a developmental mismatch caused by the transfusion of adult platelets into neonatal blood and suggested that platelet transfusions could result in a prothrombotic phenotype. However, whether this occurs in vivo and whether it predisposes transfused neonates to form microthrombi in critical organs such as the brain, lungs, or intestine (which could contribute to the higher incidences of

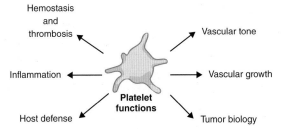

Fig. 12.1 Hemostatic and nonhemostatic functions of platelets.

bleeding, bronchopulmonary dysplasia, or the poor outcomes in NEC) is unknown.

From an immunologic perspective, the higher P-selectin expression levels in adult platelets suggest that transfused platelets would be more likely to interact with the neonatal immune system than the endogenous platelets and might have proinflammatory effects. Early findings from murine models of neonatal platelet transfusions support this hypothesis,[40,41] and the effects of platelet transfusions in neonates remain the focus of active preclinical and clinical research. Interestingly, however, a randomized trial of platelet transfusions in adult patients taking antiplatelet agents who presented with intracranial hemorrhage also found increased mortality and worse outcomes in transfused compared to nontransfused patients, suggesting that at least some of the deleterious effects of platelet transfusions are independent of developmental differences between the donor and the recipient.[42]

Potential Beneficial Effects of Platelet Transfusions

In addition to their roles in hemostasis, immune regulation, and inflammation, platelets are also important regulators of angiogenesis. They carry both pro- and antiantiogenic proteins in their alpha granules, which are released in response to specific signals in settings such as wound healing or within rapidly growing tumors.[43-45] The publication of a case report suggesting that a platelet transfusion was associated with spontaneous resolution of aggressive posterior retinopathy in a preterm neonate,[46] coupled with several studies showing an association between severe retinopathy of prematurity (ROP) and thrombocytopenia,[47-50] raised the possibility that platelets might play a role in ROP. In a 2018 study of 202 VLBW infants (24% of whom had severe ROP), any episode of thrombocytopenia at the onset of proliferative retinopathy (≥30 weeks postmenstrual age) was significantly associated with the development of severe ROP, even after adjusting for other well-known confounding factors like gestational age, sepsis, and NEC.[51] Based on this study, the authors investigated the effects of thrombocytopenia

and platelet transfusions in a well-established mouse model of oxygen-induced retinopathy. In this model, platelet depletion (using an antiplatelet antibody) at the onset of neovascular tuft formation worsened proliferative retinopathy by 30%. Platelet transfusions given at the same time, in contrast, reduced retinal neovascularization by 19.3%. This effect was associated with decreased neural retina VEGF-A protein, with no impact on VEGF-A plasma levels.[51] Additional studies suggested that the beneficial effects of platelets on retinal neovascularization were dependent on the release of their alpha granule content. Taken together, the findings in the murine model suggested that platelets might have local antiangiogenic effects on endothelial cells, leading to a downstream suppression of VEGF-A in the neural retina and to potential beneficial effects of platelet transfusions during the proliferative phase of ROP.[51] However, this has been difficult to prove in clinical practice, with some observational studies reporting an association between number of platelet transfusions and ROP.[52] In the largest randomized controlled trial of platelet transfusions in neonates (PlaNeT-2 study) there was no difference between the groups in incidence of severe ROP.[24]

Implementation of Practice Change

Despite the accumulating evidence supporting the lack of benefit and potential harm associated with platelet transfusions, translating evidence to clinical practice is difficult. These problems (as they pertain to neonatal platelet transfusions) and possible strategies to overcome them were the focus of a recent review.[53] Nevertheless, a recent publication highlighted the successful implementation of a restrictive platelet transfusion guideline in our NICU, using a combination of strategies that led to a reduction in the rate of nonindicated platelet transfusions from 12.5 to 2.9 per 100 patient admissions (Fig. 12.2).[54] Based on this example it is imperative that individual NICUs generate their own guidelines based on the available evidence, with the goal of reducing unnecessary and potentially harmful platelet transfusions.

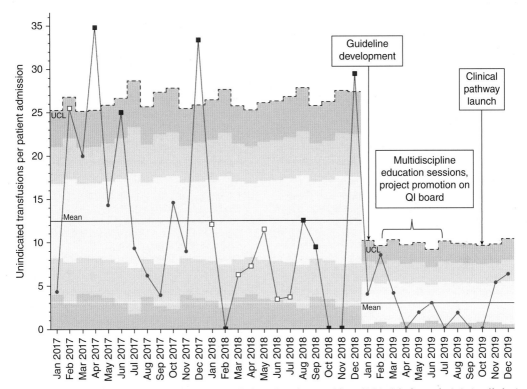

Fig. 12.2 Rate of nonindicated transfusions per 100 patient admissions. Rate decreased from 12.5 to 2.9 after project start on U-chart analysis. (Reprinted with permission from Davenport PE, Chan Yuen J, Briere J, et al. Implementation of a neonatal platelet transfusion guideline to reduce non-indicated transfusions using a quality improvement framework. *J Perinatol.* 2021;41[6]:1487-1494.)

REFERENCES

1. Castle V, Andrew M, Kelton J, et al. Frequency and mechanism of neonatal thrombocytopenia. *J Pediatr.* 1986;108(5 Pt 1):749-755.
2. Christensen RD, Henry E, Wiedmeier SE, et al. Thrombocytopenia among extremely low birth weight neonates: data from a multihospital healthcare system. *J Perinatol.* 2006;26(6):348-353.
3. Patel RM, Hendrickson JE, Nellis ME, et al. Variation in neonatal transfusion practice. *J Pediatr.* 2021;235:92-99.e4.
4. Josephson CD, Su LL, Christensen RD, et al. Platelet transfusion practices among neonatologists in the United States and Canada: results of a survey. *Pediatrics.* 2009;123(1):278-285.
5. Cremer M, Sola-Visner M, Roll S, et al. Platelet transfusions in neonates: practices in the United States vary significantly from those in Austria, Germany, and Switzerland. *Transfusion.* 2011;51(12):2634-2641.
6. Stanworth SJ, Clarke P, Watts T, et al. Prospective, observational study of outcomes in neonates with severe thrombocytopenia. *Pediatrics.* 2009;124(5):e826-e834.
7. Sparger KA, Assmann SF, Granger S, et al. Platelet transfusion practices among very-low-birth-weight infants. *JAMA Pediatr.* 2016;170(7):687-694.
8. Andrew M, Castle V, Saigal S, et al. Clinical impact of neonatal thrombocytopenia. *J Pediatr.* 1987;110(3):457-464.
9. Baer VL, Lambert DK, Henry E, et al. Severe thrombocytopenia in the NICU. *Pediatrics.* 2009;124(6):e1095-e1100.
10. Deschmann E, Saxonhouse MA, Feldman HA, et al. Association between in vitro bleeding time and bleeding in preterm infants with thrombocytopenia. *JAMA Pediatr.* 2019;173(4):393-394.
11. Josephson CD, Granger S, Assmann SF, et al. Bleeding risks are higher in children versus adults given prophylactic platelet transfusions for treatment-induced hypoproliferative thrombocytopenia. *Blood.* 2012;120(4):748-760.
12. Slichter SJ, Kaufman RM, Assmann SF, et al. Dose of prophylactic platelet transfusions and prevention of hemorrhage. *N Engl J Med.* 2010;362(7):600-613.
13. von Lindern JS, Hulzebos CV, Bos AF, et al. Thrombocytopaenia and intraventricular haemorrhage in very premature infants: a tale of two cities. *Arch Dis Child Fetal Neonatal Ed.* 2012;97(5):F348-F352.
14. Deschmann E, Saxonhouse MA, Feldman HA, et al. Association of bleeding scores and platelet transfusions with platelet counts and closure times in response to adenosine diphosphate (CT-ADPs) among preterm neonates with thrombocytopenia. *JAMA Netw Open.* 2020;3(4):e203394.
15. Del Vecchio A, Sola MC, Theriaque DW, et al. Platelet transfusions in the neonatal intensive care unit: factors predicting which patients will require multiple transfusions. *Transfusion.* 2001;41(6):803-808.
16. Garcia MG, Duenas E, Sola MC, et al. Epidemiologic and outcome studies of patients who received platelet transfusions in

the neonatal intensive care unit. *J Perinatol.* 2001;21(7): 415-420.

17. Bonifacio L, Petrova A, Nanjundaswamy S, et al. Thrombocytopenia related neonatal outcome in preterms. *Indian J Pediatr.* 2007;74(3):269-274.

18. Baer VL, Lambert DK, Henry E, et al. Do platelet transfusions in the NICU adversely affect survival? Analysis of 1600 thrombocytopenic neonates in a multihospital healthcare system. *J Perinatol.* 2007;27(12):790-796.

19. Elgendy MM, Durgham R, Othman HF, et al. Platelet transfusion and outcomes of preterm infants: a cross-sectional study. *Neonatology.* 2021;118(4):425-433.

20. Kenton AB, Hegemier S, Smith EO, et al. Platelet transfusions in infants with necrotizing enterocolitis do not lower mortality but may increase morbidity. *J Perinatol.* 2005;25(3):173-177.

21. Patel RM, Josephson CD, Shenvi N, et al. Platelet transfusions and mortality in necrotizing enterocolitis. *Transfusion.* 2019; 59(3):981-988.

22. Andrew M, Vegh P, Caco C, et al. A randomized, controlled trial of platelet transfusions in thrombocytopenic premature infants. *J Pediatr.* 1993;123(2):285-291.

23. Kumar J, Dutta S, Sundaram V, et al. Platelet transfusion for PDA closure in preterm infants: a randomized controlled trial. *Pediatrics.* 2019;143(5):e20182565.

24. Curley A, Stanworth SJ, Willoughby K, et al. Randomized trial of platelet-transfusion thresholds in neonates. *N Engl J Med.* 2019;380(3):242-251.

25. Fustolo-Gunnink SF, Fijnvandraat K, van Klaveren D, et al. Preterm neonates benefit from low prophylactic platelet transfusion threshold despite varying risk of bleeding or death. *Blood.* 2019;134(26):2354-2360.

26. Ballabh P. Pathogenesis and prevention of intraventricular hemorrhage. *Clin Perinatol.* 2014;41(1):47-67.

27. Ferrer-Marin F, Sola-Visner M. Neonatal platelet physiology and implications for transfusion. *Platelets.* 2021:1-9.

28. Franco AT, Corken A, Ware J. Platelets at the interface of thrombosis, inflammation, and cancer. *Blood.* 2015;126(5):582-588.

29. Weyrich AS. Platelets: more than a sack of glue. *Hematology.* 2014;2014(1):400-403.

30. Semple JW, Italiano Jr JE, Freedman J. Platelets and the immune continuum. *Nat Rev Immunol.* 2011;11(4):264-274.

31. Lisman T. Platelet-neutrophil interactions as drivers of inflammatory and thrombotic disease. *Cell Tissue Res.* 2018;371(3):567-576.

32. Kolaczkowska E, Kubes P. Neutrophil recruitment and function in health and inflammation. *Nat Rev Immunol.* 2013;13(3): 159-175.

33. Engelmann B, Massberg S. Thrombosis as an intravascular effector of innate immunity. *Nat Rev Immunol.* 2013;13(1):34-45.

34. Sitaru AG, Holzhauer S, Speer CP, et al. Neonatal platelets from cord blood and peripheral blood. *Platelets.* 2005;16(3-4):203-210.

35. Caparros-Perez E, Teruel-Montoya R, Palma-Barquero V, et al. Down regulation of the Munc18b-syntaxin-11 complex and beta1-tubulin impairs secretion and spreading in neonatal platelets. *Thromb Haemost.* 2017;117(11):2079-2091.

36. Esiaba I, Angeles DM, Milford TM, et al. Platelet-neutrophil interactions are lower in cord blood of premature newborns. *Neonatology.* 2019;115(2):149-155.

37. Yost CC, Schwertz H, Cody MJ, et al. Neonatal NET-inhibitory factor and related peptides inhibit neutrophil extracellular trap formation. *J Clin Invest.* 2016;126(10):3783-3798.

38. Stokhuijzen E, Koornneef JM, Nota B, et al. Differences between platelets derived from neonatal cord blood and adult peripheral blood assessed by mass spectrometry. *J Proteome Res.* 2017;16(10):3567-3575.

39. Ferrer-Marin F, Chavda C, Lampa M, et al. Effects of in vitro adult platelet transfusions on neonatal hemostasis. *J Thromb Haemost.* 2011;9(5):1020-1028.

40. Davenport P, Nolton E, Feldman H, et al. Pro-inflammatory effects of platelet transfusions in newborn mice with and without underlying inflammation. American Society of Hematology Annual Meeting, 2020.

41. Maurya P, McGrath K, Ture SK, et al. Adult, but not neonatal platelet transfusions drive a monocyte trafficking phenotype *in vitro* and *in vivo.* American Society of Hematology Annual Meeting, 2020.

42. Baharoglu MI, Cordonnier C, Al-Shahi Salman R, et al. Platelet transfusion versus standard care after acute stroke due to spontaneous cerebral haemorrhage associated with antiplatelet therapy (PATCH): a randomised, open-label, phase 3 trial. *Lancet.* 2016;387(10038):2605-2613.

43. Italiano Jr JE, Richardson JL, Patel-Hett S, et al. Angiogenesis is regulated by a novel mechanism: pro- and antiangiogenic proteins are organized into separate platelet alpha granules and differentially released. *Blood.* 2008;111(3):1227-1233.

44. Battinelli EM, Markens BA, Italiano Jr JE. Release of angiogenesis regulatory proteins from platelet alpha granules: modulation of physiologic and pathologic angiogenesis. *Blood.* 2011;118(5):1359-1369.

45. Peterson JE, Zurakowski D, Italiano Jr JE, et al. Normal ranges of angiogenesis regulatory proteins in human platelets. *Am J Hematol.* 2010;85(7):487-493.

46. Vinekar A, Hegde K, Gilbert C, et al. Do platelets have a role in the pathogenesis of aggressive posterior retinopathy of prematurity? *Retina.* 2010;30(4):S20-S23.

47. Jensen AK, Ying GS, Huang J, et al. Thrombocytopenia and retinopathy of prematurity. *J AAPOS.* 2011;15(1):e3-e4.

48. Jensen AK, Ying GS, Huang J, et al. Longitudinal study of the association between thrombocytopenia and retinopathy of prematurity. *J AAPOS.* 2018;22(2):119-123.

49. Lundgren P, Lundberg L, Hellgren G, et al. Aggressive posterior retinopathy of prematurity is associated with multiple infectious episodes and thrombocytopenia. *Neonatology.* 2017; 111(1):79-85.

50. Sancak S, Toptan HH, Gokmen Yildirim T, et al. Thrombocytopenia as a risk factor for retinopathy of prematurity. *Retina.* 2019;39(4):706-711.

51. Cakir B, Liegl R, Hellgren G, et al. Thrombocytopenia is associated with severe retinopathy of prematurity. *JCI Insight.* 2018;3(19):e99448.

52. Hengartner T, Adams M, Pfister RE, et al. Associations between red blood cell and platelet transfusions and retinopathy of prematurity. *Neonatology.* 2020:1-7.

53. Sola-Visner M, Leeman KT, Stanworth SJ. Neonatal platelet transfusions: new evidence and the challenges of translating evidence-based recommendations into clinical practice. *J Thromb Haemost.* 2022;20(3):556-564.

54. Davenport PE, Chan Yuen J, Briere J, et al. Implementation of a neonatal platelet transfusion guideline to reduce non-indicated transfusions using a quality improvement framework. *J Perinatol.* 2021;41(6):1487-1494.

Chapter 13

Novel Approaches to Identify NICU Patients Who Would Benefit From Platelet Transfusions

Emöke Deschmann, MD, MMSc, PhD

Chapter Outline

Introduction

The underlying reasons for bleeding are multifactorial and likely include a combination of hematologic (i.e., platelet, von Willebrand factor [vWF], coagulation factors) and environmental factors such as vessel wall integrity, inflammation, and hemodynamic status. However, it is unknown to what extent these components contribute to bleeding. Since platelets have a major role in primary hemostasis, a low platelet count is considered a risk factor for bleeding.[1-3]

Thrombocytopenia is common in the neonatal intensive care unit (NICU), and if severe it is treated with platelet transfusions to prevent bleeding. Approximately 5% to 15% of preterm neonates admitted to the NICUs develop major bleeding (most commonly intraventricular hemorrhage [IVH]) during their NICU stay, potentially leading to lifelong consequences.[1,3] Of thrombocytopenic neonates, 25% have one or more platelet counts below 50×10^9/L (severe thrombocytopenia), and 9% of these infants experience significant bleeding.[2] Platelet transfusions are frequently given to neonates whose platelet counts fall below an arbitrary (and highly variable) trigger, in an attempt to prevent bleeding.[2,4,5] However, several studies from the past decade have shown that platelet count is a poor predictor of bleeding in neonates,[2,3,6] suggesting that other hematologic and clinical factors (i.e., platelet function, hematocrit, vWF concentrations, gestational age, postnatal age, diagnosis, severity of illness) may be stronger determinants of bleeding risk than platelet count alone. Most of these factors are highly dynamic in neonates, whose hemostatic balance is also different from that of adults. Specifically, neonatal platelets are hyporesponsive to most agonists compared with adult platelets, and this hyporesponsiveness is more pronounced in preterm infants.[7-10] In healthy full-term and preterm neonates, the effects of hypofunctional platelets are counteracted by their higher hematocrits, mean corpuscular volumes, and concentrations of vWF (all prothrombotic factors that accelerate clotting), paradoxically leading to shorter bleeding times in neonates compared to adults.[11] Any alteration in these compensatory factors can disrupt the delicate primary hemostatic balance of neonates. Neonatal platelet function also changes over time and reaches near-adult levels by 10 to 14 days of life in preterm as well as in full-term neonates.[9,10,12,13]

The recent recognition of the central effects of platelets on inflammation also raised the question of whether platelet transfusions could be harmful to some infants, depending on the underlying etiology of the thrombocytopenia and the clinical context. This hypothesis was supported by a number of observational studies that reported an association between number of platelet transfusions and increased mortality and morbidity among NICU patients.[14-16] At least one study reported an association between number of platelet transfusion and worse outcomes in necrotizing enterocolitis (NEC),[17] and it was postulated that this could be related to inflammatory mediators released by platelets. More recently, the largest randomized controlled trial of platelet transfusions in thrombocytopenic preterm neonates showed a higher rate of bleeding and death among infants transfused for platelet counts below 50 $\times$ 10^9/L compared to those transfused for platelet counts below 25 $\times$ 10^9/L.[18]

Currently, over 75% of neonates with severe thrombocytopenia (platelet count <50 $\times$ 10^9/L) are treated with platelet transfusions to prevent bleeding; however, only 9% to 11% of these neonates develop major bleeding.[2,19] In addition, there is no evidence supporting that platelet transfusions can prevent neonatal bleeding. The facts that (1) platelet count is a poor predictor of bleeding, (2) platelet transfusions in preterm neonates have been shown to be harmful, and (3) platelet transfusions may not reduce bleeding risk in thrombocytopenic neonates highlight the need for revised and individualized approaches to neonatal platelet transfusion decisions.

Bleeding Prediction

CLINICAL FACTORS

Since IVH is a potentially devastating complication of preterm birth, and the leading type of major bleeding (responsible for >50% of major bleedings), this bleeding type has been studied most thoroughly.[20,21] Several studies have identified clinical risk factors associated with this outcome. Gestational age has been shown to be the strongest predictive factor for both incidence and severity of IVH.[22] The highest risk period for developing IVH is independent of gestational age and is within the first 24 hours after birth. Hemorrhages can progress over 48 hours or more, and at the end of the first postnatal week, 90% of IVH can be detected at their full extent.[23]

The combination of thrombocytopenia and platelet dysfunction has been proposed as an important potential contributor to the high incidence of IVH in preterm infants. Multiple studies evaluating platelet adhesion, aggregation, and activation demonstrated that neonatal platelets are hyporesponsive in vitro to most platelet agonists, compared with adult platelets.[7,8] In full-term infants, this platelet hyporeactivity is fully compensated by the high hematocrit, high mean corpuscular volume (MCV), elevated concentrations of vWF, and the predominance of ultralong vWF polymers in the neonatal blood, all factors that enhance primary hemostasis.[24] However, in preterm infants, and particularly among infants born at less than 30 weeks, the platelet hyporeactivity is more pronounced and might be less well compensated by other factors.[8-10] Supporting this, bleeding tests performed on the first day of life were longer in preterm compared with term infants, with neonates less than 33 weeks of gestation showing the longest bleeding times.[13] Platelet function in neonates is also influenced by postnatal age. Studies using flow cytometry or whole blood platelet aggregation have found that the platelet hyporeactivity is still present 3 to 4 days after birth in term as well as in preterm infants.[12] After that, the results of available studies have been somewhat inconsistent, with some reporting prolonged platelet hyporeactivity,[9,25] but most observing substantial improvement to full normalization in the platelet function by 10 to 14 days.[9,10,12] The data are supported by the findings of a bleeding time study in which, by day 10, all infants had shorter bleeding times than at birth, and gestational age–related differences at the beginning had disappeared. Little or no further shortening occurred between days 10 and 30.[13]

Accordingly, the majority of neonates who suffer clinically significant bleeding are those less than 30 weeks of gestation and less than 10 to 14 days of life.[2,6] This raises the obvious question of whether the more pronounced platelet dysfunction present in that subset of infants and precisely during that period contributes to this risk.

Clinical observations and animal studies have established that sepsis and/or inflammation significantly increase the bleeding risk in the setting of thrombocytopenia.[26,27]

In a contemporary multicenter observational study by Stanworth et al. (platelet transfusion thresholds in premature neonates [PlaNeT-1] study), neonates with severe thrombocytopenia were followed, and bleeding episodes were prospectively and systematically recorded.[2,6] The study showed that the most common form of major bleeding was grade 3 or 4 IVH; however, most of those episodes occurred before enrollment in the study and therefore before the development of severe thrombocytopenia, which suggests that other factors are important in the development of neonatal bleeding. They found that the strongest predictors of bleeding in thrombocytopenic neonates were gestational age less than 28 weeks, postnatal age less than 10 days, and the diagnosis of NEC.[2]

NEW LABORATORY TESTS

The understanding of the poor predictive value of the platelet count and of the potential risks associated with platelet transfusions highlighted the need for better tests to assess bleeding risk, to limit platelet transfusions to neonates with severe thrombocytopenia and high bleeding risk.

Hemostasis is a complex process consisting of multiple steps and affected by many factors, including both cellular and plasma components. It starts with platelet adhesion to damaged endothelium and ends in clot fibrinolysis. There are several methods available to evaluate the different aspects of hemostasis, including platelet adhesion, aggregation, coagulation, and fibrinolysis. Along these lines an ideal hemostasis assay should rather measure all these processes to predict the overall bleeding risk. There are several tests measuring one or more steps of the hemostatic process; however, there is no single test evaluating the whole course. Therefore the specific clinical problem needs to guide the choice of method.

Given the multifactorial and dynamic nature of neonatal hemostasis, it is logical that a global test of primary hemostasis would be valuable in this population, in whom many rapidly changing factors—in addition to the platelet count—determine hemostatic efficiency. A single prior study measured the effects of

neonatal thrombocytopenia on bleeding times.[28] These investigators found a moderate correlation between platelet counts and bleeding times, although there was a great variability among infants with platelet counts less than 100×10^9/L. The validity of these findings was questioned due to the limitations of the bleeding time test, particularly its poor reproducibility and operator dependency.

The platelet function analyzer-100 (PFA-100) is an in vitro test of primary hemostasis (i.e., an in vitro bleeding time) mainly used for monitoring antiplatelet therapy and to screen for platelet function disorders in adults.[29] This reproducible, nonoperator dependent test measures the time it takes for whole blood to occlude an aperture (closure time [CT]) following stimulation with collagen plus epinephrine (CT-Epi) or collagen plus adenosine diphosphate (CT-ADP). Consistent with bleeding time studies, PFA-100 CTs are shorter in neonatal compared to adult blood.[30]

A prior pilot study evaluating PFA-100 CTs in blood samples from thrombocytopenic neonates suggested that the CT-ADP would be more useful in this population than the CT-Epi, likely due to the profound hyporesponsiveness of neonatal platelets to epinephrine.[31,32] Specifically, all infants with platelet counts above 90×10^9/L had normal CT-ADPs; at platelet counts below 90×10^9/L, many infants had normal or minimally prolonged CT-ADPs, while some had markedly prolonged values. Based on these observations, a subsequent study[33] tested the hypothesis that prolonged CT-ADPs would identify thrombocytopenic neonates with inadequate primary hemostasis, who would exhibit more bleeding. The study found that the PFA-100 CT-ADP was a better marker of bleeding than the platelet count in extremely preterm neonates (<27 weeks of gestation). Consistent with other studies,[2] neonates with a gestational age less than 27 weeks also had a higher frequency of grade 2 to 4 bleeding than more mature infants. Although the reasons for their high bleeding risk are multifactorial and likely include in vivo factors, 88% of infants with grades 3 to 4 bleeding had maximally prolonged CT-ADPs, suggesting that inadequate hemostasis might contribute to severe bleeding. Breakdown of bleeding scores into grades 0 to 1 (none or mild), 2 (moderate), and 3 to 4 (major/severe) also revealed a significant correlation between median CT-ADP and bleeding severity[33] (Table 13.1).

TABLE 13.1 Correlation Between CT-ADP or Platelet Counts and Bleeding Scores

Bleeding Score	Fraction With Maximum CT-ADP	CT-ADP, sec Median (range)	Platelet Count, 10⁹/L Median (range)
0–1	18/65 (28%)	155 (70–300)	67 (13–98)
2	11/26 (42%)	271 (69–300)	56 (16–95)
3–4	7/8 (88%)	300 (183–300)	56 (25–93)
p-value	0.003*	0.006**	0.15**

*Fisher exact test.
**Wilcoxon rank-sum test.
Adapted from Deschmann E, Saxonhouse MA, Feldman HA, et al. Association between in vitro bleeding time and bleeding in
preterm infants with thrombocytopenia. *JAMA Pediatr.* 2019;173(4):393-394.

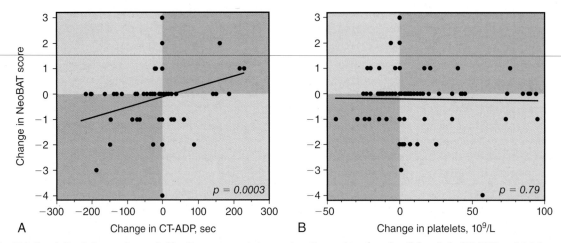

Fig. 13.1 Correlation between changes in bleeding scores and changes in collagen plus adenosine diphosphate *(CT-ADP)* or platelet counts.
One-day changes in bleeding scores correlated well with changes in CT-ADP **(A)**, but not with changes in platelet count **(B)** in infants with gestational age less than 27 weeks. *p* indicates significance of fitted regression line. (Adapted from Deschmann E, Saxonhouse MA, Feldman HA, et al. Association of bleeding scores and platelet transfusions with platelet counts and closure times in response to adenosine diphosphate [CT-ADPs] among preterm
neonates with thrombocytopenia. *JAMA Netw Open.* 2020;3[4]:e203394.)

In a secondary analysis,[34] the study found an association between changes in bleeding score (measure of clinical bleeding) and changes in the CT-ADP (Fig. 13.1A) but
not changes in platelet count (see Fig. 13.1B), suggesting
that primary hemostasis and bleeding are dynamic and
more interconnected than platelet count and bleeding in
extremely preterm neonates with thrombocytopenia.
However, the CT-ADP requires 800 μL of blood, which
severely limits its potential widespread use in small
preterm infants.

Rotational thromboelastography (ROTEM; TEM
International, Munich, Germany) and thromboelastography (TEG; Haemonetics, Braintree, MA) are both
point-of-care viscoelastic tests of hemostasis in whole
blood, which allow measurement of global clot formation and dissolution in real time (Fig. 13.2).[35] ROTEM
is a modern modification of the TEG technology (fully
automated); therefore both provide essentially the same
information on clot formation kinetics and strength,
although the results are not interchangeable. Both tests

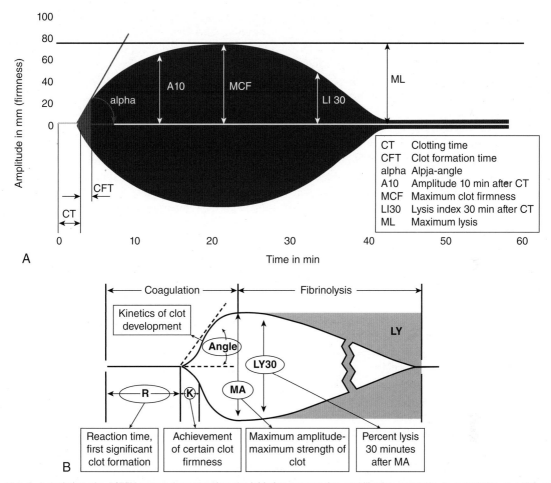

Fig. 13.2 A, A depiction of a ROTEM output demonstrating clot initiation, propagation, stabilization, and lysis. **B,** A depiction of a TEG output demonstrating clot initiation, propagation, stabilization, and lysis. *ROTEM,* Rotational thromboelastography; *TEG,* thromboelastography. (From Author X. Title of article. *Am J Hematol.* 2013;89(2):228-232. doi:10.1002/ajh.23599.)

require 340 μL whole blood. The advantage of these viscoelastic assays is that they can measure coagulation, platelet function, clot retraction, and fibrinolysis simultaneously.[36] However, viscoelastic tests are less sensitive for platelet count and assessment of primary hemostasis where platelets play major role. A single-center study investigated the role of ROTEM parameters in predicting bleeding risk in 110 critically ill neonates with thrombocytopenia (median gestational age 34 [28–38] and mean platelet count 60.7±39.8). Neonates with suspected or confirmed sepsis and/or with perinatal hypoxia were defined as critically ill neonates. The study found that two ROTEM parameters (EXTEM A5

and EXTEM A10) were strong predictors of bleeding.[37] Of note, the investigators found an incidence of IVH of 36.3% for the whole population (110 patients) and 44.2% among those with bleeding events (77 patients). However, the unusually high incidence of IVH in this patient population (with a median gestational age of 34 weeks) raises concerns regarding the generalizability of the results.

The immature platelet fraction (IPF) is a relatively new laboratory parameter measured in Sysmex XN hematology analyzers, which quantifies the percentage and the absolute number of immature platelets (formerly known as reticulated platelets) in the circulation.

Immature platelets are newly released platelets (<24 hours old), which are larger and more hemostatically active than older platelets. Thus we would predict that thrombocytopenic patients with a higher IPF% and immature platelet count (IPC; the product of IPF% × platelet count) would have a lower bleeding risk than patients with similar degrees of thrombocytopenia but lower IPF and IPC.

Two recent studies in pediatric patients with immune thrombocytopenia (ITP) tested this hypothesis.[38,39] The study by McDonnell et al. enrolled 272 pediatric patients between 2 months and 21 years with severe thrombocytopenia (platelet count <50 × 10⁹/L). These investigators found that the IPF not only differentiated ITP from bone marrow failure, but it could also identify severely thrombocytopenic patients at increased risk of bleeding (specifically, at platelet counts <10 × 10⁹/L, a low IPF was associated with the highest bleeding score, while a high IPF was associated with lower bleeding risk).[39] The second pediatric study included 57 pediatric patients with ITP, many of them in remission and some with a platelet count above 100 × 10⁹/L, with a median platelet count of 59 × 10⁹/L. This study found that moderate to severe bleeding only occurred when the platelet count was below 50 × 10⁹/L, and that higher IPF% were associated with higher bleeding scores. However, the latter finding could have reflected the fact that patients with higher platelet counts, who rarely experienced clinically significant bleeding, also had lower IPF%.[38] Thus the IPF% is likely most useful to predict bleeding risk in patients with severe thrombocytopenia. This hypothesis was supported by a study of 141 pediatric and adult patients with ITP, which showed that the inverse correlation between IPC and bleeding score was strongest at times of severe and profound thrombocytopenia (platelet count <60 × 10⁹/L and <30 × 10⁹/L, respectively), particularly in pediatric patients.[40]

Finally, one small study in adult patients with hematologic malignancies also found a higher IPC to be associated with less bleeding manifestations. In this study, 49 patients with platelet count below 50 × 10⁹/L were followed for up to 30 days, and blood samples were collected three times a week for laboratory markers of hemostasis and platelet cytometry assays. Among the checked hematologic parameters, only the IPC was associated with bleeding after adjustment for platelet count: Low IPC was associated strongly with increased bleeding, and there was an inverse correlation between IPC and the proportion of study days on which bleeding occurred.[41]

A currently ongoing study (ClinicalTrials.gov Identifier: NCT04598750) is evaluating IPF% and IPC in preterm neonates with severe thrombocytopenia as potential markers of bleeding risk.

However, these laboratory tests do not incorporate important in vivo determinants of bleeding risk, such as vessel wall integrity, inflammation, and hemodynamic status. This likely imposes a limit to the sensitivity and specificity that any in vitro test can achieve in the assessment of bleeding risk in this population.

PREDICTION MODELS

While currently platelet transfusions are given based on solely platelet counts, the evidence suggests that factors other than the degree of thrombocytopenia determine the bleeding risk. A dynamic prediction model was recently developed in attempt to predict major bleeding in preterm neonates at any time-point during the first week after the onset of severe thrombocytopenia, which incorporated the variables gestational age, postnatal age, intrauterine growth retardation, NEC, sepsis, platelet count, and mechanical ventilation.[19] This model had a good predictive performance, indicated by a median C-index of the final model of 0.74 (Fig. 13.3). While the model has not yet been prospectively validated and does not include measures of primary hemostasis, this is a promising approach to making individualized treatment decisions in this population with high bleeding risk. Probably a dynamic prediction model, including innovative laboratory tests of primary hemostasis together with clinical factors, would ultimately be the best tool for clinicians to quantify bleeding risk. It could potentially lead to a much better prediction of bleeding risk in thrombocytopenic preterm neonates and to changes in our transfusion practices resulting from incorporating this knowledge into our clinical decision making.

Transfusion Effect

Regardless of extensive donor screening, contamination of platelet suspensions with bacterial or viral pathogens (known and unknown) can still occur.[42]

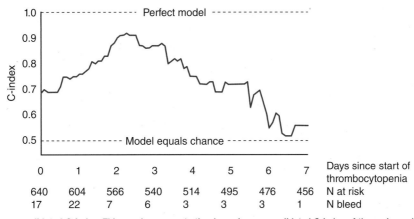

Fig. 13.3 Dynamic, cross-validated C-index. This graph represents the dynamic, cross-validated C-index of the main model. A C-index of 1 resembles a model that discriminates perfectly between patients with and without major bleeding, while a C-index of 0.5 indicates that the prediction is as good as chance. For each time-point, the number at risk at the beginning of that day has been reported, as well as the total number of major bleeds that occurred during those 24 hours. For example, at the start of day 1, the number of patients still at risk was 604, and during this day 22 neonates developed a major bleed. (From Author X. Title of article. *Haematologica.* 2019;104(11):2300-2306. doi:10.3324/haematol.2018.208595.)

Particularly, bacterial infections are more frequently associated with platelet transfusions than with any other blood product because this blood product needs to be stored at room temperature.[43] Furthermore, transfusion-transmitted infections with the potential for serious long-term consequences (i.e., Chagas disease)[44-46] are more relevant in neonates, whose expected lifespan is over 70 years. Other transfusion complications, such as transfusion-related acute lung injury (TRALI), are likely to be unrecognized and are probably underreported in neonates, who frequently have respiratory decompensations for other reasons. In the neonatal population, no study to date has demonstrated a beneficial effect of platelet transfusions. On the contrary, several publications have shown a strong association between platelet transfusions and high morbidity and mortality among NICU patients.[14,15,17,47] It is unclear from these studies whether this association simply reflects the fact that sicker patients receive more platelets, or whether platelet transfusions themselves adversely affect outcome, as has been suggested.[14] Most recently, PlaNeT-2 found an association between platelet transfusions and increased mortality and morbidity among preterm neonates: There was a significantly higher rate of death or major bleeding, and a higher rate of bronchopulmonary dysplasia when using more liberal strategy for platelet transfusions.[48] The currently available evidence strongly supports the hypothesis that platelet transfusions can be harmful to neonates and that restrictive transfusion thresholds can be safely used in the great majority of neonates. It highlights the need to make platelet transfusion decisions in neonates thoughtfully, carefully balancing the risks and benefits in each individual patient.

Limitations

Due to the observational nature of the studies described, it is important to recognize that all associations presented may be subject to residual or unmeasured confounding variables and that causal relationships have not been established. However, dynamic prediction models (described earlier) that include clinical factors such as gestational age, postnatal age, illness severity, etc., as well as laboratory measures of primary hemostasis or platelet production, are a promising novel approach toward making individualized treatment decisions. Furthermore, it is unknown if platelet transfusions given to nonbleeding neonates with thrombocytopenia will decrease their bleeding risk and the neonatal mortality. Findings from observational and randomized studies of platelet transfusions in neonates (reviewed in a different chapter) suggest that platelet transfusions have their own risks to be balanced against any potential benefits.

REFERENCES

1. Baer VL, Lambert DK, Henry E, et al. Severe thrombocytopenia in the NICU. *Pediatrics.* 2009;124(6):e1095-e1100.
2. Stanworth SJ, Clarke P, Watts T, et al. Prospective, observational study of outcomes in neonates with severe thrombocytopenia. *Pediatrics.* 2009;124(5):e826-e834.
3. von Lindern JS, van den Bruele T, Lopriore E, et al. Thrombocytopenia in neonates and the risk of intraventricular hemorrhage: a retrospective cohort study. *BMC Pediatr.* 2011;11:16.
4. Josephson CD, Su LL, Christensen RD, et al. Platelet transfusion practices among neonatologists in the United States and Canada: results of a survey. *Pediatrics.* 2009;123(1):278-285.
5. Cremer M, Sola-Visner M, Roll S, et al. Platelet transfusions in neonates: practices in the United States vary significantly from those in Austria, Germany, and Switzerland. *Transfusion.* 2011; 51(12):2634-2641.
6. Muthukumar P, Venkatesh V, Curley A, et al. Severe thrombocytopenia and patterns of bleeding in neonates: results from a prospective observational study and implications for use of platelet transfusions. *Transfus Med.* 2012;22(5):338-343.
7. Israels SJ, Odaibo FS, Robertson C, et al. Deficient thromboxane synthesis and response in platelets from premature infants. *Pediatr Res.* 1997;41(2):218-223.
8. Rajasekhar D, Barnard MR, Bednarek FJ, et al. Platelet hyperactivity in very low birth weight neonates. *Thromb Haemost.* 1997;77(5):1002-1007.
9. Sitaru AG, Holzhauer S, Speer CP, et al. Neonatal platelets from cord blood and peripheral blood. *Platelets.* 2005;16(3-4):203-210.
10. Ucar T, Gurman C, Arsan S, et al. Platelet aggregation in term and preterm newborns. *Pediatr Hematol Oncol.* 2005;22(2):139-145.
11. Andrew M, Paes B, Bowker J, et al. Evaluation of an automated bleeding time device in the newborn. *Am J Hematol.* 1990; 35(4):275-277.
12. Bednarek FJ, Bean S, Barnard MR, et al. The platelet hyporeactivity of extremely low birth weight neonates is age-dependent. *Thromb Res.* 2009;124(1):42-45.
13. Del Vecchio A, Latini G, Henry E, et al. Template bleeding times of 240 neonates born at 24 to 41 weeks gestation. *J Perinatol.* 2008;28(6):427-431.
14. Baer VL, Lambert DK, Henry E, et al. Do platelet transfusions in the NICU adversely affect survival? Analysis of 1600 thrombocytopenic neonates in a multihospital healthcare system. *J Perinatol.* 2007;27(12):790-796.
15. Del Vecchio A, Sola MC, Theriaque DW, et al. Platelet transfusions in the neonatal intensive care unit: factors predicting which patients will require multiple transfusions. *Transfusion.* 2001;41(6):803-808.
16. Garcia MG, Duenas E, Sola MC, et al. Epidemiologic and outcome studies of patients who received platelet transfusions in the neonatal intensive care unit. *J Perinatol.* 2001;21(7):415-420.
17. Kenton AB, Hegemier S, Smith EO, et al. Platelet transfusions in infants with necrotizing enterocolitis do not lower mortality but may increase morbidity. *J Perinatol.* 2005;25(3):173-177.
18. Curley A, Stanworth SJ, Willoughby K, et al. Randomized trial of platelet-transfusion thresholds in neonates. *N Eng J Med.* 2019;380(3):242-251.
19. Fustolo-Gunnink SF, Fijnvandraat K, Putter H, et al. Dynamic prediction of bleeding risk in thrombocytopenic preterm neonates. *Haematologica.* 2019;104(11):2300-2306.
20. Poryo M, Boeckh JC, Gortner L, et al. Ante-, peri- and postnatal factors associated with intraventricular hemorrhage in very premature infants. *Early Human Dev.* 2018;116:1-8.
21. Luque MJ, Tapia JL, Villarroel L, et al. A risk prediction model for severe intraventricular hemorrhage in very low birth weight infants and the effect of prophylactic indomethacin. *J Perinatol.* 2014;34(1):43-48.
22. van de Bor M, Verloove-Vanhorick SP, Brand R, et al. Incidence and prediction of periventricular-intraventricular hemorrhage in very preterm infants. *J Perinat Med.* 1987;15(4):333-339.
23. McCrea HJ, Ment LR. The diagnosis, management, and postnatal prevention of intraventricular hemorrhage in the preterm neonate. *Clin Perinatol.* 2008;35(4):777-792, vii.
24. Sola-Visner M. Platelets in the neonatal period: developmental differences in platelet production, function, and hemostasis and the potential impact of therapies. *Hematology.* 2012;2012: 506-511.
25. Hezard N, Potron G, Schlegel N, et al. Unexpected persistence of platelet hyporeactivity beyond the neonatal period: a flow cytometric study in neonates, infants and older children. *Thromb Haemost.* 2003;90(1):116-123.
26. Goerge T, Ho-Tin-Noe B, Carbo C, et al. Inflammation induces hemorrhage in thrombocytopenia. *Blood.* 2008;111(10): 4958-4964.
27. Finkelstein Y, Shenkman B, Sirota L, et al. Whole blood platelet deposition on extracellular matrix under flow conditions in preterm neonatal sepsis. *Eur J Pediatr.* 2002;161(5):270-274.
28. Andrew M, Castle V, Saigal S, et al. Clinical impact of neonatal thrombocytopenia. *J Pediatr.* 1987;110(3):457-464.
29. Kundu SK, Heilmann EJ, Sio R, et al. Description of an in vitro platelet function analyzer—PFA-100. *Semin Thromb Hemost.* 1995;21(2):S106-S112.
30. Boudewijns M, Raes M, Peeters V, et al. Evaluation of platelet function on cord blood in 80 healthy term neonates using the platelet function analyser (PFA-100): shorter in vitro bleeding times in neonates than adults. *Eur J Pediatr.* 2003;162(3):212-213.
31. Deschmann E, Sola-Visner M, Saxonhouse MA. Primary hemostasis in neonates with thrombocytopenia. *J Pediatr.* 2014;164(1): 167-172.
32. Caparros-Perez E, Teruel-Montoya R, Lopez-Andreo MJ, et al. Comprehensive comparison of neonate and adult human platelet transcriptomes. *PLoS One.* 2017;12(8):e0183042.
33. Deschmann E, Saxonhouse MA, Feldman HA, et al. Association between in vitro bleeding time and bleeding in preterm infants with thrombocytopenia. *JAMA Pediatr.* 2019;173(4):393-394.
34. Deschmann E, Saxonhouse MA, Feldman HA, et al. Association of bleeding scores and platelet transfusions with platelet counts and closure times in response to adenosine diphosphate (CT-ADPs) among preterm neonates with thrombocytopenia. *JAMA Netw Open.* 2020;3(4):e203394.
35. Whiting D, DiNardo JA. TEG and ROTEM: technology and clinical applications. *Am J Hematol.* 2014;89(2):228-232.
36. Tynngard N, Lindahl TL, Ramstrom S. Assays of different aspects of haemostasis—what do they measure? *Thromb J.* 2015; 13:8.
37. Parastatidou S, Sokou R, Tsantes AG, et al. The role of ROTEM variables based on clot elasticity and platelet component in predicting bleeding risk in thrombocytopenic critically ill neonates. *Eur J Haematol.* 2021;106(2):175-183.
38. Frelinger AL III, Grace RF, Gerrits AJ, et al. Platelet function tests, independent of platelet count, are associated with bleeding severity in ITP. *Blood.* 2015;126(7):873-879.
39. McDonnell A, Bride KL, Lim D, et al. Utility of the immature platelet fraction in pediatric immune thrombocytopenia: differentiating from bone marrow failure and predicting bleeding risk. *Pediatr Blood Cancer.* 2018;65(2).

40. Greene LA, Chen S, Seery C, et al. Beyond the platelet count: immature platelet fraction and thromboelastometry correlate with bleeding in patients with immune thrombocytopenia. *Br J Haematol*. 2014;166(4):592-600.

41. Estcourt LJ, Stanworth SJ, Harrison P, et al. Prospective observational cohort study of the association between thromboelastometry, coagulation and platelet parameters and bleeding in patients with haematological malignancies—the ATHENA study. *Br J Haematol*. 2014;166(4):581-591.

42. Strauss RG. Blood banking and transfusion issues in perinatal medicine. In: Christensen R, ed. *Hematologic Problems of the Neonate*. Philadelphia: WB Saunders; 2000:405-425.

43. Kuehnert MJ, Roth VR, Haley NR, et al. Transfusion-transmitted bacterial infection in the United States, 1998 through 2000. *Transfusion*. 2001;41(12):1493-1499.

44. Agapova M, Busch MP, Custer B. Cost-effectiveness of screening the US blood supply for *Trypanosoma cruzi*. *Transfusion*. 2010; 50(10):2220-2232.

45. Benjamin RJ, Stramer SL, Leiby DA, et al. *Trypanosoma cruzi* infection in North America and Spain: evidence in support of transfusion transmission. *Transfusion*. 2012;52(9):1913-1921.

46. Lindholm PF, Annen K, Ramsey G. Approaches to minimize infection risk in blood banking and transfusion practice. *Infect Dis Drug Targets*. 2011;11(1):45-56.

47. Bonifacio L, Petrova A, Nanjundaswamy S, et al. Thrombocytopenia related neonatal outcome in preterms. *Indian J Pediatr*. 2007;74(3):269-274.

48. Curley A, Stanworth SJ, Willoughby K, et al. Randomized trial of platelet-transfusion thresholds in Neonates. *N Eng J Med*. 2019;380(3):242-251.

Chapter 14

Evidence-Based Guidelines for Administering Fresh Frozen Plasma in the NICU

Mario Motta, MD and Brunetta Guaragni, MD

Introduction

Fresh frozen plasma (FFP) is the most commonly used hemostatic agent in neonatal intensive care units (NICUs), especially among critically ill neonates and for those who need extracorporeal life support (ECLS). Current guidelines on FFP administration in neonates are mainly based on poor-quality evidence, and therefore a lack of consensus exists on its optimal use.

Making the right diagnosis of coagulopathy in neonates and determining when to use FFP can be difficult due to the age-related changes in coagulation proteins occurring during childhood. In addition, neonatal reference values for coagulation tests are based on limited data and are obtained with specific analyzers and reagents that may differ from one NICU to another. Consequently, in the absence of normal values tailored to the NICU equipment, coagulation results may be difficult to interpret.

In this chapter we update evidence based on available studies that evaluate the use of FFP, and we summarize relevant information by ranking the quality of evidence and strength of recommendations. We also discuss the role of standard laboratory tests and viscoelastic coagulation tests in the therapeutic decision-making process for administering FFP.

Data Derived From Clinical Audits and Surveys on FFP Use in the NICU

Several clinical audits report that FFP administration continues to be a frequent intervention in NICUs with a related high level of prophylactic administration (without bleeding evidence). In retrospective reviews, the reported rate of FFP transfusion ranges from 2% to 12% of NICU admitted patients, with a significant percentage of use outside of published recommendations.[1-3] Additionally, a UK-wide prospective study of FFP transfusion practices showed that 2.3% of all patients treated with FFP were children (aged 1–15 years), and 4.4% of these were less than 1 year old. Sixty-two percent of infants who received FFP did not have clinical bleeding, and 14% of infants treated with FFP did not have coagulation tests before the FFP administration.[4] In a multicenter retrospective study involving 43 tertiary care pediatric hospitals in the United States, FFP was noted to have been administered to 2.85% of pediatric hospital admissions, and 29% of these transfusions were given to neonates.[5] A prospective study involving 17 Italian NICUs recorded FFP administration to be a relatively frequent intervention, with 8% of admitted neonates receiving one or more transfusions.[6] This study showed that a remarkably high proportion (60%) of transfusions was noncompliant with guidelines, and 63% of transfused neonates received FFP prophylactically without bleeding evidence. In a retrospective single-center[7] analysis over a period of 16 years, changes on the use of FFP transfusions and the use of clotting tests in preterm neonates were evaluated over the study period; the percentage of preterm neonates receiving FFP transfusion decreased significantly from 5.7% to 2%, and similarly the rate of neonates undergoing coagulation testing decreased from 24.3% to 8%. In this study, 56% of FFP transfusions were administered prophylactically for concomitant coagulopathy, whereas 17% of transfusions were given for clinical bleeding. Over the same period, the percentage of neonates with major bleeding did not change significantly.

Due to the high risk of bleeding, neonates undergoing ECLS are high-use recipients of hemostatic blood products. A recent survey on the use of plasma and platelet transfusions during extracorporeal membrane oxygenation (ECMO) in pediatric population (48% of the subjects were neonates) showed 60% of the plasma transfusions were given for bleeding prophylaxis and the rest (40%) were prescribed for bleeding. Indications for plasma transfusions were mainly guided by evidence of coagulopathy with clotting tests.[8] In addition, 76% of the participating centers recommended a more liberal plasma transfusion threshold for bleeding and for younger patients.

An international survey involving 17 hospitals from 15 different countries reported current neonatal and pediatric transfusion practice.[9] This survey found that plasma transfusions seem to be more dependent on the diagnosis than on clotting tests or clotting factor thresholds, although four hospitals have several coagulation factor–based thresholds for plasma transfusions.

Recommendations Derived From Clinical Studies on the Appropriate Use of Plasma in Neonates

Various controlled studies evaluated the potential usefulness of plasma transfusions in neonates across different clinical settings. The main characteristics and results of randomized controlled trials are summarized in Tables 14.1, 14.2, and 14.3. One study addressed the effectiveness of FFP in disseminated intravascular coagulation, and no differences in improvement of coagulation tests or in survival rate were observed.[10] A possible beneficial effect of FFP administration in neonates with disseminated intravascular coagulation was described only in case reports.[11,12] Four studies evaluated the hypothesis that early volume expansion obtained with FFP administration would reduce

TABLE 14.1	Controlled Studies Evaluating the Effectiveness of FFP Administration in Neonates				
Study	**Design**	**Clinical Setting**	**Intervention**	**Outcome**	
Gross et al.[10]	Single-center RCT	DIC	FFP + PLTs vs. ET vs. control	No differences in survival or resolution of DIC	
Hambleton and Appleyard[13]	Single-center RCT	Prevention of IVH in LBW neonates	FFP for 2 days vs. control	No evidence of beneficial effect	

TABLE 14.1 Controlled Studies Evaluating the Effectiveness of FFP Administration in Neonates—cont'd

Study	Design	Clinical Setting	Intervention	Outcome
Beverley et al.[14*§]	Single-center RCT	Prevention of IVH in preterm neonates	FFP for 2 days vs. control	Decreased rate of IVH
Ekblad et al.[15§]	Single-center RCT	Prevention of IVH and improvement of renal function in preterm neonates	FFP for 3 days vs. control	No evidence of beneficial effect
NNNI Trial Group[16,18*]	Multicenter RCT	Prevention of mortality, cerebral ultrasound abnormality, and disability in preterm neonates	FFP for 2 days vs. Gelofusin vs. dextrose-saline	No evidence of beneficial effect
Emery et al.[22]	Single-center RCT	Hypotension in preterm neonates	FFP vs. 20% albumin vs. 4.5% albumin	No benefit in blood pressure levels in any group
Gottuso et al.[21*]	Multicenter RCT	Prevention of mortality in LBW neonates with RDS	FFP vs. ET vs. control	No evidence of beneficial effect in FFP group, possible benefit for ET
Acunas et al.[19]	Multicenter RCT	Sepsis	FFP vs. IVIG vs. control	No evidence of immunity function improvement in FFP group

*The meta-analysis of these three studies showed no significant difference in mortality rate.[17]
§The meta-analysis of these two studies found a nonsignificant trend to reduce any grade of IVH.[17]
DIC, Disseminated intravascular coagulation; *ET*, exchange transfusion; *FFP*, fresh frozen plasma; *IVH*, intraventricular hemorrhage; *IVIG*, intravenous immunoglobulin; *LBW*, low birth weight; *PLT*, platelet; *PRBC*, peripheral red blood cell; *RCT*, randomized controlled trial; *RDS*, respiratory distress syndrome.

TABLE 14.2 Controlled Studies Evaluating the Effectiveness of FFP Administration for Extracorporeal Life Support in the Pediatric Population

Study	Design	Clinical Setting, Study Population	Intervention	Outcome
Mou et al.[23]	Single-center RCT	CPB for cardiovascular surgery, infants including neonatal patients	FFP+PRBC vs. whole blood for CPB priming	Decreased length of stay and perioperative fluid overload in FFP+PRBC group
Desborough et al.[24]	Meta-analysis of four RCTs	CPB for cardiovascular surgery, pediatric including neonatal patients	FFP during or after CPB priming vs. no plasma	No differences in blood loss and in PRBC transfusions at 24 hr
Bianchi et al.[25]	Single-center RCT	CPB for cardiovascular surgery, infants including neonatal patients	FFP for CPB priming (early) vs. FFP after cardiac surgery (late)	Decreased postoperative bleeding in early FFP
McMichael et al.[27]	Single-center RCT	Extracorporeal membrane oxygenation, pediatric including neonatal patients	Scheduled FFP (every 48 hr) vs. standard FFP administration	No differences for: • circuit life • blood product transfusions • bleedings

CPB, Cardiopulmonary bypass; *FFP*, fresh frozen plasma; *PRBC*, peripheral red blood cell; *RCT*, randomized controlled trial.

TABLE 14.3 Controlled Studies Comparing the Efficacy of Different Solution Used for Partial Exchange Transfusion

Study	Design	Inclusion Criteria	Intervention	Outcome
Deorari et al.[29]	Single-center RCT	Venous Ht >65% with symptoms	Plasma vs. normal saline	Similar changes in postexchange Ht and viscosity values
Roithmaier et al.[30]	Single-center RCT	Venous Ht >65% with symptoms	Virus-inactivated human plasma serum vs. Ringer solution	Similar reduction in postexchange Ht PV increase in serum group BV reduction in Ringer group
Krishnan et al.[31]	Single-center RCT	Venous Ht >65% with symptoms or Ht >70% alone	Plasma vs. normal saline	Similar reduction in postexchange Ht

BV, Blood volume; *Ht*, hematocrit; *PV*, plasma volume; *RCT*, randomized controlled trial.

morbidity and mortality in preterm neonates.[13-16] In one of these studies a significant reduction in the occurrence of intracranial hemorrhage (ICH) was found among neonates receiving FFP, in comparison to controls.[14] In contrast, the other three studies reported a similar rate of ICH and/or cerebral ultrasound abnormalities.[13,15,16] In addition, a meta-analysis that included these four studies showed no significant differences in the occurrence of any grade of intraventricular hemorrhage and mortality rate.[17] In the Northern Neonatal Nursing Initiative trial, the largest of these four studies, where a 2-year follow-up was performed, no significant difference of severe disability between neonates receiving FFP and controls was observed.[18] The potential benefit of FFP administration in neonates for the treatment of sepsis, respiratory distress syndrome, and hypotension was not established by controlled studies.[19-22]

Some studies reported information of blood product usage for extracorporeal life support in the pediatric population. In a randomized clinical trial on infants undergoing cardiopulmonary bypass (CPB) for heart surgery, the circuit priming with a combination of packed red cells and FFP was demonstrated to have advantage over the use of fresh whole blood about reduction in hospital stay and improvement in cumulative fluid balance.[23] In a systematic review that evaluated the use of FFP in patients undergoing cardiovascular surgery, a separate meta-analysis was obtained from four randomized clinical trials that included pediatric and neonatal patients.[24] This analysis

showed no significant differences in blood loss and in red cell transfusions at 24 hours between the prophylactic administration of FFP group and the comparison group that did not receive plasma transfusions. However, since there was a very serious risk of bias for these outcomes due to inadequate or unclear sequence generation and inadequate blinding of participants, clinicians, and/or analysts, the authors downgraded the quality of the evidence to low. In a randomized clinical trial of newborns and small infants undergoing cardiac surgery with CPB, the use of FFP in the priming solution appears slightly superior to late administration in terms of postoperative bleeding.[25] Guidelines of the Network for the Advancement of Patient Blood Management, Haemostasis and Thrombosis suggest the addition of FFP to the CPB prime in neonates undergoing cardiac surgery.[26]

In a clinical study on the effects of prophylactic FFP administration on ECMO circuit longevity, infants were randomized to receive FFP every 48 hours or usual care.[27] Scheduled administration of FFP did not increase circuit life, and there was no difference in blood product transfusions between the two groups. Patients in the intervention group had similar hemorrhagic and thrombotic complications as the control group.

Partial exchange transfusion (PET) is traditionally used as the method to lower the hematocrit and treat hyperviscosity in neonatal polycythemia. Although there is no evidence that this procedure improves long-term outcome of neonates, the standard of care for polycythemic neonates with worsening symptoms continues to be PET in many NICUs.[28] Three randomized clinical trials compared the efficacy between crystalloid solution and plasma used for PET to treat neonatal polycythemia (see Table 14.3).[29-31] Two meta-analyses that included all these three studies showed no significant difference in the reduction of postexchange hematocrit.[32,33] In addition, both crystalloid solution and plasma were reported to be effective in the improvement of symptoms.

Congenital thrombotic thrombocytopenic purpura (ADAMTS-13 deficiency) may present in neonates as isolated thrombocytopenia or combined with a severe microangiopathic hemolytic anemia (Coombs negative) and jaundice. In children and infants, a dose of 15 to 20 mL/kg body weight of FFP on 1 to 3 consecutive days resolved most uncomplicated bouts of TTP, and a prophylactic administration of FFP with an interval of 3 to 4 days prevented severe sequelae in most children.[34]

Recommendations of plasma administration in neonates, based on scientific evidence, are summarized in Box 14.1. Level of evidence and strength of recommendation are consistent with the Grading of Recommendation, Assessment, Development, and Evaluation (GRADE) Working Group (Box 14.2).[35]

Effect of FFP Dose on Clotting Times

Clinical studies have provided information about the volume of administered FFP and its effect on clotting times. In a controlled trial analyzing asphyxiated low birth weight neonates treated with two infusions of FFP (10 mL/kg) there was no improvement in either thrombotest or prothrombin time (PT), though there

BOX 14.1 CLINICAL SETTING WHERE THE USE OF FFP IS RECOMMENDED (A) OR NOT RECOMMENDED (B) IN NEONATES

(A) Use of FFP is Recommended	Level of Evidence	Strength of Recommendations
Treatment of acute bleeding in combination of:		
1 Coagulopathy¥ due to multiple coagulation factor deficiencies (i.e., DIC, liver failure)	C	1
2 Single inherited clotting factor deficiency without safe replacement product available#	C	1
3 Vitamin K deficiency*	C	1
Prophylaxis of bleeding for an invasive procedure in presence of coagulopathy	C	2
Treatment of congenital thrombotic thrombocytopenic purpura	C	1
Blood reconstitution (in conjunction with PRBC) for:		
1 Circuit priming for CPB	B	1
2 Circuit priming for ECMO	C	1
3 Exchange transfusion for hyperbilirubinemia	C	1
(B) Use of FFP is Not Recommended	Level of Evidence	Strength of Recommendations
Prevention of mortality and morbidity in preterm infants	A	1
Replacement fluid for partial exchange transfusion for polycythemia/hyperviscosity	B	1
Treatment of sepsis	C	1
Treatment of RDS	B	1
Volume replacement for hypotension	B	1
Treatment of coagulopathy without bleeding during therapeutic hypothermia for asphyxia	C	2

¥Coagulopathy is defined as coagulation tests outside the 95% confidence limits of the age-related haemostatic parameters (Table 14.4).

#Currently, this only applies to factor V; however, FFP may be also given if treatment is urgently required before the diagnosis of inherited clotting factor deficiency (i.e., haemophilia) has been confirmed.

*The administration of FFP should be combined with intravenous infusion of vitamin K. Methods for grading evidence and formulating recommendation according to the GRADE system.[35]

CPB, Cardiopulmonary bypass; *DIC*, disseminated intravascular coagulation; *ECMO*, extracorporeal membrane oxygenation; *FFP*, fresh frozen plasma; *PRBC*, peripheral red blood cell; *RDS*, respiratory distress syndrome.

BOX 14.2 CRITERIA FOR ASSIGNING GRADE OF EVIDENCE AND STRENGTH OF RECOMMENDATIONS[35]

Quality of Evidence	Type of Clinical Study	Consistency of Results
A = High	Randomized trial without important limitations	Considerable confidence in the estimate of effect
B = Moderate	Randomized trial with important limitations or exceptionally observational studies with strong evidence	Further research likely to have impact on the confidence in estimate, may change estimate
C = Low	Observational studies or case series	Further research is very likely to have impact on confidence, likely to change the estimate
Strength of recommendations	Balance between benefits and harms	
1 = Strong	Certainty of imbalance	
2 = Weak	Uncertainty of imbalance	

The grading scheme classifies the quality of evidence as high (grade A), moderate (grade B), or low (grade C) according to the study design and to the consistency of results. The strength of recommendations was further classified as either strong (1) or weak (2) according to the balance between desirable and undesirable outcomes.

was a significant change in activated partial thromboplastin time (APTT) in small for dates neonates so treated.[13] In a research consistent with the latter results, FFP infusions (10 mL/kg) administered to preterm neonates with respiratory distress syndrome and abnormally prolonged PT (>18 seconds) or APTT (>70 seconds) produced a full correction of both PT and APTT in only 7 of 23 treated neonates.[36] In another study, the volume of a single FFP transfusion was 10, 20, and more than 20 mL/kg in 71%, 23%, and 2% of cases, respectively.[2] The FFP administration converted prolonged coagulation tests, which were assessed considering specific age-related reference ranges, into the normal range for gestational age in 40% of cases. Other authors reported a single-dose infusion of 10 mL/kg in 44% and 20 mL/kg in 56% FFP-administered neonates, respectively.[3] Recovery of coagulation tests after FFP transfusion was 42% for PT and 60% for APTT.

In the UK National Comparative Audit of the use of FFP, the median overall dose of FFP administered in infants was 14 mL/kg, with 20% of them receiving a dose less than 10 mL/kg.[4] In a subsequent report,[37] authors outlined that considering only infants where FFP was administered to correct isolated abnormal coagulation values and using the Andrew et al. reference ranges for coagulation tests (Table 14.4),[38,39] the recovery of PT and APTT was obtained in 15% and 10% of cases, respectively. While in the same context of isolated coagulopathy, using the reference ranges suggested by Christensen et al. (see Table 14.4),[40] which were updated for lower gestational age, the correction

of coagulation tests after FFP administration was obtained in 68% of less than 28 weeks of gestation infants and in 59% of 28 to 34 weeks of gestation infants. In our clinical audit on the use of FFP in NICUs, the mean dose of FFP administered was 16 mL/kg; pre- and postinfusion assessment of coagulation test in neonates showed a significant reduction of both PT and APTT, suggesting that the infused volume of FFP was sufficient to affect clotting times.[6]

Assuming that FFP has an average clotting factor and inhibitor potency of 1 IU/mL, a dose of 10 mL/kg of body weight should increase clotting factor and inhibitor levels by 10 IU/dL (10%).[41] Hence the rapid infusion of at least 10 mL/kg of FFP is required to increase the plasma protein levels significantly. In an international audit of plasma transfusions in critically ill children, which included infants and neonates, 443 plasma transfusions have been reported: 56% and 44% in bleeding and nonbleeding children, respectively.[42] The median dose of plasma administered was 11 mL/kg, and the median international normalized ratio (INR) and APTT changes were -0.2 and -5, respectively. A dose-response relationship was observed only in children with a baseline INR of at least 2.5.

Considering clinical and pharmacokinetic available data, the infusion dose of FFP should be at least 10 to 15 mL/kg of body weight. Higher doses (>20 mL/kg) of FFP should be determined by the clinical situation, the underlying disease process, the half-life of the factor being replaced, and the potential of volume overload.

TABLE 14.4 Defining Coagulopathy in the Premature and Term Neonate, at Birth (A) and During the First 3 Months of Life (B), According to PT, APTT, and Fibrinogen Values

(A)

Gestational Age at Birth (wk)	PT, Upper Limit* (sec)	APTT, Upper Limit* (sec)	Fibrinogen, Lower Limit* (mg/dL)
<28[40]	>21	>64	<71
28–34[40]	>21	>57	<87
30–36[39]	>16	>79	<150
≥37 [38]	>16	>55	<167

(B)

Gestational Age at Birth (wk)	PT, Upper Limit* (sec)	APTT, Upper Limit* (sec)	Fibrinogen, Lower Limit* (mg/dL)
30–36[39]			
and postnatal age of			
5 days	>15	>74	<160
30 days	>14	>62	<150
90 days	>15	>51	<150
≥37[38]			
and postnatal age of			
5 days	>15	>60	<162
30 days	>14	>55	<162
90 days	>14	>50	<150

*The upper limit of PT and APTT, and the lower limit of fibrinogen are defined for values outside the 95% confidence limits of the age-related reference ranges.

APTT, Activated partial thromboplastin time; *PT*, prothrombin time.

Implications of Hemostasis Assessment in Therapeutic Decision Making for FFP Administration

DEVELOPMENTAL HEMOSTASIS

An understanding of physiologic hemostasis and the interpretation of coagulation tests to detect coagulopathy is required to optimize transfusion management of the neonate. The dynamic evolving process of the hemostatic system occurring during childhood was first described by Andrews and termed developmental hemostasis.[43] The fundamental principle underlying developmental hemostasis is that the levels of most coagulation proteins vary significantly with age.

Prolongation of PT and APTT in fetuses throughout intrauterine life is explained by low levels of vitamin K–dependent factors, contact factors, V and VIII coagulation factors, and fibrinogen.[44] Similarly, low levels of antithrombin, protein C, and protein S are found, which likely contribute to a satisfactory hemostatic balance.[44] An increase in the levels of coagulation factors and natural inhibitors is observed after week 34 of intrauterine life, but only factors V and VIII reached adult values at birth (Fig. 14.1).[44]

During the first 6 months of life, the concentration of these coagulation factors gradually increases until it reaches values close to the adult ones.[45] As for the fibrinolytic system, the plasma concentration of plasminogen is reduced at birth, while the tissue plasminogen activator and the plasminogen activator inhibitor are increased.[45] This variation of procoagulant and anticoagulant proteins, which is observed in both full-term and preterm infants, defines a dynamic equilibrium of the hemostatic system that, in normal conditions, functions regularly.

STANDARD COAGULATION TESTS

The abovementioned age-related changes in protein levels lead to corresponding changes in standard

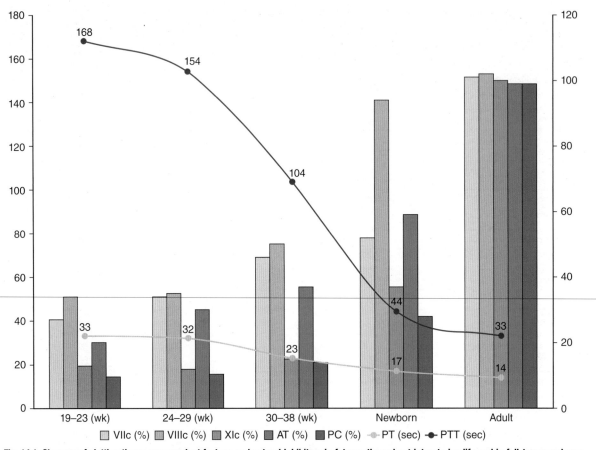

Fig. 14.1 Changes of clotting times, procoagulant factors, and natural inhibitors in fetuses throughout intrauterine life and in full-term newborns and adults. Mean values at different age (*wk*, week of intrauterine life) are presented in seconds *(sec)* for prothrombin time *(PT)* and activated partial thromboplastin time *(APTT)*, and in percentage *(%)* for coagulation factors and natural inhibitor factors. *AT*, Antithrombin; *PC*, protein C. (From Reverdiau-Moalic P, Delahousse B, Body G, et al. Evolution of blood coagulation activators and inhibitors in the healthy human fetus. *Blood.* 1996;88(3):900-906.)

coagulation screening tests such as the PT and the APTT (see Fig. 14.1). Given the age-dependent specificity of hemostasis, the evaluation and interpretation of coagulation test in newborns should be based on appropriate reference ranges for gestational and postnatal age.[38-40] Moreover, as the PT and APTT tests are performed on citrated platelet-poor plasma with the addition of exogenous reagents, both clot formation times will vary depending on the reagents and methodology used in the test. A consensus statement of the International Society on Thrombosis and Hemostasis recommends that diagnostic laboratories processing pediatric samples use age-, analyzer-, and reagent-appropriate reference ranges.[46]

Abnormal coagulation tests, defined as levels at which the results are outside the 95% confidence limits of the age-related hemostatic parameter, are shown in Table 14.4. In neonates, the presence of abnormal coagulation tests have significant limitations as predictors of bleeding and do not necessarily correlate with clinically relevant disease.[2,6,40,47] In addition, there is a lack of evidence demonstrating that FFP administration to nonbleeding neonates with abnormal coagulation tests actually reduces their risk of a subsequent hemorrhage.[48,49] Therefore the appropriate use of FFP should be considered for the treatment of active bleeding in newborns with confirmatory tests of coagulopathy rather than for the prevention of bleeding in those with abnormal standard coagulation tests (see Box 14.1).

Routine screening of clotting tests on admission to NICU was reported to increase the prophylactic use of FFP administered to correct isolated abnormal coagulation values without associated bleeding.[37] Therefore routine coagulation testing on admission is not indicated because this practice might lead to increased FFP transfusion without benefit.

Concern has been raised about the risk of bleeding among neonates with perinatal asphyxia and undergoing therapeutic hypothermia.[50] Coagulopathy is one of the consequences of perinatal asphyxia, and combined hypothermia might increase hemostatic dysfunction.[51-55] Abnormal clotting tests, including PT and APTT, with concomitant reduction of pro- and anticoagulant proteins have been described in asphyxiated neonates treated with whole body cooling.[56] A meta-analysis evaluating the effect of therapeutic hypothermia in encephalopathic asphyxiated newborns showed no significant effect on coagulopathy and no significant major thrombosis or hemorrhage in cooled neonates vs. noncooled neonates.[57] A recent retrospective study presented data on 76 neonates treated with hypothermia for hypoxic ischemic encephalopathy, and 54% of them had bleeding episodes.[58] Thirty-three (43.4%) neonates received FFP transfusion, 28.9 % and 14.5% for bleeding associated with coagulopathy and for isolated abnormal clotting tests without bleeding, respectively. In this study, neonates with bleeding, compared to nonbleeding neonates, had longer coagulation tests, including INR and APTT, and lower platelet count and fibrinogen level. Receiver operating characteristic curve analyses of fibrinogen level, platelet count, and INR resulted as statistically significant; however, both specificity and sensitivity in predicting bleeding episodes were low. Although there are no accepted guidelines, current evidence does not support the use of FFP in asphyxiated cooled neonates with isolated abnormal clotting tests in the absence of bleeding (see Box 14.1). Considering that therapeutic hypothermia is the current standard of care for hypoxic ischemic encephalopathy after perinatal asphyxia, further studies are needed to evaluate the effect of hypothermia on neonatal hemostatic function and to investigate the efficacy of intervention against hemorrhage in this clinical setting.

The subgroup analysis of the international audit on FFP administration showed no difference in INR values prior to plasma transfusion and no difference in INR reduction following transfusion in children supported by ECMO who were transfused for bleeding vs. nonbleeding indications.[8] This survey concluded that since children supported by ECMO receive large volumes of plasma with significant variation in practice, clinical interventional studies are necessary to provide evidence to direct the transfusion of hemostatic products in this setting.

Risk factors associated with blood loss and blood product transfusions were investigated in children and infants undergoing open heart surgery.[59] Younger patient age was found to be the variable most significantly associated with bleeding and transfusions. Lower platelet count during CPB was also significantly associated with bleeding and transfusion, whereas preoperative prothrombin time was not.

VISCOELASTIC TESTS OF COAGULATION

Due to the complexity of the coagulation process, standard laboratory tests are unable to measure all the individual elements involved in hemostatic function. Consequently, first line coagulation tests must be interpreted with caution. As occurring in adults, in newborns one of the main limitations of the standard coagulation tests is their poor predictive power for the risk of bleeding.[6,40] Viscoelastic tests of coagulation such as thromboelastography (TEG, Haemonetics Corp, Braintree, MA, USA) and rotational thromboelastometry (ROTEM, TEM International, Munich, Germany) may be able to overcome some of these limitations.[60] They differ from conventional coagulation tests as they analyze the viscoelastic properties of the clot by evaluating the entire hemostatic process, its development, stabilization, and dissolution (Fig. 14.2). These analyses provide comprehensive information on the interaction between plasma coagulation proteins, platelets, and blood cells during clot formation and more closely reflect what occurs in vivo than do standard tests.

Interest in and experience with viscoelastic tests in neonates has been increasing over the years, and its use seems promising in the diagnosis and treatment of acquired coagulopathies. There are published studies that proved the reproducibility and reliability of the

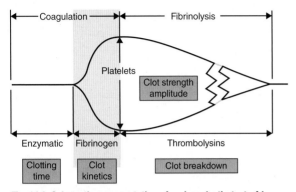

Fig. 14.2 Schematic representation of a viscoelastic test of hemostasis. The viscoelastic analysis determines all phases of hemostasis:
- The clotting time represents the time to initial fibrin formation and is associated with the enzymatic reactions.
- The clot kinetics represent the rate of clot buildup and is associated with the fibrinogen function or the interactions between the enzymatic pathways and platelet activation.
- The clot strength (attainment of maximum amplitude), which mainly indicate platelet function (80–90%); fibrinogen also contributes (10–20%).
- The clot breakdown is related to the activity of thrombolysins.

viscoelastic coagulation tests to assess hemostasis in the neonatal population by developing local, age-, analyzer-, and reagent-appropriate reference ranges.[61-64] There are also studies assessing viscoelastic test parameters to find a possible correlation between coagulopathy and clinical bleeding. The thromboelastographic profiles of 49 premature neonates with and without ICH were measured at birth, and no significant differences of TEG and standard coagulation tests values between the two groups were observed.[65] Similar results were obtained in a retrospective study comparing TEG parameters between a group of 24 bleeding preterm neonates (22 of them had ICH) with a group of 94 nonbleeding preterm neonates.[62] Together these two studies suggest that the onset of ICH in preterm neonates is usually not associated with coagulopathy, thus FFP administration is unlikely to prevent ICH. In contrast, a prospective observational study presented normative ranges for citrated-modified and heparinase-modified TEG parameters in term neonates and established cut points for TEG parameters associated to clinical bleeding in term infants.[66] Though as their bleeding group was comprised of neonates with severe disease, including hypoxic ischemic encephalopathy and respiratory failure requiring ECMO, they could

not exclude whether any of these conditions intrinsically would affect the TEG parameters. Research was conducted on the effect of cooling on the coagulation of 24 neonates undergoing therapeutic hypothermia for perinatal asphyxia.[67] TEG assays were simultaneously performed at 33.5°C and 37°C for comparison. TEG results were affected by temperature indicating more impaired coagulation at lower temperature. In addition, TEG parameters were predictive of clinical bleeding with temperature-dependent cut points, while standard coagulation tests were not predictive of bleeding. These findings suggest that TEG assays should be carried out under temperature-regulated conditions for neonates undergoing therapeutic hypothermia, and they may be a more suitable method to assess bleeding risk and optimize transfusion treatment in this population.

Forty-six neonates with congenital diaphragmatic hernia and supported by ECMO between 2008 and 2018 were retrospectively reviewed.[68] From 2015 anticoagulation management was implemented and standardized by including routine TEG monitoring. TEG assay led to a significant increase in platelets transfusions and a decrease of cryoprecipitate administration but did not change the use of FFP. Additionally, comparing the pre-2015 and the post-2015 group, a significant reduction in the incidence of hemothorax was found. These findings highlight that, in neonates undergoing ECMO, the TEG assay is an additional tool that could provide useful information for the rapid diagnosis of hemorrhagic conditions and could help clinicians in administering correct and timely transfusions.

A study examined blood samples from 44 neonates undergoing CPB by using research and clinical assays to evaluate the heparin-protamine balance and to determine a possible association with postoperative bleeding.[69] Thirty-six percent of patients had excessive postoperative bleeding, and none of the coagulation tests (including ROTEM) predicted this complication, suggesting that in this setting the hemorrhagic events involve several factor and causes. A single-center observational study investigated ROTEM parameters in full-term and preterm neonates with confirmed and suspected sepsis.[70] A hypocoagulable state was found in septic neonates compared to those with suspected sepsis or to healthy neonates. This hypercoagulable profile was even more intense in septic neonates with clinically bleeding events than in those without. By assessing 332 critically ill full-term and preterm neonates, the same authors developed and internally validated a predictive model for neonatal bleeding.[71] In that study, the neonatal bleeding assessment tool (NeoBAT)[72] was utilized to record hemorrhagic events occurring within 24 hours of the ROTEM testing. ROTEM parameters, platelet counts, and creatinine levels were identified as the most robust predictors of hemorrhage and were included into a Neonatal Bleeding Risk (NeoBRis) index. This multivariable prediction model showed excellent performance, suggesting that, after its external validation, it will help clinicians detect the 24-hour bleeding risk and will support timely individualized transfusions.

Best Evidence-Based Practice for Administering FFP in the NICU

Clinical audits continue to report a frequent use of FFP in NICUs outside evidence-based recommendations, raising important questions about cost and risk. The two main reasons for poor adherence to guidelines are the lack of clinical trials evaluating FFP efficacy in many specific circumstances and the significant limitation of standard coagulation tests as predictors of bleeding. In this context:

- NICUs should implement evidence-based guidelines for the use of FFP to minimize the adverse effects of transfusion and wastage of products (level of evidence C; strength of recommendations 1).
- The use of FFP in neonatology should primarily be for neonates with active bleeding and associated coagulopathy (grading of recommendations related to specific conditions is reported in Box 14.1).
- The results of standard coagulation tests should be interpreted with appropriate reference ranges for gestational and postnatal age (see Table 14.4) (level of evidence B; strength of recommendations 1).
- The dose of FFP should be at least 10 to 15 mL/kg of body weight (level of evidence C; strength of recommendations 1).
- Routine coagulation testing on NICU admission is not indicated because this practice might lead to increased FFP transfusion without

benefit (level of evidence C; strength of recommendations 2).

The promising results of preliminary studies on viscoelastic tests in neonatology show that these assays may overcome the limitations of standard coagulation tests with the advantages to be a bedside tool capable of evaluating the entire hemostatic process with a minimum amount of blood. However, there are currently insufficient data to support or refute the routine use of TEG and ROTEM to guide hemostatic treatment vs. usual care in bleeding neonates.

REFERENCES

1. Baer VL, Lambert DK, Schmutz N, et al. Adherence to NICU transfusion guidelines: data from a multihospital healthcare system. *J Perinatol.* 2008;28(7):492-497.
2. Puetz J, Darling G, McCormick KA, et al. Fresh frozen plasma and recombinant factor VIIa use in neonates. *J Pediatr Hematol Oncol.* 2009;31(12):901-906.
3. Altuntas N, Yenicesu I, Beken S, et al. Clinical use of fresh-frozen plasma in neonatal intensive care unit. *Transfus Apher Sci.* 2012;47(1):91-94.
4. Stanworth SJ, Grant-Casey J, Lowe D, et al. The use of fresh-frozen plasma in England: high levels of inappropriate use in adults and children. *Transfusion.* 2011;51(1):62-70.
5. Puetz J, Witmer C, Huang YS, et al. Widespread use of fresh frozen plasma in US children's hospitals despite limited evidence demonstrating a beneficial effect. *J Pediatr.* 2012;160(2):210-215.e1.
6. Motta M, Del Vecchio A, Perrone B, et al. Fresh frozen plasma use in the NICU: a prospective, observational, multicentred study. *Arch Dis Child Fetal Neonatal Ed.* 2014;99(4):F303-F308.
7. Houben NAM, Heeger LE, Stanworth SJ, et al. Changes in the use of fresh-frozen plasma transfusions in preterm neonates: a single center experience. *J Clin Med.* 2020;9(11):3789.
8. Nellis ME, Saini A, Spinella PC, et al. Pediatric plasma and platelet transfusions on extracorporeal membrane oxygenation: a subgroup analysis of two large international point-prevalence studies and the role of local guidelines. *Pediatr Crit Care Med.* 2020;21(3):267-275.
9. Bruun MT, Yazer MH, Spinella PC, et al. Vox Sanguinis International Forum on paediatric indications for blood component transfusion: summary. *Vox Sang.* 2019;114(5):523-530.
10. Gross SJ, Filston HC, Anderson JC. Controlled study of treatment for disseminated intravascular coagulation in the neonate. *J Pediatr.* 1982;100(3):445-448.
11. Yuen P, Cheung A, Lin HJ, et al. Purpura fulminans in a Chinese boy with congenital protein C deficiency. *Pediatrics.* 1986;77(5):670-676.
12. Branson HE, Katz J, Marble R, et al. Inherited protein C deficiency and coumarin-responsive chronic relapsing purpura fulminans in a newborn infant. *Lancet.* 1983;2:(8360):1165-1168.
13. Hambleton G, Appleyard WJ. Controlled trial of fresh frozen plasma in asphyxiated low birthweight infants. *Arch Dis Child.* 1973;48(1):31-35.
14. Beverley DW, Pitts-Tucker TJ, Congdon PJ, et al. Prevention of intraventricular haemorrhage by fresh frozen plasma. *Arch Dis Child.* 1985;60:710-713.

15. Ekblad H, Kero P, Shaffer SG, et al. Extracellular volume in preterm infants: influence of gestational age and colloids. *Early Hum Dev.* 1991;27(1-2):1-7.

16. Northern Neonatal Nursing Initiative (NNNI) Trial Group. A randomized trial comparing the effect of prophylactic intravenous fresh frozen plasma, gelatin or glucose on early mortality and morbidity in preterm babies. *Eur J Pediatr.* 1996;155(7):580-588.

17. Osborn DA, Evans N. Early volume expansion for prevention of morbidity and mortality in very preterm infants. *Cochrane Database Syst Rev.* 2004;(2):CD002055.

18. Northern Neonatal Nursing Initiative (NNNI) Trial Group. Randomised trial of prophylactic early fresh-frozen plasma or gelatin or glucose in preterm babies: outcome at 2 years. *Lancet.* 1996;348(9022):229-232.

19. Acunas BA, Peakman M, Liossis G, et al. Effect of fresh frozen plasma and gammaglobulin on humoral immunity in neonatal sepsis. *Arch Dis Child Fetal Neonatal Ed.* 1994;70(3):F182-F187.

20. Krediet TG, Beurskens FJ, van Dijk H, et al. Antibody responses and opsonic activity in sera of preterm neonates with coagulase-negative staphylococcal septicemia and the effect of the administration of fresh frozen plasma. *Pediatr Res.* 1998;43(5):645-651.

21. Gottuso MA, Williams ML, Oski FA. The role of exchange transfusion in the management of low-birth-weight infants with and without severe respiratory distress syndrome. *J Pediatr.* 1976;89(2):279-285.

22. Emery EF, Greenough A, Gamsu HR. Randomised controlled trial of colloid infusions in hypotensive preterm infants. *Arch Dis Child.* 1992;67(10 Spec No):1185-1188.

23. Mou SS, Giroir BP, Molitor-Kirsch EA, et al. Fresh whole blood versus reconstituted blood for pump priming in heart surgery in infants. *N Engl J Med.* 2004;351(16):1635-1644.

24. Desborough M, Sandu R, Brunskill SJ, et al. Fresh frozen plasma for cardiovascular surgery. *Cochrane Database Syst Rev.* 2015;(7):CD007614.

25. Bianchi P, Cotza M, Beccaris C, et al. Early or late fresh frozen plasma administration in newborns and small infants undergoing cardiac surgery: the APPEAR randomized trial. *Br J Anaesth.* 2017;118(5):788-796.

26. Faraoni D, Meier J, New HV, et al. Patient blood management for neonates and children undergoing cardiac surgery: 2019 NATA guidelines. *J Cardiothorac Vasc Anesth.* 2019;33(12):3249-3263.

27. McMichael ABV, Zimmerman KO, Kumar KR, et al. Evaluation of effect of scheduled fresh frozen plasma on ECMO circuit life: a randomized pilot trial. *Transfusion.* 2021;61(1):42-51.

28. Ozek E, Soll R, Schimmel MS. Partial exchange transfusion to prevent neurodevelopmental disability in infants with polycythemia. *Cochrane Database Syst Rev.* 2010;(1):CD005089.

29. Deorari AK, Paul VK, Shreshta L, et al. Symptomatic neonatal polycythemia: comparison of partial exchange transfusion with saline versus plasma. *Indian Pediatr.* 1995;32(11):1167-1171.

30. Roithmaier A, Arlettaz R, Bauer K, et al. Randomized controlled trial of Ringer solution versus serum for partial exchange transfusion in neonatal polycythaemia. *Eur J Pediatr.* 1995;154(1):53-56.

31. Krishnan L, Rahim A. Neonatal polycythemia. *Indian J Pediatr.* 1997;64:541-546.

32. Dempsey EM, Barrington K. Crystalloid or colloid for partial exchange transfusion in neonatal polycythemia: a systematic review and meta-analysis. *Acta Paediatr.* 2005;94(11):1650-1655.

33. de Waal KA, Baerts W, Offringa M. Systematic review of the optimal fluid for dilutional exchange transfusion in neonatal polycythaemia. *Arch Dis Child Fetal Neonatal Ed.* 2006;91(1):F7-F10.

34. Hassenpflug WA, Budde U, Schneppenheim S, et al. Inherited thrombotic thrombocytopenic purpura in children. *Semin Thromb Hemost.* 2014;40(4):487-492.

35. Atkins D, Best D, Briss PA, et al. Grading quality of evidence and strength of recommendations. *BMJ.* 2004;328(7454):1490-1494.

36. Johnson CA, Snyder MS, Weaver RL. The effects of fresh frozen plasma infusions on coagulation screening tests in neonates. *Arch Dis Child.* 1982;57(12):950-952.

37. Catford K, Muthukumar P, Reddy C, et al. Routine neonatal coagulation testing increases use of fresh-frozen plasma. *Transfusion.* 2014;54:1444-1445.

38. Andrew M, Paes B, Milner R, et al. Development of the human coagulation system in the full-term infant. *Blood.* 1987;70(1):165-172.

39. Andrew M, Paes B, Milner R, et al. Development of the human coagulation system in the healthy premature infant. *Blood.* 1988;72(5):1651-1657.

40. Christensen RD, Baer VL, Lambert DK, et al. Reference intervals for common coagulation tests of preterm infants (CME). *Transfusion.* 2014;54(3):627-632.

41. Hellstern P, Muntean W, Schramm W, et al. Practical guidelines for the clinical use of plasma. *Thromb Res.* 2002;107(1):S53-S57.

42. Karam O, Demaret P, Shefler A, et al. Indications and effects of plasma transfusions in critically ill children. *Am J Respir Crit Care Med.* 2015;191(12):1395-1402.

43. Andrew M. The relevance of developmental hemostasis to hemorrhagic disorders of newborns. *Semin Perinatol.* 1997;21(1):70-85.

44. Reverdiau-Moalic P, Delahousse B, Body G, et al. Evolution of blood coagulation activators and inhibitors in the healthy human fetus. *Blood.* 1996;88(3):900-906.

45. Monagle P, Massicotte P. Developmental haemostasis: secondary haemostasis. *Semin Fetal Neonatal Med.* 2011;16(6):294-300.

46. Ignjatovic V, Kenet G, Monagle P, Perinatal and Paediatric Haemostasis Subcommittee of the Scientific and Standardization Committee of the International Society on Thrombosis and Haemostasis. Developmental hemostasis: recommendations for laboratories reporting pediatric samples. *J Thromb Haemost.* 2012;10(2):298-300.

47. Venkatesh V, Khan R, Curley A, et al. How we decide when a neonate needs a transfusion. *Br J Haematol.* 2013;160(4):421-433.

48. Van de Bor M, Briet E, Van Bel F, et al. Hemostasis and periventricular-intraventricular hemorrhage of the newborn. *Am J Dis Child.* 1986;140(11):1131-1134.

49. Tran TT, Veldman A, Malhotra A. Does risk-based coagulation screening predict intraventricular haemorrhage in extreme premature infants? *Blood Coagul Fibrinolysis.* 2012;23(6):532-536.

50. Bauman ME, Cheung PY, Massicotte MP. Hemostasis and platelet dysfunction in asphyxiated neonates. *J Pediatr.* 2011;158(suppl 2):e35-e39.

51. Shah P, Riphagen S, Beyene J, et al. Multiorgan dysfunction in infants with post-asphyxial hypoxic-ischaemic encephalopathy. *Arch Dis Child Fetal Neonatal Ed.* 2004;89(2):F152-F155.

52. Sarkar S, Barks JD, Bhagat I, et al. Effects of therapeutic hypothermia on multiorgan dysfunction in asphyxiated newborns: whole-body cooling versus selective head cooling. *J Perinatol.* 2009;29(8):558-563.

53. Rohrer MJ, Natale AM. Effect of hypothermia on the coagulation cascade. *Crit Care Med.* 1992;20(10):1402-1405.

54. Wolberg AS, Meng ZH, Monroe III DM, et al. A systematic evaluation of the effect of temperature on coagulation enzyme

activity and platelet function. *J Trauma*. 2004;56(6):1221-1228.

55. Mitrophanov AY, Rosendaal FR, Reifman J. Computational analysis of the effects of reduced temperature on thrombin generation: the contributions of hypothermia to coagulopathy. *Anesth Analg*. 2013;117(3):565-574.

56. Oncel MY, Erdeve O, Calisici E, et al. The effect of whole-body cooling on hematological and coagulation parameters in asphyxic newborns. *Pediatr Hematol Oncol*. 2013;30(3):246-252.

57. Jacobs SE, Berg M, Hunt R, et al. Cooling for newborns with hypoxic ischaemic encephalopathy. *Cochrane Database Syst Rev*. 2013;(1):CD003311.

58. Forman KR, Diab Y, Wong EC, et al. Coagulopathy in newborns with hypoxic ischemic encephalopathy (HIE) treated with therapeutic hypothermia: a retrospective case-control study. *BMC Pediatr*. 2014;14:277.

59. Williams GD, Bratton SL, Ramamoorthy C. Factors associated with blood loss and blood product transfusions: a multivariate analysis in children after open-heart surgery. *Anesth Analg*. 1999;89(1):57-64.

60. Radicioni M, Mezzetti D, Del Vecchio A. Thromboelastography: might work in neonatology too? *J Matern Fetal Neonatal Med*. 2012;25(4):S18-S21.

61. Edwards RM, Naik-Mathuria BJ, Gay AN, et al. Parameters of thromboelastography in healthy newborns. *Am J Clin Pathol*. 2008;130(1):99-102.

62. Motta M, Guaragni B, Pezzotti E, et al. Reference intervals of citrated-native whole blood thromboelastography in premature neonates. *Early Hum Dev*. 2017;115:60-63.

63. Ghirardello S, Raffaeli G, Scalambrino E, et al. The intra-assay reproducibility of thromboelastography in very low birth weight infants. *Early Hum Dev*. 2018;127:48-52.

64. Radicioni M, Massetti V, Bini V, et al. Impact of blood sampling technique on reproducibility of viscoelastic coagulation monitor (VCM) system test results in the neonate. *J Matern Fetal Neonatal Med*. 2021;25:1-7.

65. Radicioni M, Bruni A, Bini V, et al. Thromboelastographic profiles of the premature infants with and without intracranial hemorrhage at birth: a pilot study. *J Matern Fetal Neonatal Med*. 2015;28(15):1779-1783.

66. Sewell EK, Forman KR, Wong ECC, et al. Thromboelastography in term neonates: an alternative approach to evaluating coagulopathy. *Arch Dis Child Fetal Neonatal Ed*. 2017;102(1):F79-F84.

67. Forman KR, Wong E, Gallagher M, et al. Effect of temperature on thromboelastography and implications for clinical use in newborns undergoing therapeutic hypothermia. *Pediatr Res*. 2014;75(5):663-669.

68. Phillips RC, Shahi N, LeopoldD, et al. Thromboelastography-guided management of coagulopathy in neonates with congenital diaphragmatic hernia supported by extracorporeal membrane oxygenation. *Pediatr Surg Int*. 2020;36(9):1027-1033.

69. Peterson JA, Maroney SA, Zwifelhofer W, et al. Heparin-protamine balance after neonatal cardiopulmonary bypass surgery. *J Thromb Haemost*. 2018;16(10):1973-1983.

70. Sokou R, Giallouros G, Konstantinidi A, et al. Thromboelastometry for diagnosis of neonatal sepsis-associated coagulopathy: an observational study. *Eur J Pediatr*. 2010;177(3):355-362.

71. Sokou R, Piovani D, Konstantinidi A, et al. A risk score for predicting the incidence of hemorrhage in critically ill neonates: development and validation study. *Thromb Haemost*. 2021;121(2):131-139.

72. Venkatesh V, Curley A, Khan R, et al. A novel approach to standardised recording of bleeding in a high risk neonatal population. *Arch Dis Child Fetal Neonatal Ed*. 2013;98(3):F260-F263.

Chapter 15

Pathophysiologic Importance of Platelets in Neonatal Necrotizing Enterocolitis

Sharada H. Gowda, MD and Akhil Maheshwari, MD, FAAP, FRCP (Edin), FIAH

Chapter Outline

Introduction

The onset of necrotizing enterocolitis (NEC) is associated with decreased platelet counts in most patients within 24 hours, and the severity of this thrombocytopenia (defined as platelet counts $<150 \times 10^9/L$) typically correlates with the severity and extent of intestinal injury. The platelet counts usually continue to drop until 3 days after disease onset.[1-4] Patients with the most severe, surgical NEC may develop thrombocytopenia with platelet counts below $100 \times 10^9/L$ within 24 hours of the diagnosis, and those with severe disease may show counts in the range of 30 to $60 \times 10^9/L$.[1-3,5-7] Some infants with surgical NEC may show decreased platelet counts prior to the onset of diagnostic abdominal signs. Platelet counts may also provide predictive information for the outcome; severe thrombocytopenia ($<50 \times 10^9/L$) may predict the need for surgical intervention, NEC-related gastrointestinal complications such as cholestatic liver disease and short bowel syndrome, prolonged length of hospital stay, and mortality.[2,3,5,6,8] Overall, NEC is a leading cause of acquired acute and subacute thrombocytopenia in neonatal intensive care units (NICUs) in the United States and many other countries.

Ververidis et al.[5] followed 58 patients with NEC and noted that 54 (93%) developed thrombocytopenia. Ragazzi et al.[6] described a strong correlation between the extent of disease and the drop in platelet counts. Kenton et al.[4] reviewed 91 patients; severe thrombocytopenia ($<50 \times 10^9/L$) frequently occurred within the first 24 hours of onset of severe NEC. Hutter,[2] O'Neill,[1] and Patel[3] described similar findings in surgical NEC. Baer et al.[9,10] reviewed a large cohort of 11,281 neonates treated in level III NICUs and identified NEC to be the leading cause of platelet counts below $50 \times 10^9/L$ in 273 (2.4%). At our center, we reviewed the medical records of infants with confirmed NEC (stages II and III) from a 12-year period and found almost all of these infants had a fall in platelet counts within 24 hours (unpublished data).

Hutter et al.[2] studied fatal NEC. Patients who died of NEC had lower platelet nadirs ($46.5 \times 10^9/L$) than the survivors ($69.3 \times 10^9/L$). Ververidis et al.[5] also

185

reported that their 16/58 (27.6%) infants with fatal acute NEC had lower nadirs in platelet counts than the survivors. Severe thrombocytopenia has been seen as a predictor of mortality in NEC in several other studies; the odds ratios (ORs) of death were as high as sixfold in some cohorts. Thrombocytopenic infants also developed post-NEC complications more often, such as cholestasis and fivefold increase in short bowel syndrome.[3-6]

The pathogenesis of NEC-related thrombocytopenia is not clear. There is anecdotal clinical evidence for platelet consumption seen in the rapid reduction in platelet counts after the onset of NEC and in the short-lived rise in platelet concentrations following transfusions.[11] However, a compensatory increase in megakaryopoiesis is not seen in all infants.[12,13] Brown et al.[13] evaluated thrombopoiesis among six infants with NEC; they measured circulating megakaryocyte progenitors, reticulated platelets (RPs), platelet counts, and plasma thrombopoietin levels. Infants with NEC had thrombocytopenia but no change in plasma thrombopoietin levels. In another study, Cremer et al.[12] evaluated 12 patients with fatal surgical NEC. These infants had lower platelet counts and immature platelet fractions (IPF) than the survivors. The reasons for dampened thrombopoiesis in some patients are unclear, although one speculation is that activated platelets might have released platelet factor 4, which is a known inhibitor of megakaryopoiesis.[14]

There have been some speculations on the pathophysiology of NEC-related thrombocytopenia. In the necrotic bowel, bacterial products and tissue factor/thromboplastin released from dying cells are believed to stimulate the vascular endothelium, which may then stimulate platelets to release or induce the expression of inflammatory cytokines, platelet-activating factor, coagulation factors, and arachidonic acid metabolites.[11,15-17] These mediators may then further activate the endothelium to form a feed-forward loop.[1,17] The site of platelet consumption in NEC remains to be identified but has been presumed to be in microthrombi within inflamed bowel.[11,15] To understand the mechanism(s) of NEC-related thrombocytopenia there has been a need for developmentally appropriate preclinical models where the progression of intestinal injury can be timed. We sought to address this gap by developing a neonatal mouse model of intestinal injury.[18-20]

DATA FROM MURINE MODELS

We developed neonatal murine models using wild type and genetically modified pups to investigate the mechanism(s) of NEC-related thrombocytopenia.[18,21] The incidence of NEC peaks in premature infants at a postmenstrual age (gestational age at birth + postnatal age at onset of NEC) of approximately 32 weeks,[22-24] and therefore we postulated that the pathoanatomy of NEC may represent a generic injury response of the intestine during a specific developmental epoch rather than reflecting the effects of specific pathogenic trigger(s).[18] In this context we tested the immunogen trinitrobenzene sulfonic acid (TNBS; 2 doses of 50 mg/kg body weight in 30% w/v ethanol), in 10-day-old C57BL/6J mice by gavage and rectal instillation.[18-21,25] TNBS is useful because it can be standardized and titrated for causing injury in different batches of mouse pups and it induces a consistent, timeable, clearly localized, and bacteria-dependent inflammatory injury that resembles NEC in many ways (vide infra).[18-20,26]

TNBS has been previously used in adult mice to induce colitis,[27] where it caused subacute inflammation with basal cryptitis in distal parts of the colon. However, there were concerns about the artificial nature of the injury caused by TNBS, which is a nitroaryl oxidizing agent derived from picric acid, and that the possibility of direct chemical damage could not be excluded. However, in P10 mice there were several reassuring factors that the mucosal damage was not due to a corrosive action. The instilled volumes of the TNBS solution were very small (1.5 µL/g body weight), its aqueous solution was not injurious, and no bowel injury occurred in germ-free animals.[18] Here, the intestinal injury seems to occur when its alcoholic solvent created small foci of mucosal damage, and consequent translocation of luminal bacteria led to the recruitment and inflammatory activation of gut macrophages. The histopathologic changes also closely resembled those seen in NEC.[18-20,26]

In P10 mice, TNBS induced an acute, temporally predictable necrotizing ileocolitis that resembled human NEC and was distinct from the more subacute inflammation in the distal colon in adult rodents that was mediated via recruitment of Th1-Th17 lymphocytes.[27] In neonates, TNBS caused a rapidly progressive intestinal injury with a strong ileocecal predilection, with prominent necrosis, macrophage-rich infiltrates, and systemic inflammation mediated via signaling networks shared with human NEC.[18-20,25] The rapid and highly predictable progression of bowel injury in the neonatal model made it useful for studying NEC complications such as thrombocytopenia.[21] The histopathologic evidence of intestinal injury could be easily seen at 12 hours, and thrombocytopenia ensued soon thereafter.[18-21]

We examined the platelet volume indices (mean platelet volume [MPV], platelet-to-large cell ratio, and platelet distribution width [PDW]) and the IPF, indicating increased thrombopoiesis. Consistent with human NEC,[9,28] the affected mice showed larger MPVs and IPFs in the bloodstream. The megakaryocyte number, ploidy, and CD41 expression were also higher, indicating increased megakaryocyte differentiation and platelet production. The results favored increased platelet consumption, not impaired production, as the likely mechanism of thrombocytopenia.[21] Although we did not investigate the mechanism(s) that could increase platelet production during NEC, lipopolysaccharides are known to stimulate megakaryocyte differentiation and platelet production in conjunction with inflammatory cytokines such as interleukin-6.[29] These findings are consistent with the clinical observations of Brown et al.,[13] who showed a modest increase in circulating RPs and megakaryocytic precursors in infants with NEC.

1. We had anticipated platelet activation to be a delayed, secondary consequence of bacterial translocation through the damaged mucosa. However, the mouse model showed it to be a thrombin-mediated, early pathogenetic event beginning as early as 3 hours after initiation of intestinal injury. Platelets can be an important source of inflammatory factors (Fig. 15.1). Although the platelet counts were unchanged at 3 hours, there were morphologic signs of activation (Fig. 15.2) and increased expression of the activated conformation of the integrin α_{IIb}/β_3 (Fig. 15.3) (detected in our studies as reactivity to the antibody clone JON/A).[30] There was less ATP release following collagen stimulation (a sign of exhausted stores due to prior release), fewer dense granules, and increased aggregability upon collagen exposure; all these changes preceded obvious mucosal injury or endotoxemia.[26] Unlike dense granules, the α-granule

discharge was seen later, at 6 hours or more. Our mechanistic studies showed that platelet activation was triggered by thrombin, which in turn was activated by tissue factor (TF) released from intestinal macrophages.[26] This TF was preformed and stored in microvesicles in neonatal, but not adult, gut macrophages (Fig. 15.4). The changes seen in plasma thrombin activity were also age specific and seen only in neonates, not adults. Compared to adults, neonatal platelets were also more sensitive to thrombin due to higher expression of several downstream signaling mediators and the deficiency of endogenous thrombin antagonists.[26] These characteristics reflected higher expression of Toll-like receptor 4.

The higher sensitivity of neonatal platelets to thrombin than those from adults seems to be developmentally regulated. Neonatal platelets expressed several thrombin-signaling proteins at higher levels than in adults,[31] including the platelet glycoprotein-1b beta chain (GP1bβ), vasodilator-stimulated phosphoprotein, guanine nucleotide-binding protein subunit alpha 13 (G13), guanine nucleotide-binding protein (g[q] subunit α), cytosolic phospholipase A-2 (PLA2), phospholipase A2-activating protein (PLA2AP), and the synaptosomal-associated protein 23 (SNAP23). Neonatal platelets also expressed higher levels of the ras homolog gene family member A (RhoA), the Rho GDP-dissociation inhibitor 1 (ARHGDIA), and the Rho GDP-dissociation inhibitor 2 (ARHGDIB). Human infants also carried low plasma levels of antithrombin, which may be accentuated during critical illness and may potentiate the effects of thrombin generated during tissue injury.[32] These findings are of translational importance because the administration of antithrombin perfluorocarbon nanoparticles,[33] which can bind thrombin in nascent blood clots and prevent progressive activation of the coagulation cascades, were protective against intestinal injury.

The platelet counts and the timing of onset of thrombocytopenia were inversely related to the severity of intestinal injury.[1-3,5,6] Pups with mild injury showed some reduction in platelet counts at 18 hours and a nadir at 24 hours. In moderate-severe injury, platelet counts began dropping at 12 to 15 hours until 18 to 24 hours; survivors showed some recovery of

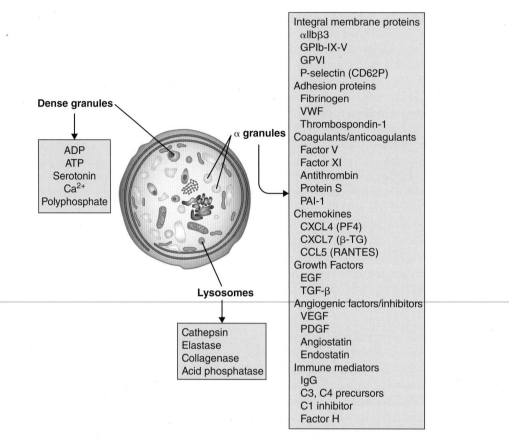

Fig. 15.1 **Platelet granules: the most frequently seen categories include the dense and α granules, and lysosomes.** The schematic also shows the major contents of each type of these granules. In the murine model, inflammatory intestinal injury was associated with rapid degranulation of dense granules. *CXCL*, CXC-chemokine ligand; *EGF*, epidermal growth factor; *GP*, glycoprotein; *IgG*, immunoglobulin G; *PAI-1*, plasminogen activator inhibitor-1; *PDGF*, platelet-derived growth factor; *PF4*, platelet factor 4; *RANTES*, regulated upon activation, normal T-cell expressed, and secreted; *TGF-β*, transforming growth factor-β; *VEGF*, vascular endothelial growth factor; *VWF*, von Willebrand factor. (Reproduced with permission and after minor modifications from Hoffman R, Benz EJ, Silberstein LE, et al. Molecular basis of platelet function. In: Rand ML, Israels SJ, eds. *Hematology: Basic Principles and Practice*. Elsevier; 2017:1870-1884.e2.)

platelet counts between 24 and 48 hours. Interestingly, mice with severe injury showed a transient rise in platelet counts at the 6-hour time point, probably reflecting the release of platelets from storage.

To determine the mechanism of thrombocytopenia, we compared the platelet indices in pups with intestinal injury with those in controls. The MPV is the quotient of the plateletcrit (ratio of platelet volume to the whole blood volume) and the platelet counts (= plateletcrit [%]/platelet count [× 10^9/L] × 10^5). The PDW is the range of platelet volumes at 20% frequency (peak of the frequency histogram = 100%),

and the platelet–large cell ratio (P-LCR) is the proportion of large platelets (>12 fL) in the total platelet population. The median MPV increased from 6.6 fL (range 6.1–8.3) in controls and increased to 7.5 (6.6–7.7), 7.2 (6.5–9.6), and 7.6 (6.4–9.9) fL in mice with mild, moderate, and severe intestinal injury. The MPV increased despite the drop in plateletcrits due to the concomitant drop in platelet counts. The PDW and P-LCR also increased in intestinal injury. The increase in platelet volume indices in murine intestinal injury indicated an increased number of larger, younger platelets in the circulation.[34,35] Pups with

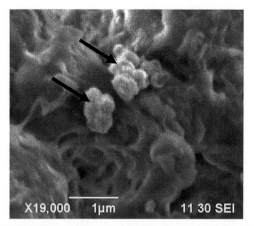

Fig. 15.2 Platelet activation is an early event during necrotizing enterocolitis *(NEC)*-like injury. In the murine model of NEC, platelets were seen in the intestine as early as 3 hours after initiation of the intestinal injury protocol. The scanning electron micrograph shows platelets with discrete, irregular shape changes that imparted a lobular appearance *(arrows)* consistent with activation.

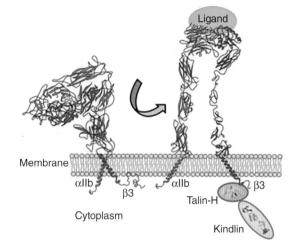

Fig. 15.3 Model showing the activation of $\alpha_{IIb}\beta_3$ granules. Signaling pathways induced by platelet agonists result in talin and kindlin binding to the cytoplasmic tail of $\beta3$ and inside-out signaling such that the integrin is transformed from its low-affinity bent conformation on the resting platelet to its high-affinity extended conformation on the activated platelet. The extended conformation has the ligand binding site exposed, allowing for the binding of fibrinogen or von Willebrand factor, and thus for platelet aggregation. Binding of these ligands initiates outside-in signaling, triggering further intracellular signal transduction and platelet responses. This model is based on the crystal structure of the extracellular domain of $\alpha_v\beta_3$, and the cytoplasmic tails on the nuclear magnetic resonance structure of $\alpha_{IIb}\beta_3$. (Reproduced with permission and after minor modifications from Hoffman R, Benz EJ, Silberstein LE, et al. Molecular basis of platelet function. In: Rand ML, Israels SJ, eds. *Hematology: Basic Principles and Practice.* Elsevier; 2017:1870-1884.e2.)

intestinal injury showed significantly increased IPFs, rising from a baseline of 7.4% (range 2.9–11.9%) to 9.4% (range 3.1–33.5). Pups with intestinal injury also showed increased number and ploidy of megakaryocytes in the bone marrow.[36]

In the murine model, platelet depletion protected against neonatal intestinal injury. We subjected some mouse pups to antibody-mediated platelet depletion

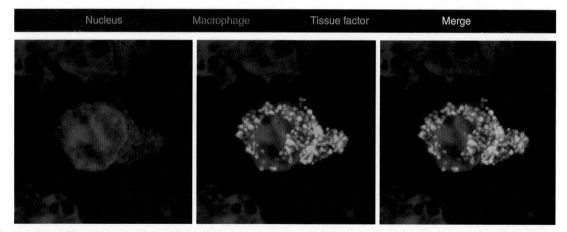

Fig. 15.4 Neonatal intestinal macrophages contain tissue factor in cytoplasmic granules. Representative fluorescence photomicrographs (200×) of uninflamed premature intestine show immunoreactivity for TF *(green)* in intestinal macrophages (antibody HAM56⁺, *red*). The image on right showed a merged picture. Nuclei were stained using DAPI (4′,6-diamidino-2-phenylindole), which is a blue-fluorescent DNA stain that exhibits 20-fold enhancement of fluorescence upon binding to AT regions of double-stranded DNA.

before inducing intestinal injury (intraperitoneal administration of rat monoclonal anti-GP1bα, 0.05 μg/g body weight),[21] and this reduced the severity of bowel injury and improved survival without increasing the severity of hemorrhages into the injured intestine.[37] These mice also showed less systemic inflammation, as evident from lower plasma C-reactive protein, CXCL2, and serum amyloid A, inflammatory markers known to be associated with human NEC and murine NEC-like injury.[38] These findings in the animal model suggested that thrombocytopenia could be a secondary, protective event.

The use of mouse pups on postnatal day 10 (P10) to study NEC-like injury was acceptable because the murine neonatal intestine resembles the human midgestation intestine until P14 to P16.[39,40] However, the transition from fetal (hepatic) to adult (bone marrow) megakaryopoiesis may occur between P5 and P14.[41] We confirmed our findings by measuring platelet counts, platelet volume indices, and IPF in a small cohort of P3 mice; the findings were similar. We concluded that murine NEC-like injury resembled human NEC at least in terms of decreased platelet counts. There was evidence of increased megakaryocyte differentiation and thrombopoiesis, which suggested that peripheral consumption of platelets was the likely mechanism of thrombocytopenia in these animals, not decreased platelet production.

PLATELET TRANSFUSIONS IN NEC

Platelet transfusions are frequently administered to infants with NEC because these critically ill patients are perceived to be at risk of life-threatening hemorrhagic complications.[10,42-47] Most of these platelet transfusions are administered prophylactically to correct the low platelet counts, not to treat actual bleeding.[44,46,48] The data on the efficacy and safety of these platelet transfusions remain scant.[43,44]

In the United States, platelet transfusion practices vary considerably across centers.[43] The threshold for platelet transfusions in many centers may be perceived as relatively liberal as compared to the clinical practice at other states or in other parts of the world.[44] Baer et al.[47] audited the practice and reported that up to 50% of extremely low birth weight (ELBW) infants received one or more platelet transfusions during their hospital stay. In another study, Petäjä et al.[49] reviewed all platelet transfusions and found that 60% of platelet transfusions in neonates were given outside of their established guidelines, at platelet counts higher than recommended.

There are emerging concerns about the possibility of harm from transfused platelets, which might get activated and release preformed vasoconstrictors and inflammatory mediators.[50,51] There is also increasing information linking platelet transfusions with suboptimal outcomes in NEC,[52-54] but some clinicians continue to favor relatively liberal transfusion thresholds because it is unclear whether the inferior outcomes in the recipients truly reflect harm from transfused platelets or are merely the confounding effect of higher severity of illness in these patients.[43,44] In a recent study, preterm infants with severe thrombocytopenia had higher mortality or major bleeding when they received platelet transfusion(s) at a platelet-count threshold of below 50×10^9/L than those transfused at platelet counts below 25×10^9/L.[55] Our findings from a preclinical study also support the idea that moderately low platelet counts may not always need prompt and aggressive correction in premature infants.

There is increasing evidence that links platelet transfusions in critically ill infants with adverse outcomes.[10,52,54,56] In their studies, Baer et al.[54] and Garcia et al.[53] found that in infants with NEC, the number of platelet transfusions predicted mortality. Kenton et al.[52] reported that platelet transfusions predicted complications such as cholestasis and short bowel syndrome. More recently, Del Vecchio et al.[57] showed that one platelet transfusion for NEC or other indications increased the relative risk of death by 10.4-fold than those who did not receive any such transfusions. Neonates who had received more than four platelet transfusions had a relative risk of death that was 29.9 times that of those who had not received a transfusion.

Despite all the observational data about increased mortality, it is difficult to know whether platelet transfusions were directly harmful.[52,54] Baer et al.[54] performed a sensitivity analysis on regression data[58] and showed that unknown factors accounted for only a part of the observed mortality, and therefore platelet transfusions likely had a direct contribution to harm. The association between platelet transfusions and adverse outcomes in NEC is difficult to evaluate because withholding a potentially life-saving therapy from a critically ill infant creates an ethical dilemma, and most infants tolerate such treatment without obvious harm. A few studies have compared the current vs. more conservative transfusion thresholds in critically ill infants and have shown no difference in outcomes.[47,59-61]

The issue of overtreatment and potential harm is now being asked frequently in critical care for adult and elderly patients.[62,63] However, it is emotionally difficult to withhold a potentially effective treatment from an ill infant at high risk of death.[64,65] These questions are also not asked frequently because with the small doses/volumes, drugs and transfusions are not the most important determinants of the cost of neonatal care[7]; tailored, multispecialty provisions such as surfactant administration, assisted ventilation, and parenteral nutrition and the length of hospital stay are much more important.[66] Moreover, despite the high cost of care for some patients, neonatal intensive care is still believed to be cost effective and accounts for only a small fraction of the overall health care budgets.[66,67] For all these reasons, neonatal studies designed to examine the impact of withholding interventions that do not cause obvious, immediate harm are frequently questioned about statistical power.[68] The care providers want to be absolutely certain. Furthermore, considering the fragility of these patients, such studies are usually designed to compare only incremental reductions and therefore take longer.[69]

Possible Therapeutic Interventions for Platelet Transfusion-Related Worsening of NEC

Ongoing studies suggest that several possibilities to prevent platelet activation may deserve evaluation:

(a) Low platelet counts were associated with less severe intestinal injury. These findings emphasize the need for further evaluation of lower thresholds for platelet transfusion.

(b) Considering the importance of tissue factor in intestinal injury, we examined whether blocking the extrinsic pathway of coagulation could be therapeutically effective. We treated some mice with PCI-27483 (N-aminoiminomethyl benzimidazol aminosulfonyl dihydroxy biphenyl acetyl aspartic acid), a small molecule inhibitor of factor VIIa in the VIIa/TF complex,[70] before inducing intestinal injury. This pretreatment blocked the early rise in plasma thrombin activity during intestinal injury. Further evaluation is needed.

(c) In our NEC model, TLR4$^{-/-}$ mice were protected against both NEC-related thrombocytopenia and NEC-like injury. TLR4 inhibitors such as TAK-242 or monoclonal anti-TLR4 antibodies such as NI-0101 may bring new therapeutic possibilities.[71,72]

(d) Bivalirudin and bivalirudin-tagged nanoparticles[73] were effective in our animal model and may prevent/ameliorate both thrombocytopenia and neonatal intestinal injury.[26] These nanoparticles improved survival. Notably, animals treated with bivalirudin nanoparticles showed some leukocyte infiltration and submucosal edema but did not have major mucosal damage. Other strategies such as clot-targeted micellar formulation or combination with other low molecular weight heparin agents such as enoxaparin may also deserve evaluation.[74,75]

(e) The effects of bivalirudin were recapitulated by D-phenylalanyl-prolyl-arginyl chloromethyl ketone (PPACK), another synthetic inhibitor of thrombin-mediated platelet activation and may deserve evaluation.[76]

(f) In other ongoing studies on anemia/transfusion-related NEC, we have found macrophage depletion to be beneficial.[77] This may be another approach to reduce the levels of tissue factor and consequent platelet activation.

Alternative Potential Therapies for Thrombocytopenia

Recombinant cytokines and growth factors such as interleukin-11, thrombopoietin, and thrombopoietin-mimetic agents such as romiplostim and eltrombopag may reduce the need for platelet transfusions but have a delayed impact.[78] There may also be a risk of thrombotic/thromboembolic complications. These could be useful in selected cases with persistent thrombocytopenia secondary to short bowel syndrome and cholestasis.[35,79] Newer thrombopoietin receptor agonists such as avatrombopag may also need consideration.[80] Melatonin, which can inhibit platelet activation, may also be useful in some patients.[81]

Summary

Thrombocytopenia is frequently seen in infants with NEC. The platelet counts typically drop within 24 to 72 hours of the onset of NEC, and its severity is proportional to the severity and stage of NEC. The likely mechanisms of thrombocytopenia may be due to platelet consumption in the microthrombi in the intestinal microvasculature. Our preclinical models suggest that activated macrophages in the neonatal intestine may bind platelets and evoke the release of secondary inflammatory mediators. There is a need for continued clinical studies to develop a consensus regarding most appropriate thresholds for platelet transfusions. Carefully designed studies may be helpful in the evaluation of the safety and efficacy of platelet transfusions in NEC.

REFERENCES

1. O'Neill Jr JA. Neonatal necrotizing enterocolitis. *Surg Clin North Am.* 1981;61:1013-1022.
2. Hutter Jr JJ, Hathaway WE, Wayne ER. Hematologic abnormalities in severe neonatal necrotizing enterocolitis. *J Pediatr.* 1976;88:1026-1031.
3. Patel CC. Hematologic abnormalities in acute necrotizing enterocolitis. *Pediatr Clin North Am.* 1977;24:579-584.
4. Kenton AB, O'Donovan D, Cass DL, et al. Severe thrombocytopenia predicts outcome in neonates with necrotizing enterocolitis. *J Perinatol.* 2005;25:14-20.
5. Ververidis M, Kiely EM, Spitz L, et al. The clinical significance of thrombocytopenia in neonates with necrotizing enterocolitis. *J Pediatr Surg.* 2001;36:799-803.
6. Ragazzi S, Pierro A, Peters M, et al. Early full blood count and severity of disease in neonates with necrotizing enterocolitis. *Pediatr Surg Int.* 2003;19:376-379.
7. Hilsenrath P, Nemechek J, Widness JA, et al. Cost-effectiveness of a limited-donor blood program for neonatal red cell transfusions. *Transfusion.* 1999;39:938-943.
8. Miner CA, Fullmer S, Eggett DL, et al. Factors affecting the severity of necrotizing enterocolitis. *J Matern Fetal Neonatal Med.* 2013;26:1715-1719.
9. Baer VL, Lambert DK, Henry E, et al. Severe thrombocytopenia in the NICU. *Pediatrics.* 2009;124:e1095-e1100.
10. Dohner ML, Wiedmeier SE, Stoddard RA, et al. Very high users of platelet transfusions in the neonatal intensive care unit. *Transfusion.* 2009;49:869-872.
11. Sola MC, Del Vecchio A, Rimsza LM. Evaluation and treatment of thrombocytopenia in the neonatal intensive care unit. *Clin Perinatol.* 2000;27:655-679.
12. Cremer M, Weimann A, Szekessy D, et al. Low immature platelet fraction suggests decreased megakaryopoiesis in neonates with sepsis or necrotizing enterocolitis. *J Perinato.l* 2013;33:622-626.
13. Brown RE, Rimsza LM, Pastos K, et al. Effects of sepsis on neonatal thrombopoiesis. *Pediatr Res.* 2008;64:399-404.
14. Lambert MP, Rauova L, Bailey M, et al. Platelet factor 4 is a negative autocrine in vivo regulator of megakaryopoiesis: clinical and therapeutic implications. *Blood.* 2007;110:1153-1160.
15. Hyman PE, Abrams CE, Zipser RD. Enhanced urinary immunoreactive thromboxane in neonatal necrotizing enterocolitis. A diagnostic indicator of thrombotic activity. *Am J Dis Child.* 1987;141:686-689.
16. Hsueh W, Caplan MS, Qu XW, et al. Neonatal necrotizing enterocolitis: clinical considerations and pathogenetic concepts. *Pediatr Dev Pathol.* 2003;6:6-23.
17. Maheshwari A. Immunologic and hematological abnormalities in necrotizing enterocolitis. *Clin Perinatol.* 2015;42:567-585.
18. MohanKumar K, Kaza N, Jagadeeswaran R, et al. Gut mucosal injury in neonates is marked by macrophage infiltration in contrast to pleomorphic infiltrates in adult: evidence from an animal model. *Am J Physiol Gastrointest Liver Physiol.* 2012;303:G93-G102.
19. MohanKumar K, Namachivayam K, Chapalamadugu KC, et al. Smad7 interrupts TGF-β signaling in intestinal macrophages and promotes inflammatory activation of these cells during necrotizing enterocolitis. *Pediatr Res.* 2016;79:951-961.
20. MohanKumar K, Namachivayam K, Cheng F, et al. Trinitrobenzene sulfonic acid-induced intestinal injury in neonatal mice activates transcriptional networks similar to those seen in human necrotizing enterocolitis. *Pediatr Res.* 2016;81:99-112.
21. Namachivayam K, MohanKumar K, Garg L, et al. Neonatal mice with necrotizing enterocolitis-like injury develop thrombocytopenia despite increased megakaryopoiesis. *Pediatr Res.* 2017;81:817-824.
22. Sharma R, Hudak ML, Tepas JJ III, et al. Impact of gestational age on the clinical presentation and surgical outcome of necrotizing enterocolitis. *J Perinatol.* 2006;26:342-347.
23. Yee WH, Soraisham AS, Shah VS, et al. Incidence and timing of presentation of necrotizing enterocolitis in preterm infants. *Pediatrics.* 2012;129:e298-e304.
24. Llanos AR, Moss ME, Pinzòn MC, et al. Epidemiology of neonatal necrotising enterocolitis: a population-based study. *Paediatr Perinat Epidemiol.* 2002;16:342-349.
25. MohanKumar K, Namachivayam K, Ho TT, et al. Cytokines and growth factors in the developing intestine and during necrotizing enterocolitis. *Semin Perinatol.* 2016;41:52-60.
26. Namachivayam K, MohanKumar K, Shores DR, et al. Targeted inhibition of thrombin attenuates murine neonatal necrotizing enterocolitis. *Proc Natl Acad Sci U S A.* 2020;117:10958-10969.
27. Alex P, Zachos NC, Nguyen T, et al. Distinct cytokine patterns identified from multiplex profiles of murine DSS and TNBS-induced colitis. *Inflamm Bowel Dis.* 2009;15:341-352.
28. Christensen RD, Henry E, Wiedmeier SE, et al. Thrombocytopenia among extremely low birth weight neonates: data from a multihospital healthcare system. *J Perinatol.* 2006;26:348-353.
29. Wu D, Xie J, Wang X, et al. Micro-concentration lipopolysaccharide as a novel stimulator of megakaryocytopoiesis that synergizes with IL-6 for platelet production. *Sci Rep.* 2015;5:13748.
30. Sitaru AG, Holzhauer S, Speer CP, et al. Neonatal platelets from cord blood and peripheral blood. *Platelets.* 2005;16:203-210.

31. Stokhuijzen E, Koornneef JM, Nota B, et al. Differences between platelets derived from neonatal cord blood and adult peripheral blood assessed by mass spectrometry. *J Proteome Res*. 2017;16:3567-3575.

32. Manco-Johnson MJ. Neonatal antithrombin III deficiency. *Am J Med*. 1989;87:S49-S52.

33. Wilson AJ, Zhou Q, Vargas I, et al. Formulation and characterization of antithrombin perfluorocarbon nanoparticles. *Methods Mol Biol*. 2020;2118:111-120.

34. Abe Y, Wada H, Tomatsu H, et al. A simple technique to determine thrombopoiesis level using immature platelet fraction (IPF). *Thromb Res*. 2006;118:463-469.

35. Sparger KA, Li N, Liu Z, et al. Developmental differences between newborn and adult mice in response to romiplostim. *Blood*. 2013;122:3542.

36. Sola-Visner MC, Christensen RD, Hutson AD, et al. Megakaryocyte size and concentration in the bone marrow of thrombocytopenic and nonthrombocytopenic neonates. *Pediatr Res*. 2007;61:479-484.

37. MohanKumar K, Killingsworth CR, McIlwain RB, et al. Intestinal epithelial apoptosis initiates gut mucosal injury during extracorporeal membrane oxygenation in the newborn piglet. *Lab Invest*. 2014;94:150-160.

38. Ng PC. Biomarkers of necrotising enterocolitis. *Semin Fetal Neonatal Med*. 2014;19:33-38.

39. Walthall K, Cappon GD, Hurtt ME, et al. Postnatal development of the gastrointestinal system: a species comparison. *Birth Defects Res B Dev Reprod Toxicol*. 2005;74:132-156.

40. Nanthakumar NN, Dai D, Meng D, et al. Regulation of intestinal ontogeny: effect of glucocorticoids and luminal microbes on galactosyltransferase and trehalase induction in mice. *Glycobiology*. 2005;15:221-232.

41. Liu ZJ, Hoffmeister KM, Hu Z, et al. Expansion of the neonatal platelet mass is achieved via an extension of platelet lifespan. *Blood*. 2014;123:3381-3389.

42. Stanworth SJ, Clarke P, Watts T, et al. Prospective, observational study of outcomes in neonates with severe thrombocytopenia. *Pediatrics*. 2009;124:e826-e834.

43. Josephson CD, Su LL, Christensen RD, et al. Platelet transfusion practices among neonatologists in the United States and Canada: results of a survey. *Pediatrics*. 2009;123:278-285.

44. Cremer M, Sola-Visner M, Roll S, et al. Platelet transfusions in neonates: practices in the United States vary significantly from those in Austria, Germany, and Switzerland. *Transfusion*. 2011;51:2634-2641.

45. Baer VL, Lambert DK, Schmutz N, et al. Adherence to NICU transfusion guidelines: data from a multihospital healthcare system. *J Perinatol*. 2008;28:492-497.

46. Murray NA, Howarth LJ, McCloy MP, et al. Platelet transfusion in the management of severe thrombocytopenia in neonatal intensive care unit patients. *Transfus Med*. 2002;12:35-41.

47. Baer VL, Henry E, Lambert DK, et al. Implementing a program to improve compliance with neonatal intensive care unit transfusion guidelines was accompanied by a reduction in transfusion rate: a pre-post analysis within a multihospital health care system. *Transfusion*. 2011;51:264-269.

48. Stanworth SJ. Thrombocytopenia, bleeding, and use of platelet transfusions in sick neonates. *Hematology Am Soc Hematol Educ Program*. 2012;2012:512-516.

49. Petaja J, Andersson S, Syrjala M. A simple automatized audit system for following and managing practices of platelet and plasma transfusions in a neonatal intensive care unit. *Transfus Med*. 2004;14:281-288.

50. Collins CE, Cahill MR, Newland AC, et al. Platelets circulate in an activated state in inflammatory bowel disease. *Gastroenterology*. 1994;106:840-845.

51. Thomas MR, Storey RF. The role of platelets in inflammation. *Thromb Haemost*. 2015;114:449-458.

52. Kenton AB, Hegemier S, Smith EO, et al. Platelet transfusions in infants with necrotizing enterocolitis do not lower mortality but may increase morbidity. *J Perinatol*. 2005;25:173-177.

53. Garcia MG, Duenas E, Sola MC, et al. Epidemiologic and outcome studies of patients who received platelet transfusions in the neonatal intensive care unit. *J Perinatol*. 2001;21:415-420.

54. Baer VL, Lambert DK, Henry E, et al. Do platelet transfusions in the NICU adversely affect survival? Analysis of 1600 thrombocytopenic neonates in a multihospital healthcare system. *J Perinatol*. 2007;27:790-796.

55. Curley A, Stanworth SJ, Willoughby K, et al. Randomized trial of platelet-transfusion thresholds in neonates. *N Engl J Med*. 2019;380(3):242-251.

56. Del Vecchio A. Evaluation and management of thrombocytopenic neonates in the intensive care unit. *Early Hum Dev*. 2014; 90(2):S51-S55.

57. Del Vecchio A, Sola MC, Theriaque DW, et al. Platelet transfusions in the neonatal intensive care unit: factors predicting which patients will require multiple transfusions. *Transfusion*. 2001;41:803-808.

58. Lin DY, Psaty BM, Kronmal RA. Assessing the sensitivity of regression results to unmeasured confounders in observational studies. *Biometrics*. 1998;54:948-963.

59. Gerday E, Baer VL, Lambert DK, et al. Testing platelet mass versus platelet count to guide platelet transfusions in the neonatal intensive care unit. *Transfusion*. 2009;49:2034-2039.

60. Borges JP, dos Santos AM, da Cunha DH, et al. Restrictive guideline reduces platelet count thresholds for transfusions in very low birth weight preterm infants. *Vox Sang*. 2013;104:207-213.

61. Kahvecioglu D, Erdeve O, Alan S, et al. The impact of evaluating platelet transfusion need by platelet mass index on reducing the unnecessary transfusions in newborns. *J Matern Fetal Neonatal Med*. 2014;27:1787-1789.

62. Hubbeling D. Overtreatment: is a solution possible? *J Eval Clin Pract*. 2022;28(5):821-827.

63. Hofmann B. Acknowledging and addressing the many ethical aspects of disease. *Patient Educ Couns*. 2022;105(5):1201-1208.

64. Slaughter JL, Cua CL, Notestine JL, et al. Early prediction of spontaneous patent ductus arteriosus (PDA) closure and PDA-associated outcomes: a prospective cohort investigation. *BMC Pediatr*. 2019;19:333.

65. Doron MW, Veness-Meehan KA, Margolis LH, et al. Delivery room resuscitation decisions for extremely premature infants. *Pediatrics*. 1998;102:574-582.

66. Cheah IGS. Economic assessment of neonatal intensive care. *Transl Pediatr*. 2019;8:246-256.

67. Lassman D, Hartman M, Washington B, et al. US health spending trends by age and gender: selected years 2002-10. *Health Aff (Millwood)*. 2014;33:815-822.

68. Oakes LM. Sample size, statistical power, and false conclusions in infant looking-time research. *Infancy*. 2017;22:436-469.

69. Darmstadt GL, Walker N, Lawn JE, et al. Saving newborn lives in Asia and Africa: cost and impact of phased scale-up of interventions within the continuum of care. *Health Policy Plan*. 2008;23:101-117.

70. Gomez-Outes A, Suárez-Gea ML, Lecumberri R, et al. New parenteral anticoagulants in development. *Ther Adv Cardiovasc Dis*. 2011;5:33-59.

71. Ono Y, Maejima Y, Saito M, et al. TAK-242, a specific inhibitor of Toll-like receptor 4 signalling, prevents endotoxemia-induced skeletal muscle wasting in mice. *Sci Rep.* 2020;10:694.

72. Gao W, Xiong Y, Li Q, et al. Inhibition of Toll-like receptor signaling as a promising therapy for inflammatory diseases: a journey from molecular to nano therapeutics. *Front Physiol.* 2017;8:508.

73. Myerson J, He L, Lanza G, et al. Thrombin-inhibiting perfluorocarbon nanoparticles provide a novel strategy for the treatment and magnetic resonance imaging of acute thrombosis. *J Thromb Haemost.* 2011;9:1292-1300.

74. She ZG, Liu X, Kotamraju VR, et al. Clot-targeted micellar formulation improves anticoagulation efficacy of bivalirudin. *ACS Nano.* 2014;8:10139-10149.

75. Brophy DF, Martin EJ, Gehr TW, et al. Enhanced anticoagulant activity of enoxaparin in patients with ESRD as measured by thrombin generation time. *Am J Kidney Dis.* 2004;44:270-277.

76. Schmaier AH, Meloni FJ, Nawarawong W, et al. PPACK-thrombin is a noncompetitive inhibitor of alpha-thrombin binding to human platelets. *Thromb Res.* 1992;67:479-489.

77. MohanKumar K, Namachivayam K, Song T, et al. A murine neonatal model of necrotizing enterocolitis caused by anemia and red blood cell transfusions. *Nat Commun.* 2019;10(1):3494.

78. Ghanima W, Cooper N, Rodeghiero F, et al. Thrombopoietin receptor agonists: ten years later. *Haematologica.* 2019;104: 1112-1123.

79. Cremer M, Sallmon H, Kling PJ, et al. Thrombocytopenia and platelet transfusion in the neonate. *Semin Fetal Neonatal Med.* 2016;21:10-18.

80. Bussel JB, Kuter DJ, Aledort LM, et al. A randomized trial of avatrombopag, an investigational thrombopoietin-receptor agonist, in persistent and chronic immune thrombocytopenia. *Blood.* 2014;123:3887-3894.

81. Lansink MO, Gorlinger K, Hartmann M, et al. Melatonin does not affect disseminated intravascular coagulation but diminishes decreases in platelet count during subacute endotoxaemia in rats. *Thromb Res.* 2016;139:38-43.

Index

Note: Pages numbers followed by *f* indicate figures, by *t* tables, and by *b* boxes.